"Peter Eckman's accomplishment in *The Compleat Acupuncturist* is truly remarkable. It is a grand synthesis that certainly ranks as one of the most significant texts on pulse diagnosis in the history of the medicine. Beyond the wealth of technical information or theory communicated there is the inspiration that, if we apply ourselves diligently as Peter has, that we too may awaken to the heart of the medicine and an inspiring synthesis of our own. Peter's text reaffirms my conviction that Chinese medicine, having become a world medicine, is flourishing."

—*Lonny Jarrett, M.Ac., author of* Nourishing Destiny:
The Inner Tradition of Chinese Medicine

"I'm truly amazed at [Peter Eckman's] scholarship—and at [his] ability to draw so many threads together. I also think it is extraordinarily well-written, and very easy to read, even though the subject matter is far from easy."

—*Nora Franglen, Founder of the School of Five Element Acupuncture (SOFEA)
and author of* The Handbook of Five Element Practice, Keepers of the Soul,
Patterns of Practice *and* The Simple Guide to Five Element Acupuncture

"I am most grateful when scholars dare to take on interdisciplinary topics, as Peter Eckman has done with this project. I predict that this type of synthesis and integration will be one of the main features of the twenty-first century, and Peter is truly ahead of the game with this project!"

—*Heiner Fruehauf, Ph.D., L.Ac., Founding Professor, School of Classical
Chinese Medicine, National College of Natural Medicine, Portland, Oregon*

"Peter Eckman's book on pulse diagnosis will become an instant classic as there has certainly never been anything like it before. His intellectual rigour, combined with his vast clinical experience, has enabled him to integrate several different styles of pulse diagnosis into a coherent whole. All practitioners who place a high value on pulse diagnosis should read this book."

—*Peter Mole, acupuncturist and Dean of the College of
Integrated Chinese Medicine, Reading, UK*

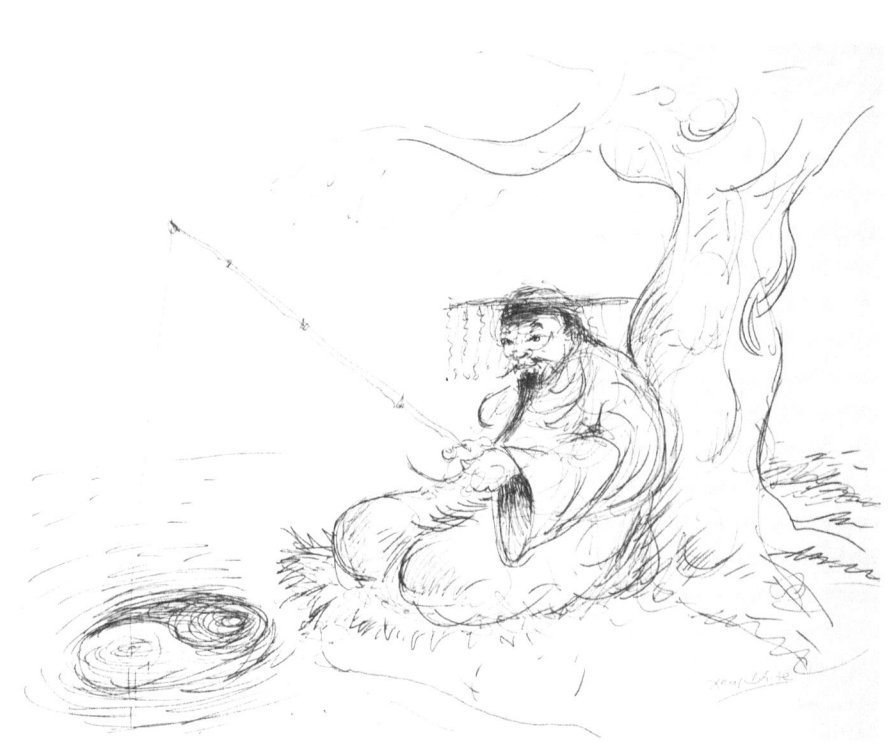

THE COMPLEAT ACUPUNCTURIST

A Guide to Constitutional and
Conditional Pulse Diagnosis

Peter Eckman, M.D., Ph.D., M.Ac.

Foreword by William Morris

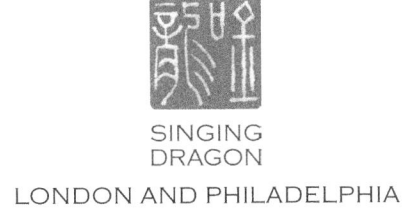

SINGING
DRAGON
LONDON AND PHILADELPHIA

Every effort has been made to trace copyright holders and to obtain their permission for the use of copyright material. The author and the publisher apologize for any omissions and would be grateful if notified of any acknowledgements that should be incorporated in future reprints or editions of this book.

First published in 2014
by Singing Dragon
an imprint of Jessica Kingsley Publishers
73 Collier Street
London N1 9BE, UK
and
400 Market Street, Suite 400
Philadelphia, PA 19106, USA

www.singingdragon.com

Copyright © Peter Eckman 2014
Foreword copyright © William Morris 2014

Library of Congress Cataloging in Publication Data
Eckman, Peter, author.
  The compleat acupuncturist : a guide to constitutional and
conditional pulse diagnosis / Peter Eckman ;
foreword by William Morris.
     p. ; cm.
  Includes bibliographical references and index.
  ISBN 978-1-84819-198-3 (alk. paper)
  I. Title.
  [DNLM: 1. Acupuncture Therapy--Case Reports. 2. Body
Constitution--physiology--Case Reports. 3.
Medicine, East Asian Traditional--Case Reports. 4. Pulse--Case Reports. WB 369]
  RM184
  615.8'92--dc23
                         2013023984

British Library Cataloguing in Publication Data
A CIP catalogue record for this book is available from the British Library

ISBN 978 1 84819 198 3
eISBN 978 0 85701 152 7

Printed and bound in Great Britain

CONTENTS

FOREWORD

Peter Eckman is a high-level syncretic thinker. Encountering his book, *Closing the Circle*, brought me to a deepened view of my practice.[1] His weave upon various forms of Chinese medical thought provided a seed for my own approach. Then, *In the Footsteps of the Yellow Emperor*[2] brought the world an in-depth view of J. R. Worsley, whose system of "Leamington style acupuncture" influenced generations of Western practitioners. Clearly these syncretic works foreshadowed *The Compleat Acupuncturist*.

Fascinated by Eckman's approach to inquiry, I dove into this alchemical work of love. Through the crucible of practice, he has transmuted his unique views.

Features that distinguish creative from reproductive knowledge are several. Well-built original thought occurs seldom. Creativity must have roots in discipline, if not to suffer critique. Alternatively, reproductive knowledge reproduces, as accurately as possible, conversations entrusted within the literature of Chinese medicine. Creativity has awareness of roots. They are watered in foundational dialogs forming a discipline. Such dialog comes in three forms: lineage, literature, and school systems.[3] Lineages form the primary roots of this book. Eckman's attention to contemporary practitioners who validate literature in practice makes it real.

Three features make this book important. First, it identifies constitutional thought; second, a method of inquiry; and, third, it synthesizes across cultures. The disparate techniques of pulse diagnosis achieve a resolution and a deepened perspective in this work.

---

1   Eckman, P. and Kutchins, S., *Closing the Circle: Lectures on the Unity of Traditional Oriental Medicine*. Fairfax, CA: Shen Foundation, 1983.

2   Eckman, P., *In the Footsteps of the Yellow Emperor: Tracing the History of Traditional Acupuncture*. San Francisco, CA: Cypress Books, 1996.

3   Scheid, V., *Chinese Medicine in Contemporary China: Plurality and Synthesis*. Durham, NC: Duke University Press, 2002.

Explanations are presented clearly for assessing the constitution. These are critical if we are to raise our view above the mud of the sign-symptom terrain and its consequent reactionary thought. I often see practitioners reacting to symptoms point by point. They have lost the center. They have lost the root. Their consequent treatments are scattered and may involve the combination of an array of different treatment principles. As the patient mentions each new symptom, another point is blithely added.

Resolution of conflicting methods of pulse diagnosis is explored here, gained by comparing and creatively interpreting multiple views on the placement of the examiner's fingers. This resolution was arrived at through a passionate exploration of Ayurvedic pulse diagnosis, the Korean teachings of Sa Am, Kuon Dowon, and Yoo Tae Woo, together with the teachings of J. R. Worsley and the great archivist Wang Shu-he, who authored the *Pulse Classic* and recovered the teachings of the Saint of Medicine, Zhang Zhong-jing.

Method is embedded in this endeavor. Peter Eckman is engaged in a transdisciplinary effort, which spans from my own neoclassical interpretations of Han Dynasty lore to his direct reception of Korean constitutional and Ayurvedic thought in the area of pulse diagnosis. I believe that he has gleaned new insight that is worthy of the pursuit.

The transdisciplinarean path can present challenges in an era of classicism. Peering through the texts provides one point of view. Peter has stood at the crossroads of Korean, American, and European roots of transmission, and has a kernel of wisdom here that he has baked in practice.

Having mentioned the term transdisciplinary, it appears prudent to discuss this notion, since I believe this book to be a pre-eminent expression of that form of inquiry. In *Acupuncture Today* I proposed a research method entitled "post-paradox" where I reframe the discussion called "transdisciplinarity" into a model of discussion that may be more readily accepted by the public.[4] I believe that, for the current work by Peter Eckman, the transdisciplinary frame is the best concept.

There are some important features of the transdisciplinary view that I would like to explicate as they relate to this work. Transdisciplinary thought suggests that which is at once between, across, and beyond disciplines, by using the prefix "trans." The transdisciplinary view maintains a goal of understanding the present world as a unity of knowledge.[5] The transdisciplinary view includes levels of reality, the logic of an included middle (the center of paradox), and complexity. These malleable logics can bring a change in perspective.[6] It

4   Morris, W., "Post-paradox: Room for View." *Acupuncture Today*, 13 (8), 2012.

5   Nicolescu, B., *Manifesto of Transdisciplinarity*. Albany, NY: State University of New York Press, 2002.

6   CIRET, "Charter of Transdisciplinarity," 1994. Available at http://ciret-transdisciplinarity.org/chart. php, accessed June 18, 2013.

resolves disparities, embracing both from a third place.[7] The keystone of the transdisciplinary view lies within the unification of the meanings that traverse and lie beyond different lineages. New knowledge emerges when lineages encounter each other, inviting a new vision of theory and practice.

Reaching a new height of inquiry into the problem of constitutional diagnosis, Peter Eckman has resolved a problem in the practice of pulse diagnosis, one that has plagued acupuncture practice since its devolution in the 1950s. He has also resolved disparities of technique in the practice of pulse diagnosis. This resolution has come about through developing a cognitive framework for choosing the placement of one's fingers.

This is a brilliant and original contribution to the practice of pulse diagnosis. I look forward to using it in my practice.

> William Morris, Ph.D., DAOM, author of *Li Shi-zhen*
> *Pulse Studies: An Illustrated Guide* and *Transformation:*
> *Treating Trauma with Acupuncture and Herbs*

---

7   Morin, E., *On Complexity* (ed. A. Montuori). Cresskill, NJ: Hampton Press, 2008.

APOLOGIA[1]

The archaic language of the title is intended to convey the author's somewhat "tongue in cheek" approach to the notion of "completeness." It is certainly not the intention to claim that this treatise covers all or even most of what informs the practice of the art and science of acupuncture, nor that the author is asserting any special claim of mastery. Rather, the idea of "compleatness" refers to the goal of integrating various notions of Oriental medical theory and practice from such diverse sources as India, Korea, and Japan, including their interpretation by Western practitioners, into the discussion of a subject that is often tacitly limited to the Chinese tradition. As will be repeatedly emphasized in the text, the author is not arguing for the superiority of any one style of acupuncture practice, nor disparaging any of the traditions that may not receive as much attention as others in this book. It is the author's view that, ultimately, all the teachings and traditions of Oriental medicine are aspects of the same shared perception of the nature of reality, in health and illness, and are to be honored for their part in elucidating the nature of the whole.

Another reason for choosing the word "compleat" is that it suggests, to the author at least, the archetypal symbol of the circle, with all its associations, and harkens back to the initial publication some 30 years ago of *Closing the Circle*,[2] jointly written with Stuart Kutchins. The present treatise can be seen as the fruit of the premises first presented there, manifesting here as a practical approach to the clinical practice of acupuncture, in this case based on the art and science of pulse diagnosis.

---

1   From the Greek, meaning the defense of a position against attack.

2   Eckman, P. and Kutchins, S., *Closing the Circle: Lectures on the Unity of Traditional Oriental Medicine.* Fairfax, CA: Shen Foundation, 1983.

This treatise is also an attempt to create a more unified theoretical foundation for Oriental medicine.[3] Whether it will be possible for someone to discover a unifying theory that covers both Eastern and Western medicine is a subject best left for future investigators.

---

3   "Most of the really great breakthroughs in science are unifications. Newton's laws of motion unified the sky and Earth as ruled by the same physics; that was radically different from the earlier Aristotelian concept, in which the two realms were separate. Einstein's laws of relativity unified space and time." Owen J. Gingerich (a science historian at Harvard), quoted in Chang, K., "Quakes, Tectonic and Theoretical." *New York Times*, January 15, 2011. Available at www.nytimes.com/2011/01/16/weekinreview/16chang.html, accessed June 18, 2013.

DEDICATION

To Korea, Land of the Morning Calm,[1] and its wondrous teachers from the medieval Buddhist monk Sa Am, to my mentors in Seoul, Kuon Dowon and Yoo Tae Woo, whose illumination blazed a trail for me to follow. I am also deeply grateful to Puramo Chong for allowing me to spend a week in his clinic, and subject him to my penchant for "pilpul."[2]

And, equally dedicated to India, too often ignored in discussions of Oriental medicine. Though I never had an Indian mentor, Mary Jo Cravatta did her best to transmit to me her Indian teachers' diagnostic methods. I hope she will smile at the unorthodox applications to which I have applied them.

As for teachers of the Chinese traditions, I am indebted to Jeffrey Yuen and Jimmy Chang for their classes on the pulse,[3] to Radha Thambirajah,[4] whom I interviewed in England, and whose book on energetics in acupuncture helped guide me to my current understanding, and to Wang Qi, who helped clarify terms and passages in the Chinese classics.

Working my way West, I have already published a book largely devoted to the work of Jack Worsley, but I would like to take this opportunity to acknowledge the work of George Soulié de Morant, who insisted on pulse diagnosis as the necessary basis for a scientific understanding of traditional acupuncture,[5] and who bravely put forth his own discoveries of what the pulse

---

1   The sobriquet "Land of the Morning Calm" was adopted by Korea from a poetic description of their country by Sir Rabindranath Tagore (1861–1941), a Nobel laureate noted for his ability to integrate science, philosophy, religion, poetry, and music into a coherent appreciation of what is. Tagore based his understanding of these things on the ancient Vedic texts, paralleling my own interpretation of the contemporary flowering of Korean acupuncture as being based on the much earlier revelations of the Ayurvedic Rishis. India and Korea alike deserve a greater share of attention from modern devotees of Oriental medicine, and it is the author's hope that this book will contribute to such a renaissance.

2   A Yiddish word that refers to Rabbinical discourses, often self-deprecatingly described as "hairsplitting."

3   Yuen, 2006–2008 and Chang, 2006.

4   Ms. Thambirajah was trained in the Five Element tradition in China, during the Cultural Revolution in the 1960s, at the Shanghai Military Medical College. The military forces were relatively free from the codification of Traditional Chinese Medicine (TCM) taking place in the civilian realm.

5   Soulié de Morant, G., *L'acuponcture Chinoise*. Paris: Maloine, 1972.

can reveal, an approach that has encouraged me to pursue a similar course. His disciple Jean Niboyet's discussion of pulses that arrive ahead of or behind their expected positions has subliminally contributed to my personal approach of separately examining the Yin and Yang status of each of the 12 Organs/ Officials/Meridians.[6]

With apologies to Sir Izaak Walton for stealing the title from *The Compleat Angler*. In 1653 Walton wrote:

> in this Discourse I do not undertake to say all that is known, or may be said of it, but I undertake to acquaint the Reader with many things that are not usually known to every Angler; and I shall leave gleanings and observations enough to be made out of the experience of all that love and practise this recreation, to which I shall encourage them. For Angling may be said to be so like the Mathematicks, that it can never be fully learnt; at least not so fully but that there will still be more new experiments left for the trial of other men that succeed us.[7]

> Tis not all fishing to fish.[8]

There is a famous passage in the classics, which describes the sensation an acupuncturist experiences upon the arrival of De Qi,[9] comparing it to that of a fish taking the bait.[10] I'm sure Sir Izaak would have appreciated the metaphor.

---

6   Niboyet, J., *Compléments d'acupuncture*. Paris: Editions Dominique Wapler, 1955.

7   Walton, I., *The Compleat Angler*. London: J. M. Dent, 1906, from the Epistle to the Reader, p.5.

8   Ibid., www.giga-usa.com/index.html.

9   De Qi is the experience of the interaction of the needle and the recipient's body at the moment when the therapeutic event happens. De Qi may be felt by the practitioner, the recipient, or both.

10   "Ode to the Streamer Out of the Dark." In *The Golden Needle and Other Odes of Traditional Acupuncture* (R. Bertschinger, trans.). Edinburgh: Churchill Livingstone, 1991, pp.17–53.

INTRODUCTION

This work is essentially a hypothetical treatise, intended to present a new perspective on acupuncture and Oriental medicine, based on the author's clinical experience of approximately 40 years. It is with great hesitation that this material is being committed to print, for it is really a work in progress, and the ideas presented are still evolving, even as they are being chronicled. Some of the ideas come from the insights of one of my esteemed teachers, Kuon Dowon in Seoul, who is now in his nineties, and still actively in practice. Dr. Kuon,[1] the originator of Korean Constitutional Acupuncture (also called Eight Constitutions Medicine), has been talking about writing a text on his style of practice for well over two decades, and, while I wish him the longest possible life, I cannot help but worry that his unique knowledge will not survive him. I think I understand his hesitation—there are still missing pieces, and perhaps even some imperfections in his methodology, which, like my own, is in a state of continual evolution. It is with this situation in mind that I have chosen to communicate these ideas, recognizing that further experience may necessitate even drastic changes in approach, but the risk of failing to transmit what strike me as some startling insights into the underlying coherence of the various branches of Oriental medicine is too great a burden (I'm wearing my Confucian hat here) for me to ignore. The unpublished material that I personally learned from Dr. Kuon is not mine to reveal during his lifetime, but the road he opened up for me has led to ample insights worthy of communication.

When I originally started writing this treatise, my focus was entirely on the topic of *constitutional pulse diagnosis*, for reasons I will explain in the Prologue. In my quest to better understand the way the constitution manifests in the pulse, however, I discovered that the pulses reflecting the current condition also contain

---

1   Kuon Dowon was born in 1921. His seminal work (a prior self-published report was issued in 1962) was presented to the 13th International Congress of Acupuncture, held in Vienna in 1965, and published as "A Study of Constitution-Acupuncture" in the *Journal of the International Congress of Acupuncture and Moxibustion*, 10, pp.149–167, in 1965. Although Kuon was not able to attend the Congress himself, his paper was presented by Johannes Bischko, the Dean of Austrian acupuncture. Kuon now refers to his methodology as Eight Constitutions Medicine, and the author was fortunate to have studied with him and observed his practice over the years 1987–1988, during which time significant new developments took place, as yet unpublished.

within themselves information about the constitution. Thus these two topics are inseparable, and I found that I would need to address conditional pulse diagnosis (which is more or less the kind of pulse diagnosis used by the vast majority of acupuncturists) as well. In attempting to clarify my own understanding of *conditional pulse diagnosis*, I came to new insights and developed new methodologies that were equally as important as the quest for a better understanding of constitutional diagnosis. I now found that I had enough material on both these subjects to merit a much larger treatise. Finally, I realized that a purely theoretical work would be much less useful than one that included case histories as examples of how to apply these theoretical constructs. Therefore I have decided to present this material in three sections: Part One on constitutional pulse diagnosis, Part Two on conditional pulse diagnosis, and Part Three on clinical case histories.

Much of this material may seem obscure to practitioners trained in the modern version of Traditional Chinese Medicine (TCM) or other traditional styles of acupuncture, but I am hopeful that those with the patience to carefully investigate these findings will be well rewarded by the clinical results such as I have myself experienced. Both the theoretical and practical material presented here can be incorporated into any of the extant styles of traditional acupuncture, be they Chinese, Korean, Japanese, French, English, or other. As readers of my previous publications are undoubtedly aware, I am a staunch believer in the basic theories of traditional Oriental medicine, and so all of the material I am presenting here is either directly or indirectly an outgrowth of that tradition, and wherever possible, I will provide classical citations. Should readers have any questions or experiences to share after studying and applying this material, I will do my best to respond to emails addressed to: HEALINGMOUNTAIN@ aol.com. Please be sure to mention acupuncture in the subject line, so that your message is not inadvertently deleted. If there is sufficient interest, a workshop may be arranged to demonstrate the various techniques of pulse diagnosis herein described, as well as for discussing the more didactic material.

My most recent publication, *In the Footsteps of the Yellow Emperor: Tracing the History of Traditional Acupuncture* (1996, 2007), while warmly received, also elicited a plea from one of the elders of Japanese acupuncture, the late Tobe Soshichiro, publisher of the prestigious journal *Ido No Nippon*, for a more clinically oriented presentation of my work. In a way, the seed he planted is responsible for the work before you, as I have never forgotten his request. May it, in small part, repay him for the incredible generosity he displayed to many a budding acupuncturist in his venerable career. As for the timing of this treatise, many students over the years have asked if there was any way in which they could learn my style of practice, to which I have given more or less the same answer as Kuon Dowon, "I'm working on it." But recently, on a nostalgic day spent sharing reminiscences and plans with my old friend and dear colleague Chieko Maekawa in Kona Hawaii, she **insisted** (in her inimitable Japanese way) that I begin transmitting my knowledge **now**! Hai, Chieko-san.

PROLOGUE

Although my initial training in acupuncture was from Korean teachers back in 1973,[1] I quickly realized that there was much about the subject that I would have to discover elsewhere, both on account of the language difficulties and the inherent limitations of the clinically based training program hastily developed by the West Coast Medical Group's cadre of Korean teachers. And so, I shortly enrolled in the College of Chinese Acupuncture in England, which was the only place in the world teaching Five Element style acupuncture in English, being the creation of J. R. Worsley, a true visionary. His style of acupuncture, which I have described previously,[2] is one which holds a powerful fascination for Westerners such as myself, being more spiritually, psychologically, and emotionally oriented than the other styles of acupuncture accessible to English speaking students. To be a successful practitioner of this approach, one needs to develop several sets of skills. Most important is the ability to develop rapport with patients, so that they might be willing to reveal their most deeply felt needs, and not merely one or another superficial discomfort, which acupuncture has a reputation for addressing successfully. As a practicing physician, I found it relatively easy to establish this kind of relationship with most of my patients. The harder skills to develop were those dependent on sensory discriminations: specifically the ability to reliably detect and classify very subtle changes in my patients' tone of voice, body odor, facial coloration, and emotional flexibility when under stress. I continued to study with Professor Worsley through three degree programs (Lic.Ac., B.Ac., and M.Ac.) and beyond, but was never satisfied with the reliability of my perceptions of these subtle colors, sounds,

---

1   West Coast Medical Group-Acupuncture was started in 1973 by an entrepreneurial physician, who hired Korean practitioners to instruct doctors in this art/science, who would then work in his clinics. The didactic program lasted a scant two weeks, but the subsequent ongoing clinical training was a unique apprenticeship opportunity, for which I am ever grateful.

2   Eckman, P., *In the Footsteps of the Yellow Emperor: Tracing the History of Traditional Acupuncture*. San Francisco, CA: Cypress Books, 1996. Revised edition, San Francisco, CA: Long River Press, 2007. Hereafter, *Footsteps*.

odors, and emotions to guide me to the crucial diagnostic assessment known as the Causative Factor or CF. To recap material from *Footsteps*, the CF is that one of the Five Elements whose state of chronic imbalance is ultimately at the root of each person's symptoms or difficulties in life, and which must be addressed if they are to recover their balance and experience "holistic" healing. I perceived that I was not alone in having difficulty with these sensory based diagnoses. It was rare that there was ever close to unanimity among my classmates in diagnosing patients in the classroom setting, and, more often than I care to remember, Professor Worsley determined the CF to be in an Element chosen by a minority of us students. Over the years, I myself have been a recipient of acupuncture treatment from multiple practitioners, including several whom I would label "Masters" (representing diverse styles of traditional acupuncture). Interestingly, I have ended up with each one of the Five Elements being diagnosed as the core of my energetic imbalance, in different instances, by at least one of these seasoned practitioners. Such variability in core diagnostic assessment tells me that this is one area in which a more reliable methodology is needed, and has specifically impelled me to search for a more accurate guide to the diagnosis of the CF or constitution. (It has also highlighted, for me, the question of the relationship of the constitution to the present condition. Successful treatments may involve either or both of these diagnostic assessments, and the relationship between the two has never been addressed, to my satisfaction, in English at least.) These comments are not meant to disparage the power or validity of Worsley's (or anyone else's) style of acupuncture teaching or practice, for as one of Worsley's senior students was fond of saying, "Give me 20 treatments, and then I will know the CF."[3] I am still awed by the depth and power of Five Element Acupuncture (FEA),[4] but I have never lost the drive to pursue a more reliable approach to CF diagnosis, nor to discover the connection between the CF and the presenting symptoms, signs, or illnesses.

I have investigated many hypothetical means for identifying the CF including physiognomy, electrical conductivity at key acupuncture points, and analysis of fingerprint patterns, among others, all of which have been promulgated by different authorities as reliable diagnostic indicators. In my experience they have not yielded the requisite diagnostic precision nor accuracy. In addition, they lacked the personal cultivation of sensory based skills that was quite appealing to me in Worsley's approach, even though I had found it so difficult to master the methods he taught. Upon reflection, it occurred to me that Worsley's diagnostic methodology was inherently difficult

---

3   Attributed to Julia Measures by Thea Elijah, in an article on "Color, Sound, Odor and Emotion" at www. perennialmedicine.com/wp-content/uploads/2011/11/5%20Element%20Treatment%20Protocols. pdf, p.6.

4   I'm adopting the more widely used terminology Five Element Acupuncture (FEA) for what I called Leamington Acupuncture (LA) in *Footsteps*.

to standardize, making it more of what I would call an art than a science.[5] While I have great respect for master artists, I felt a need to approach the problem from the standpoint of someone not necessarily gifted with such talents, but rather as one dedicated to the pursuit of rational knowledge; that is, from its (Asian) scientific side. One of my other teachers, Yoo Tae Woo, was an inspiration in this regard, having systematized a diagnostic approach that I will describe in Chapter 3, but also having taught feedback methods to reliably demonstrate the efficacy, or lack thereof, of his treatment strategies. So, in summary, I was searching for a sensory based diagnostic methodology which lent itself to rigorous standardization, systematization, and feedback verification, all of which would contribute to a more reliable identification of the CF, and therefore a more reliable approach to acupuncture treatment.

The astute reader may have realized by now that I have not mentioned the most well known and highly regarded of the traditional diagnostic methods in Oriental medicine, namely examination of the pulse. Despite its long history, however, in my opinion the basic tenets of pulse diagnosis have lacked that rigorous specificity that would satisfy my self-imposed criteria. Texts on pulse diagnosis are few to begin with, and generally have very little discussion of the actual mechanics involved in examining the pulse. In my studies with numerous teachers, I've observed quite a range of variability in finger placement, for example. I might also note that attempts to make Five Element diagnoses on the basis of the pulse can be found in practically the earliest stratum of acupuncture literature, specifically in certain passages in the *Neijing* and *Nanjing*,[6] but this has not led to the development of a method of CF diagnosis based on pulse qualities, to the best of my knowledge. Nevertheless, I have intuitively believed that the key to recognizing the CF must somehow be inscribed in the pulse,

---

5   It is my firm belief that medicine, both Western and Eastern, is best practiced as an amalgamation of science and art. I will touch on the question of the science underlying Oriental medicine at other points in this treatise.

6   The *Neijing* and *Nanjing* are two of the most important foundational classical texts of Chinese acupuncture. The former is commonly translated as *The Yellow Emperor's Classic of Internal Medicine*, while the latter is commonly translated as *The Classic of Difficulties*. The former text is in turn composed of two parts: *Suwen* (*Simple Questions*) and *Lingshu* (*Spiritual Axis*). The *Neijing* provides a set of pulse qualities which correspond to the Five Elements and their associated Zang Organs in a number of chapters, including: *Suwen* 19 and 23 and *Lingshu* 4. This schema is elaborated into a primitive "constitutional" model in the *Nanjing*, in chapters 4, 10, and 13. It would appear that its authors are saying the pulse quality at any location reveals the origin of the energetic imbalance manifesting there, which is akin to saying the root can be discerned in the branch via the pulse quality, per the following paradigm: tense or wiry indicates Wood, strong or hooked indicates Fire, relaxed or slippery indicates Earth, rough or sticky indicates Metal, and deep or stonelike indicates Water. These basic pulse qualities (or variants thereof in several cases) are presented as parallel concepts to the five colors, sounds, odors, and emotions, which are the crucial diagnostic indicators used in determining the CF in FEA. In spite of this classical reference, these pulse qualities were not incorporated into the diagnostic methodology developed by Worsley for his style of acupuncture, nor have any of his disciples claimed to be able to successfully use these pulse qualities to identify the CF. This point was impressed on my thinking following an email correspondence with Lonny Jarrett, one of the leading inheritors of Worsley's teachings, who has also made deep and extensive studies of the pulse.

but that the criteria for examining the pulse needed more rigor, plus a broader way of conceptualizing pulse diagnosis. So, with this belief in the back (or front at times) of my mind, I have held this question like a Zen koan, hoping someday to break through the conventional assumptions that keep us from seeing nature's truths, which cannot always be discovered by logical means. This book reports my progress in this quest, and while it hardly qualifies as "enlightenment," I like to think that it counts at least as a mini "satori."

To reiterate, I had originally conceived of this book as strictly focused on constitutional pulse diagnosis, but such a limitation clashed with the observations of the pulse that I found to be necessary in formulating specific treatments for my patients. As soon as I decided to include illustrative case histories, I realized that I would need to show how constitutional diagnosis is used as a foundation in treatment formulation. Furthermore, to describe my methods of treatment formulation in turn necessitated introducing much more material on several topics, including Ayurvedic pulse diagnosis, Korean Hand Acupuncture, and the evaluation of the Yin and Yang states of the Organs/Officials/Meridians, than I had originally planned, since treatment, while based on the constitution, must also take into account the patient's current condition. This change in scope not only allows me to present a wealth of pulse lore that is generally unavailable in English, but it also gives me another opportunity to introduce some personal discoveries about the meaning of pulses that are both clinically useful, and illustrate my creative approach to this ancient art, which I trust will serve as an inspiration to others. I hope the presentation does not come across as too choppy, shuttling back and forth between the related, but distinct, domains of diagnosis and treatment. The discovery of this pulse based method of both constitutional and conditional diagnosis has in turn opened the door to many other insights about energetic diagnosis based on the pulse, and has transformed my clinical practice of acupuncture. Among the topics that I will also address in this book are the following: how to decide, from the pulse, whether a given treatment should be applied on the left side, the right side, or bilaterally; how to tell whether Tonification or Sedation (Dispersion) is indicated; which one of the Elemental Command Points (Wu Shu Xue) on the CF Meridian is most appropriate to treat (Element in Element); and how to tell whether Entry/Exit blocks are present, including between Meridians of the same Element (such as Gall Bladder/Liver, for example). Emotional and/or mental distress, which is by its very nature a Shen (Spirit) level phenomenon, will be discussed using a reinterpretation of the "Seven Dragons for Seven Devils" methodology taught in Five Element Acupuncture, broadening and demystifying the nature of this protocol, while simultaneously grounding it in pulse diagnostic criteria. These are all bread and butter issues for practitioners of Five Element Acupuncture (or should be), but can be readily incorporated into any other treatment style.

I should add that some of these clinical theories are entirely novel ideas that have not been previously discussed in the literature of either Ayurvedic medicine or acupuncture, and should definitely not be taken as dogma, but are being presented in order to share my experiences with the wider acupuncture profession. It is my hope that these new approaches will prove as effective in their hands as they have in my own. I beg the reader's indulgence in attending to such a detailed exposition of my thoughts about pulse diagnosis. Perhaps it would have been possible to write a simpler clinical manual devoted only to presenting the newly discovered acupuncture techniques themselves, but I feel that sharing the process of my thinking is just as valuable a contribution, in the hope that other practitioners might find herein the confidence to follow their own pathways into the unknown.

Perhaps a good place to begin is with some thoughts about pulse diagnosis itself. Before starting the formal presentation, I would like to say a few words that presage some of the material to be presented in the text, but which are at the very edge of my own thinking at this time, while I am writing, and will, I hope, serve as an indication of how I have gone about the process of developing a wider understanding of what the pulse reveals, and how it can be used in practice. I should also point out that this digression, even before I have begun, does not even touch on the issues of constitution and condition, but by illustrating how I think, I believe it will make the subsequent material easier for some readers to approach.

Let me start by noting that pulse diagnosis is an infinitely complex subject, but one that has preoccupied me for many years. It captures, in a microcosm, all of the general principles of traditional Oriental medicine, and therefore serves as an excellent practice for honing one's understanding of these principles. In my previous publications, *Closing the Circle* and *Footsteps*, I made some observations that I would like to recapitulate here. First, in *The Circle*, which was an exploration of the relationship of Five Element and TCM styles of practice, I classified acupuncture as a relatively Yang form of treatment (non-material) in comparison to herbal medicine, which I classified as relatively Yin (material). At the time, I did not see a particular way in which this distinction might illuminate pulse diagnosis, but it remained dormant, waiting for the right catalyst. Then, in *Footsteps*, I reviewed the history of both acupuncture and herbal medicine, and documented that they have often followed distinct lines of development in different historical periods and locales. At that time, I did not see a useful connection between these observations in the two publications, but as I have thought about these matters, and continued both my reading, tutorial education, and clinical experience, the following ideas have emerged.

I have often been struck by the relative lack of discussion about the exact positions for the examiner's fingers in palpating the Cun, Guan, and Chi[7] pulses of the radial artery.[8] Although it is not commonly noted, there is quite a bit of variation in the finger positions of examiners in palpating these three pulse positions.

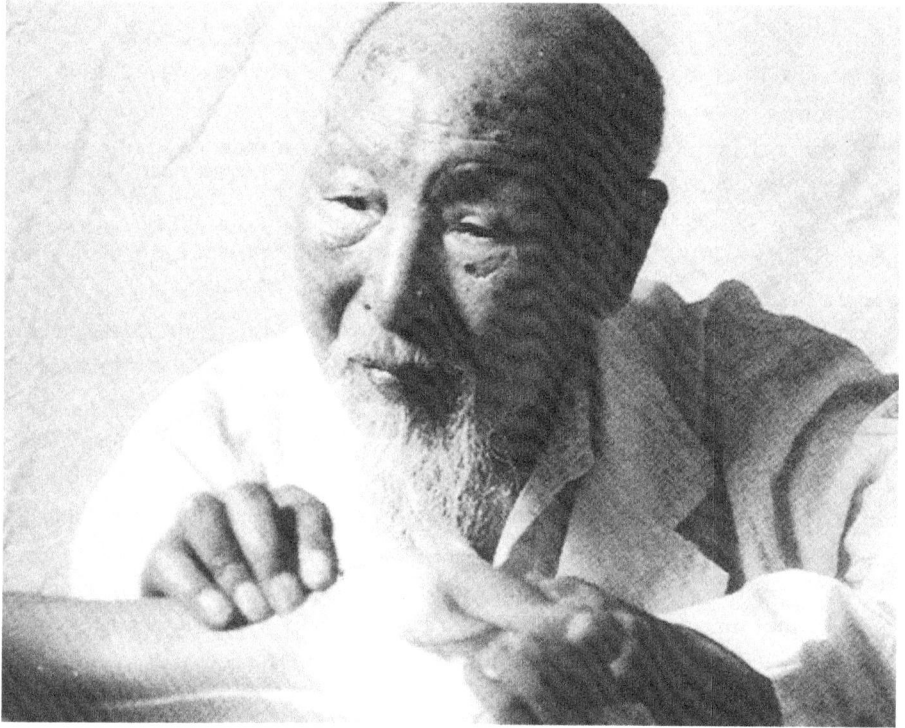

Figure P.1 Palpating fingers adjacent[9]

I will make a general characterization here, which may be extended, with variations where necessary, to other styles of pulse taking. In Worsley's Five Element style, the middle finger is placed directly over the prominence of the radial styloid process as the Guan location. The index finger is then placed next to it distally, locating the Cun position, and the ring finger is placed proximally, locating the Chi position. Worsley did not teach or practice herbal medicine, so his style is a stereotypical acupuncture oriented approach to pulse diagnosis.

---

7   Cun, Guan, and Chi have been translated as Inch, Bar, and Cubit respectively. Most contemporary publications in English retain the Chinese terms, as I have done.

8   See Figures P.1 and P.2 for examples of quite different finger placements.

9   Photo archived by Subhuti Dharmananda, reprinted with permission.

Another teacher I studied with, Jimmy Chang[10] (who has influenced many contemporary pulse teachers, including Will Morris), is emphatic that the middle finger placement for the Guan position must be substantially proximal to the prominence of the styloid process,[11] and the index and ring fingers must follow suit and also be placed slightly more proximally. In my studies with Chang, I noted that his treatment recommendations were almost entirely herbal in nature, so I am going to characterize his methodology as stereotypically reflective of herbal practice. Putting all the above findings together, it is possible to characterize Worsley's pulse diagnosis as relatively Yang compared to Chang's pulse diagnosis, which is relatively Yin.[12] (In fact, away from the center of the body is classified as Yang, while towards the center of the body is classified as Yin.)[13] Another piece of the puzzle popped into my mind when I remembered reading several books by Niboyet[14] in which he mentioned that pulses which are felt "in front" of their normal position are Excess (Yang), while those that are "behind" their normal position are Deficient (Yin). This idea is reminiscent of Ayurvedic pulse lore, where Vata pulses are felt most distally and Kapha pulses are felt most proximally, reflecting their energetic tendencies to be mobile (Yang) or static (Yin). It is clear that both Worsley's style and Chang's style are clinically useful, even if they are at least partially incongruent. The

---

10   Chang, J. and Brinkman, M., *Pulsynergy*. Privately published, 1995. Jimmy Wei-Yen Chang was originally trained in Taiwan by apprenticeship, and began practice as an acupuncturist. He later switched to the practice of herbal medicine before emigrating to California. He is a highly regarded teacher of herbal medicine and its reliance on pulse diagnosis, and has a close business relationship with the Evergreen Herb Company.

11   According to Chang, the peak of the styloid is exactly the location separating index and middle fingers. See Chang and Brinkman, 1995, p.12.

12   Will Morris has pointed out that John Shen and Heiner Fruehauf's teacher both used distal finger placement, even though their treatments were largely herbal. Obviously one can practice excellent herbal medicine or acupuncture using either of these finger positions alone, because there is always Yang in Yin and Yin in Yang. Herbs treat both Yin and Yang, as does acupuncture. What I'm proposing is a way to get a bit more specific information about the Yin and Yang status of each Organ. So far it has proved useful in my practice.

13   The Yang locations are taught in most English language acupuncture texts including *The Essentials of Chinese Acupuncture*. Beijing: Foreign Languages Press, 1980; O'Connor, J. and Bensky, D., trans. and eds., *Acupuncture: A Comprehensive Text*. Chicago, IL: Eastland Press, 1981; and Kaptchuk, T., *The Web That Has No Weaver*. New York: Congdon and Weed, 1983. By contrast, the Yin locations are also taught by Jeffrey Yuen (personal observation). He uses the *ulnar* styloid to locate the Guan position, and this turns out to be proximal to the *radial* styloid location. Leon Hammer, a disciple of Shen's, in *Chinese Pulse Diagnosis*. Seattle, WA: Eastland Press, 2001, p.62, begs the question by basing his finger positions on the Cun location, right at the proximal edge of the scaphoid bone, but because he positions the Guan and Chi locations immediately adjacently, this would appear to be consistent with the Yang locations, as suggested in footnote 12. My observation of numerous other practitioners from different traditions also shows a third common practice, where the Cun, Guan, and Chi locations are not immediately adjacent to each other, but are separated by gaps of varying length between the examining fingers.

14   *Essai sur l'acupuncture Chinoise pratique*. Paris: Editions Dominique Wapler, 1951, and *Compléments d'acupuncture*. Paris: Editions Dominique Wapler, 1955, both in French and not yet translated into English.

resolution of this conundrum occurred to me after reading and contemplating the material in an excellent book by Radha Thambirajah, *Energetics in Acupuncture*.[15] She points out, right from the beginning (Chapter 1), that Yin and Yang are the basis of acupuncture practice, and that it is not simply a question of recognizing Yin and Yang Organ systems/Meridians (Zang Fu/Jing Luo), but that each of these has its own Yin and Yang aspects. For instance, there is Heart Yin and Heart Yang, Small Intestine Yin and Small Intestine Yang, etc., each of which can be either Excess, Deficient, or Balanced. I had a revelation, of sorts, suspecting that the Worsley pulses might reflect the Yang of their related Organs/Meridians, while the Chang pulses might reflect the Yin of these same Organs/Meridians. Ms. Thambirajah was also helpful in explaining how the Command Points of each Meridian differentially affect both the Yin and the Yang aspects of their related Organ system, and how they can be used to restore a proper Yin/Yang balance to each Organ/Meridian.[16] I have used her recommendations in conjunction with the aforementioned procedure of separately palpating the Yang and Yin conditions of each of the 12 Organs/Meridians, and have found that this approach gives excellent clinical results, which I will illustrate in the case history chapter. In treatment, I have followed classical acupuncture principles, that Deficiency should be Tonified and Excess should be Dispersed, and that when possible, any Excess should be "transferred" to places that are Deficient. Five Element relationships are very important in this regard, and will be described in the body of the text. The notion of separate Yin and Yang pulses, as well as the methodology for transferring Qi between Organs/Meridians, are aspects of the conditional pulse diagnosis, and will be discussed in Chapter 13. Using this idea of Yang and Yin pulse diagnostic positions, and employing treatments based on them, is only one of many approaches to acupuncture treatment that I practice. The text presents many others. This brief discourse should not substitute for a careful study of the full range of pulse diagnostic material presented in the text as a whole, but I hope it will give both an indication of the need for flexibility in employing pulse diagnosis, and at the same time explicate the essentially rational character of

15   Thambirajah, R., *Energetics in Acupuncture*. Edinburgh: Churchill Livingstone, 2010.

16   Thambirajah teaches the doctrine (which she learned in China) that the Control Cycle (Xiang Ke) operates from Yang Organ to Yin Organ and vice versa, which is contrary to the teachings of Worsley about transferring Qi via the Control Cycle. Worsley's teachings derive directly from those of his French teacher, Lavier. It is interesting to note that Lavier initially presented the Control Cycle relationships as acting from Yang Organ to Yin Organ and vice versa, exactly as per Thambirajah, but later taught the Yin Organ to Yin Organ version that Worsley adopted (see *Footsteps*, p.158). The Korean "Four Needle Technique" originated by the medieval monk Sa Am uses Yin Organ to Yin Organ and Yang Organ to Yang Organ Control Cycle relationships. Thus it would appear that both versions capture valid aspects of Five Element energetics. My belief is that it is important to use each protocol within the style of practice to which it pertains; however, I have found that in transferring Qi via the Creative and Control Cycles (Xiang Sheng and Xiang Ke), Thambirajah's method gives more precise results in balancing not only the Elements, but also Yin and Yang.

this diagnostic methodology. My personal belief is that Oriental medicine, and its individual components, including pulse diagnosis, is based on a scientific point of view, but that is a topic for a separate treatise.

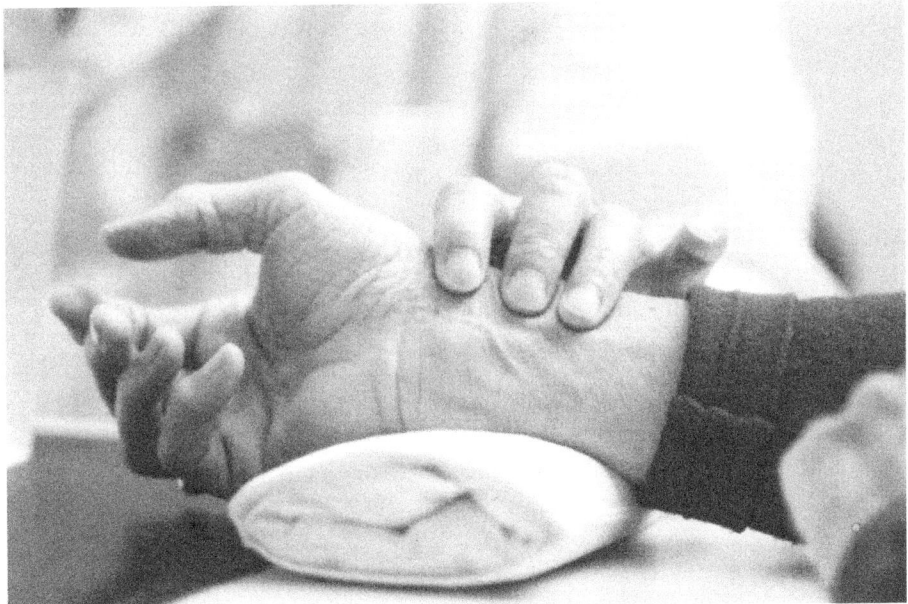

Figure P.2 Palpating fingers spread[17]

I have mentioned that the acupuncture and the herbal traditions have not always agreed in matters of doctrinal detail, including pulse diagnosis. Is there any other interpretation of this divergence than my hypothesis that they were focused on either the Yang or the Yin aspect of the Organs/Meridians? As with all issues in Oriental medicine, a good place to start is by once again applying Yin/Yang theory to the topic. In my opinion, there are two different perspectives, which can be called "somatotopic" and "energetic," representing the Yin and Yang approaches respectively. The somatotopic approach focuses on the representation of the various structures of the body (and their malfunctions) at their corresponding locations in the radial pulse. This perspective is dominant in the modern version of TCM, which I see as being strongly influenced by herbal medical teachings (a Yin treatment modality), and is also prominent in Hammer's text based on John Shen's teachings,[18] but it has clearly been discussed from the beginning of Chinese medical literature in the *Neijing*. The image of the Three Heaters, seen in tongue diagnosis, is an example of this somatotopic

---

17   Image: www.acupuncturebrooklyn.com.
18   *Chinese Pulse Diagnosis*. See also Shen, J., *Chinese Medicine*. New York: Educational Solutions, 1980, in which all the treatments are herbal in nature.

approach, and in radial pulse diagnosis it shows up as assigning the pulses of the Large and Small Intestines to the Lower Heater (Chi position). By contrast, the energetic perspective locates the pulses of the Large and Small Intestines in the more distal Cun position, with their coupled Organs, the Lungs and Heart. These relationships are based on Five Element theory, which is clearly in the energetic, rather than the structural, realm. This energetic perspective on pulse diagnosis is also to be found in the early texts of Chinese medicine, most clearly described in the *Nanjing* and *Maijing*, and forms the basis for the pulse teachings of the more specifically acupunctural styles of treatment such as that taught by Worsley in England (see Figure P.3).

	Left wrist		A	**Right wrist**	
Distal	Small Intestine	Heart		Lung	Large Intestine
Middle	Gall Bladder	Liver		Spleen	Stomach
Proximal	Bladder	Kidneys		Life Gate	Three Heater

	Superficial	**Deep**	B	**Deep**	**Superficial**
Distal	Pericardium	Heart		Lungs	Sternum
Middle	Gall Bladder	Liver		Spleen	Stomach
Proximal	Large Intestine Bladder	Kidney		Kidney	Three Heater Life Gate Small Intestine

Figure P.3 Energetic (A) and somatotopic (B) positions

It is not a question of which perspective is the correct one, as they are both correct. They merely describe the Yin and Yang aspects of pulse manifestations. The fact that both somatotopic and energetic factors influence the palpated pulse makes interpretation more challenging than is often appreciated, but my experience is that paying careful attention to the procedures developed for each tradition of pulse diagnosis can go a long way towards minimizing the confusion. Acupuncture, being a more Yang modality than herbal medicine, naturally resonates with the energetic perspective, and it will be seen to be the predominant theoretical basis for the varieties of pulse diagnostic techniques and theories that I will be discussing. Having mentioned resonance, there is one further comment about my own point of view that I would like to make explicit.

There are many styles of pulse diagnosis, and each represents a unique tradition and conceptual point of view. My own point of reference, in all things pertaining to Oriental medicine, is the concept of resonance, or Gan Ying, in Chinese. To me, the pulses transmit energetic waves of resonant information propagated from the Interior. Most approaches to pulse diagnosis don't allude to Gan Ying at all, and are presented as a priori beliefs, without any attempt to explain their underlying principles. In my mind, pulse taking is very similar to playing a musical instrument, like a violin. If you want to perceive relevant and accurate information, your fingers must be placed in *exactly* the right place to evoke a resonant response. If your finger placement is slightly off, the note may still be recognizable (with some effort), but it will not produce the same feeling as would listening to a master violinist.

Many of the chapters to follow will introduce methods of pulse diagnosis that will be unfamiliar to most readers. Each of these methods is different from the others, and it is crucial to pay careful attention to the descriptions of how to feel each of these types of pulse. I have experimented with these procedures for many years, and it is only after trying out many variations that I have confirmed the accuracy of the descriptions I'm providing. This is the logical place for others to start, if they wish to incorporate any of these new methods, but I certainly encourage experimentation afterwards, as I am confident that there are refinements that are just waiting to be discovered in these and other pulse taking practices.

ACKNOWLEDGMENTS

There are six main strands that form the framework of the material presented here. The first is the style of Five Element Acupuncture, which I studied under the tutelage of the late J. R. Worsley in England (from 1974 to 1985). I have previously outlined this material under the rubric of Leamington Acupuncture (LA) in *Footsteps*, and familiarity with that book, or any other text on Five Element Acupuncture (FEA), would be most helpful in understanding and applying the new material in this text. Central to Worsley's teachings was the concept of the Causative Factor (CF), which some commentators have speculated was inspired by Worsley's exposure to Korean influences.[1] It is fitting therefore that the next two strands in my personal fabric are both Korean.[2] I studied Korean Constitutional Acupuncture at the clinic of its originator, Kuon Dowon, from 1987 to 1988. Kuon's constitutional typology was reminiscent of Worsley's CF, and I could not help but search for the relationship between them. This presented some difficulty, as Kuon's approach encompasses eight types while Worsley's encompasses five. I also studied Korean Hand Acupuncture under its originator, Yoo Tae Woo, from 1985 to 1994 in both Seoul and the USA. Yoo's system likewise involves a constitutional theory but, alas, it only recognizes three types! My effort to discern the relationship between these different notions of constitution was unsuccessful for many years, despite keeping it always in mind, although I had experienced quite satisfactory results from each of these styles of practice, regardless of the conflicting nature of their theories and methods. Dr. Yoo asked me to edit the English edition of his introductory textbook,[3] and perhaps the many hours I spent trying to properly organize Yoo's material for a Western readership was responsible for my first fruitful insight. In any case, one day it dawned on me that Yoo's three constitutional types were strikingly similar to the three constitutional types described by the traditional

---

1   Bob Duggan, personal communication.
2   I have had helpful input from a number of other Korean teachers whom I'd like to thank, H. B. Kim, Byoung Kim, Joseph Kim, David Lee, and Chae Lew being the most important.
3   Yoo Tae Woo, *Koryo Hand Acupuncture*, vol. 1 (ed. P. Eckman). Seoul: Eum Yang Mek Jin, 1988.

Ayurvedic system of medicine of India, with which I had only a superficial acquaintance. I published a journal article on this observation,[4] hoping that someone with greater knowledge of Ayurveda could further develop this line of inquiry, but such was not to be the case. Finally, I decided that I would have to learn more about Ayurveda myself, and began studying (from 2003 to 2008) with Mary Jo Cravatta D.C., a highly skilled pulse diagnostician in the Ayurvedic lineage sponsored by the late Maharishi Mahesh Yogi. The Maharishi originally brought Dr. J. R. Raju from India to the USA to teach one of the esoteric methods of pulse diagnosis that had been maintained in India by oral tradition. In addition I read Dr. Vasant Lad's book on Ayurvedic pulse diagnosis,[5] and subsequently had a lengthy interview with him via telephone.[6] My penultimate strand was supplied by another Korean, Puramo Chong, whom I discovered via the Internet, and whose clinic I visited in 2005. Dr. Chong is an expert in Sasang Constitutional Medicine (SCM), a subject which I will explore in detail in the main body of the text, but in addition he was willing to share with me some unpublished (in English) speculations of other Korean constitutional practitioners, and I began to visualize a solution to the riddle of constitution in a form somewhat like the periodic chart of the elements. That is to say, I could perceive the outline of the general theory of constitutions, but there were undiscovered gaps (like undiscovered elements in the periodic chart) whose existence I could predict. This was a most desirable result, because if I could find the predicted constitutions, it would be the strongest validation of my constitutional hypothesis I could desire. As I continued my research, the missing constitutions began showing up where they were expected, but the reliability and reproducibility of the pulse findings were not convincingly superior to those of color, sound, odor, and emotion, a diagnostic methodology that I had aimed to supersede. Finally, after taking a pulse seminar with Joseph Adams,[7] and reading the materials written by his teacher Will Morris (together with my own studies under Jeffrey Yuen and Jimmy Chang), I carefully reviewed the information contained in the oldest Chinese text on pulse diagnosis, the *Maijing* (*Pulse Classic*), which first became available in English in 1997.[8] Amazingly, I discovered therein a methodology that has proven (with some creative interpretation) to be a highly reliable guide to constitutional analysis, based on the Six Energetic Levels. By combining all

---

4   Eckman, P., "Ayurveda and Korean Hand Acupuncture: A Brief Introduction to Some Similarities between Constitutional Typologies." *Amer. J. Acup.*, 23 (2), 1995, pp.153–158.

5   Lad, V., *Secrets of the Pulse: The Ancient Art of Ayurvedic Pulse Diagnosis*. Albuquerque, NM: Ayurvedic Press, 1996.

6   Lad's style of pulse diagnosis, like Raju's, was learned by direct transmission from his teacher, and thus represents an oral tradition. Neither of these styles of Ayurvedic pulse diagnosis is to be found in the classical texts.

7   Adams, J., "Pulse Diagnosis," seminar, Berkeley, CA, 2008.

8   Wang Shu-he, *The Pulse Classic* (Yang Shou-zhong, trans.). Boulder, CO: Blue Poppy Press, 1997.

of the foregoing methods, I found it possible to greatly improve the accuracy of my constitutional diagnoses, as the findings from each method support those of all the others. Having established a firmer grounding for CF determination, I next turned my attention to a better understanding of the reflections in the pulse of the patient's current condition. I have developed what I consider to be a unique point of view about this topic, which I have already presented as separate Yin and Yang pulse examinations. I will reprise this topic in a chapter of its own, dedicated to reintegrating Yin/Yang theory into what has primarily been a Five Element discussion. This book summarizes my investigations up to the present, so, without further ado, I offer the work as it currently stands.

As always, there are way too many people to thank individually for their help in this project, but I am especially grateful to the following: Marlene Elbin has been "pestering" me to teach for a number of years, and this book started as a way to try to organize my thoughts for such an endeavor. Carol Ferraro, inspired by *Footsteps*, began writing a book about her spiritual approach to chiropractic about the same time as I started this book, and we have egged each other on at our quasi-weekly folkdance sessions. Stuart Kutchins has shared my odyssey and fascination with Korean acupuncture, virtually from beginning to end, and has lent body and mind to helping me refine my thoughts (I'm talking guinea pig here). Jane Grissmer spurred me to keep my focus on traditional acupuncture theory by inviting me to teach a class at the Tai Sophia institute on "Classical Chinese Medical Literature," and, while I was not able to discuss any of the Korean or Indian pulse material which forms such a large part of this text, I was able to explore the ramifications of Gan Ying resonance theory as the underlying basis for all of Oriental medicine, and that focus has silently been my beacon throughout this treatise. I will not attempt to elaborate on resonance theory here, but hope to present a separate treatise on this subject in the future. I am deeply grateful to Will Morris for writing the Foreword and for his ebullient encouragement. Lonny Jarrett was kind enough to read and annotate the manuscript, which gave me much to think about. Both Neal White and Elisabeth Waller-White offered their unconditional assistance in the artistic and production/distribution realms, where I dare not tread, and I cannot thank them enough. Finally, the love of my life, my wife Marina, has returned a smile to the face of this aging Baby Boomer, giving me the energy to finish the book you are about to begin.

There is one further remark I feel impelled to include here. What I am presenting is primarily a diagnostic methodology. This methodology can be employed by practitioners of various traditions and at various levels of understanding of the deepest natures of their human patients, in health and in illness. On the one hand, such a methodology can be applied in an almost mechanical manner, to arrive at a diagnosis. On the other hand, to serve as a vehicle for healing on a deep level, it is necessary to appreciate the dimensions, from physical to mental to emotional to spiritual, which acupuncture treatment has the capacity to impact. Whenever I find myself getting too caught up in the mechanical details of diagnosis, I reread some of the voluminous, but unpublished, material written by my incomparable friend and colleague, Thea Elijah. I have found no better way to immediately reconnect with the spiritual root that gives life to the technical matters I'm describing. And so I must thank her, and acknowledge the importance of her friendship in helping me remember where I'm trying to go.

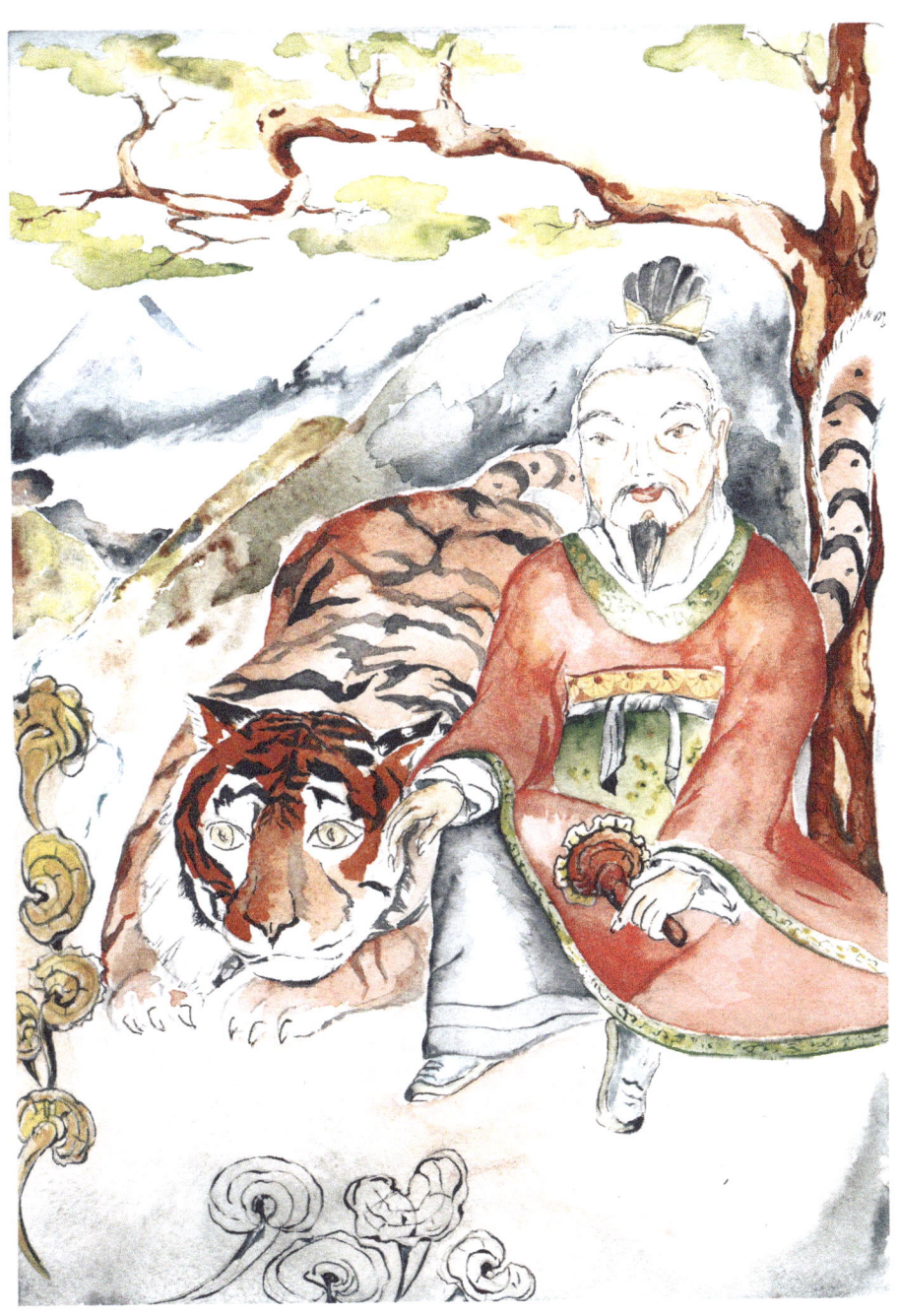

San-shin, the Mountain Spirit, an ancient Deity said to inspire
the unique medical and cultural thought of Korea

Image: Marina Chentsova Eckman.

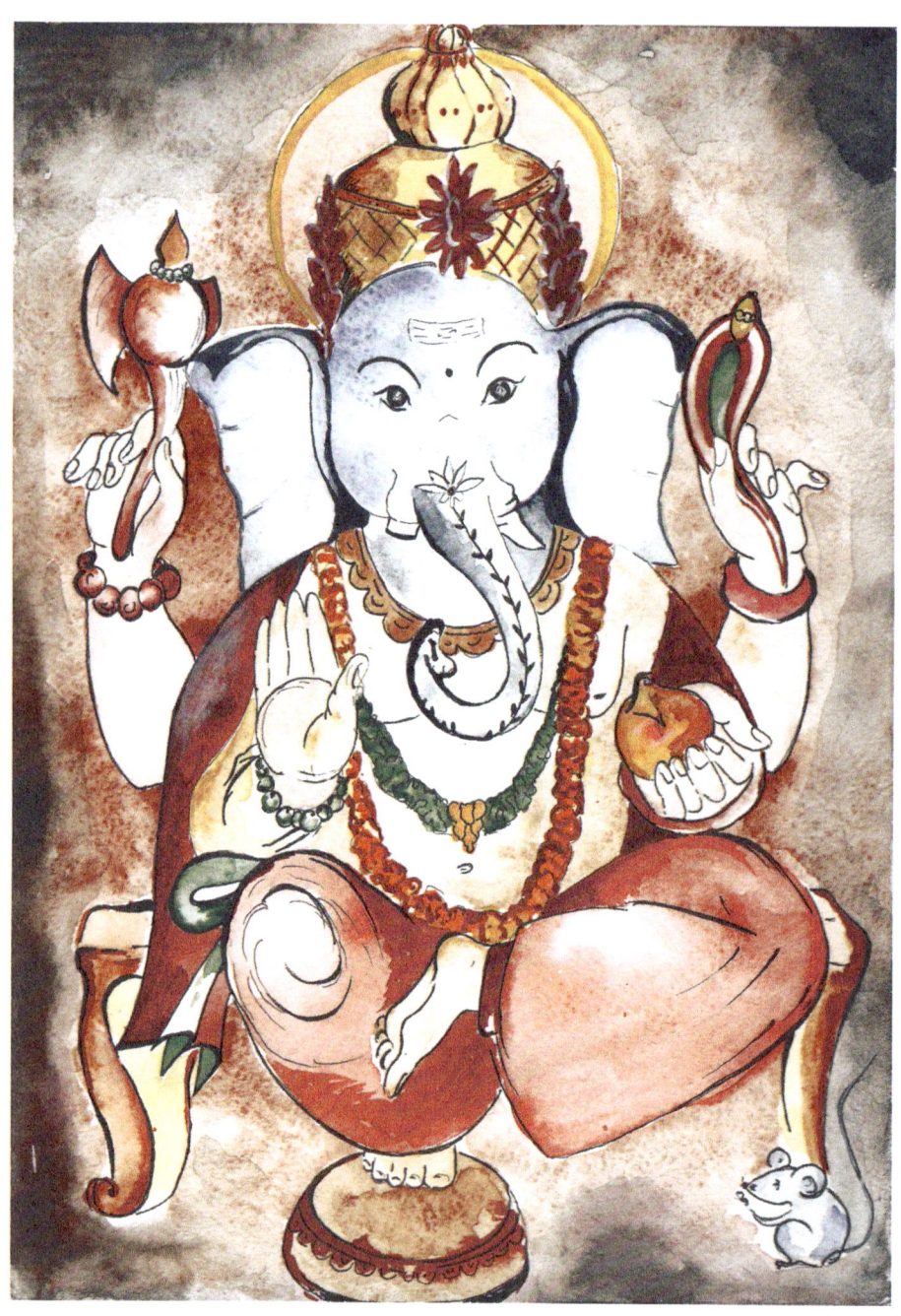

Ganesha, the Remover of Obstacles, revered in India as the Patron of Arts and Sciences and as the Deity of Intellect and Wisdom
Image: Marina Chentsova Eckman.

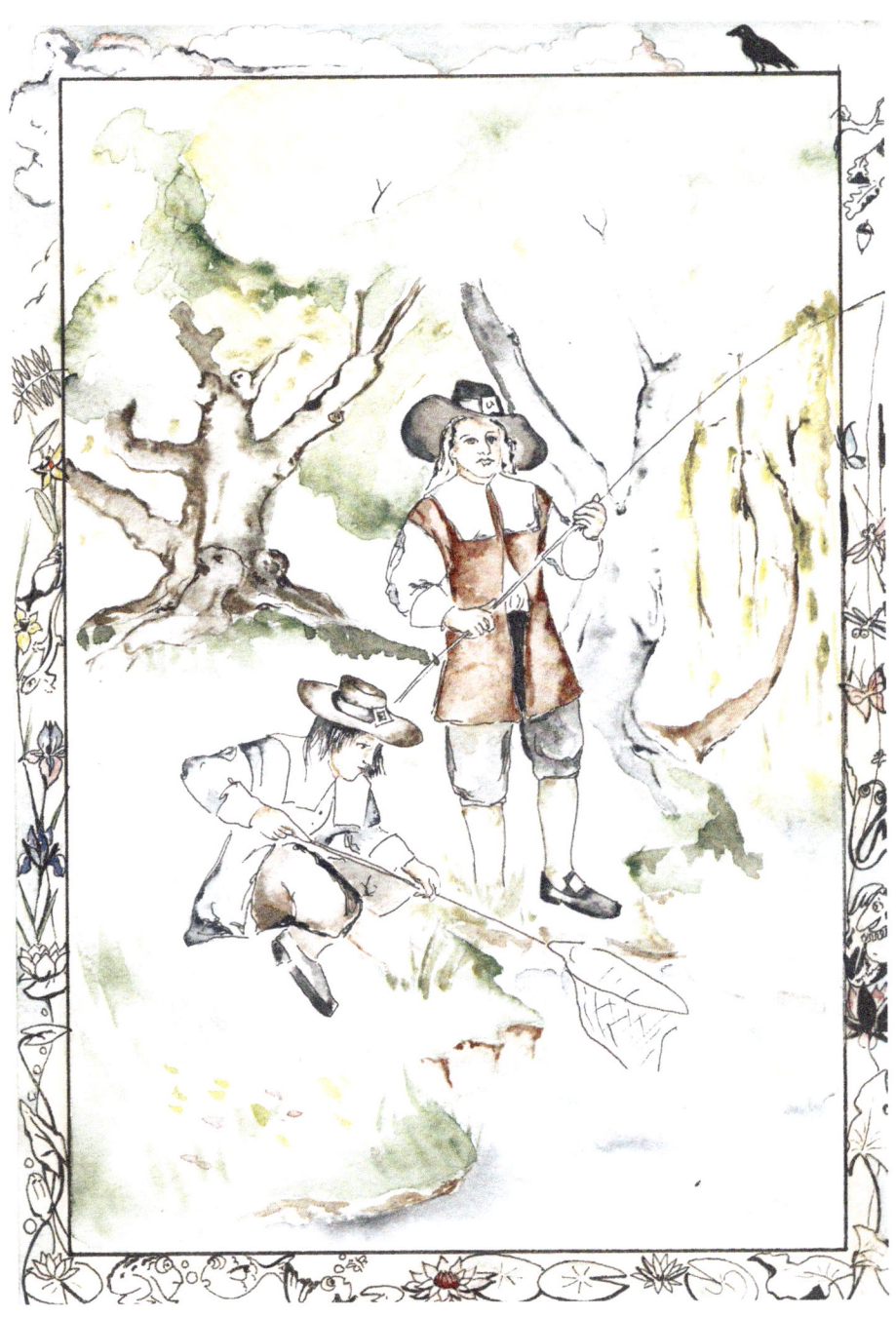

Sir Izaak Walton
Image: Marina Chentsova Eckman.

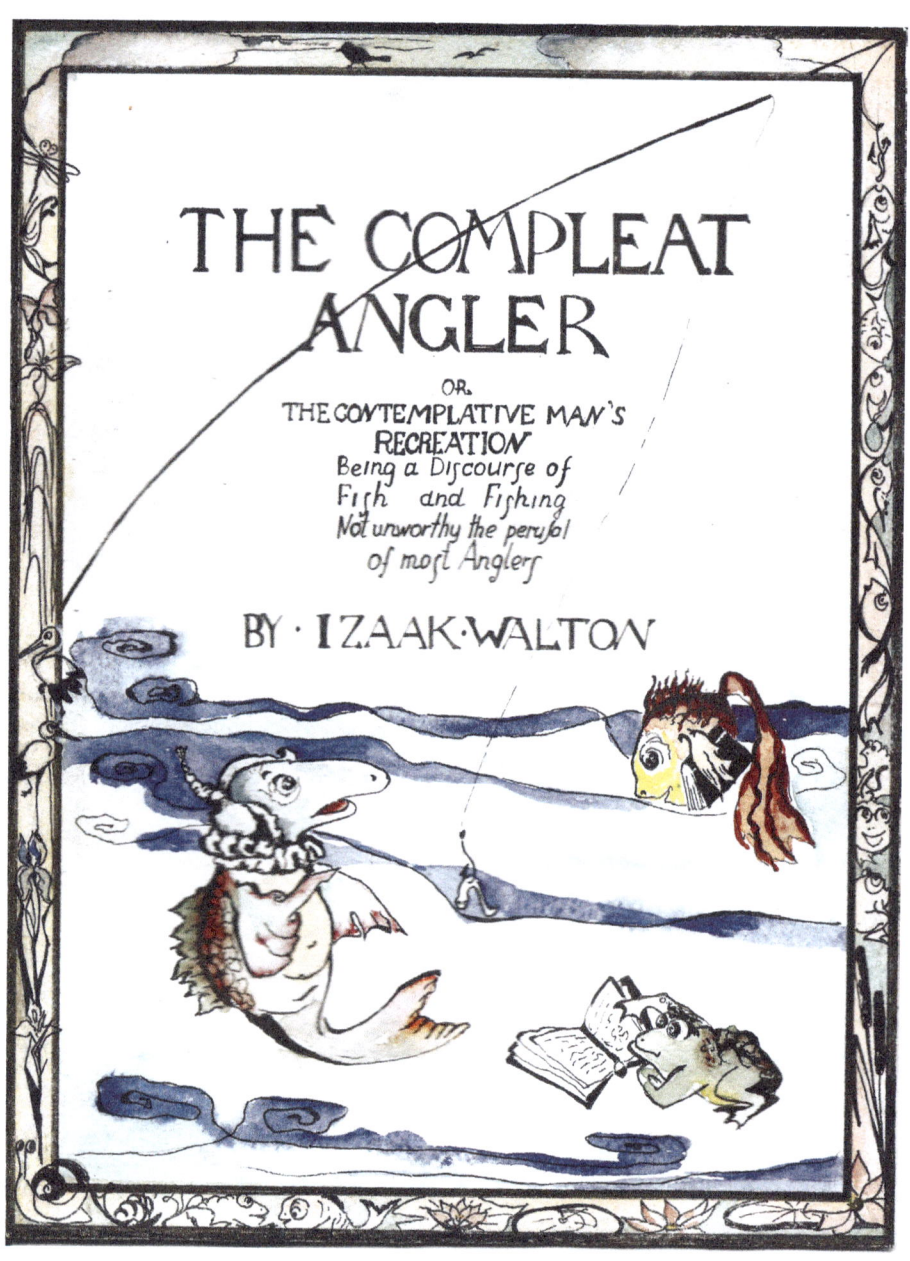

The Contemplative Man's Recreation in 1653

Image: Marina Chentsova Eckman. Cover for Walton's classic originally published in London in 1653.

PART ONE

CONSTITUTIONAL PULSE DIAGNOSIS

CHAPTER I

CONSTITUTION AND CONDITION

Regardless of the therapeutic modality employed, all treatment can be thought of as primarily concerned with either the manifested condition (symptoms, diseases, syndromes, etc.) or with the original energetic disturbance that allowed the current presentation to develop. There are several technical terms that describe this distinction, roots and branches being the one most commonly employed in Oriental medicine. It provides a fitting image: If the branches or leaves on a tree are attacked by some injurious factor, a gardener may apply localized treatments, even to the extent of pruning them, in order to allow a new round of growth from the presumably healthy roots to occur, and all will be well. On the other hand, if the very roots are attacked, even if the leaves and branches continue to appear healthy for a while, the tree itself may be doomed unless the roots can be restored to a healthy state, so the best gardeners will never disregard the health of the roots, whether or not there are problems showing up in the branches or leaves. Traditionally, this line of thought can be taken a step further: If the roots are maintained in perfect health, then the branches and leaves will be supplied with the optimal requirements to withstand many an injurious factor, and there are those who claim that a well guarded root will lead to a state of immunity to illness. This is an example of the hierarchical nature of many of the relationships in living beings: The roots can be thought of as more significant than the branches, which are relatively more expendable. Thus it may seem counter-intuitive that the roots are usually unseen (hidden in the ground for most plants), while the branches are easily observed, and where any abnormality may be readily detected. Human beings are not really different from trees in this regard: What is easily seen as an abnormality or symptom may be much less crucial to the survival of the individual than the unseen phenomena (the root imbalance) which may ultimately determine their fate. For didactic purposes I have presented the notion of roots and branches as separable aspects of a living organism, but this is not really the case. In fact, there is a constant interplay, back and forth, between the roots and branches, in both plants and people, as in all living beings. Thus it is not necessarily true that simply treating a diseased branch will fail to cure an illness, even if there are less than perfectly healthy roots. The branches are always sending influences back to the roots, and, in some circumstances, the beneficial influences that treated branches can now send back to the roots may be enough to also heal the roots. For this reason, I believe it is wrong to dismiss symptomatic treatment as insufficient at best, and outright harmful at worst. Each situation needs to be evaluated on its own merits. At the same time it would be a capital mistake to forget the natural hierarchy between roots and branches. When in doubt, take care of the roots.

We live in a world of multiple medical systems whose variants occur in both the spatial and temporal realms. It is common to contrast modern Western medicine with traditional Oriental medicine, for example. In tracing each of these lineages backwards in time, we come across the curious finding that distinguishing East and West may not be so simple. How are we to classify ancient Greece? Was it East or West? Hippocrates (see Figure 1.1) is known as the "Father of Western medicine," but in fact both his notions and those of Galen, who followed in his footsteps, are in many ways closer to those of Oriental medicine, being based on Humoral and Elemental theories of balance. I make this observation for several reasons, the first of which is to introduce the topic of constitutional theories, the Hellenic (Greek) Four Temperaments (Sanguine, Phlegmatic, Choleric, and Melancholic) being perhaps the most well-known example of constitutional types with which the Western reader might be familiar (see Figure 1.2).[1] The second reason for starting with ancient Hellenic (Greek) thought is to shine a light on the obvious similarities between it and the traditional medical systems known as Unnani (Arabic/Persian), Ayurveda (Indian), and that of China. In *Footsteps*, I made the claim that the various versions of Oriental medicine I surveyed were all branches off a common trunk of shared beliefs. When I finished that book in 1996, I had not yet realized that this common trunk also includes Hellenic, Unnani, and Ayurvedic medicine, and this subsequent realization was crucial to my current understanding of both constitutions and conditions. I should point out that the concepts of Humors and Elements can be applied to either a root or a branch, and likewise to one's constitution or one's condition. It is always imperative to specify how these terms are being applied in each case.

---

1   These temperaments are correlated with the Four Humors: Blood, Phlegm, Yellow Bile, and Black Bile.

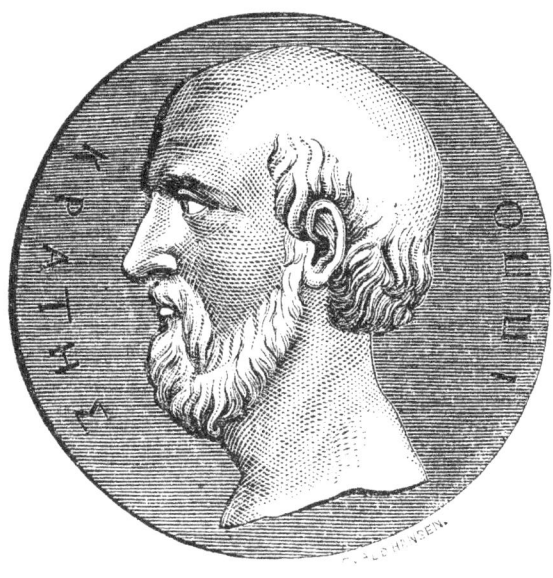

Figure 1.1 Hippocrates, exemplar of Eastern or Western medicine?[2]

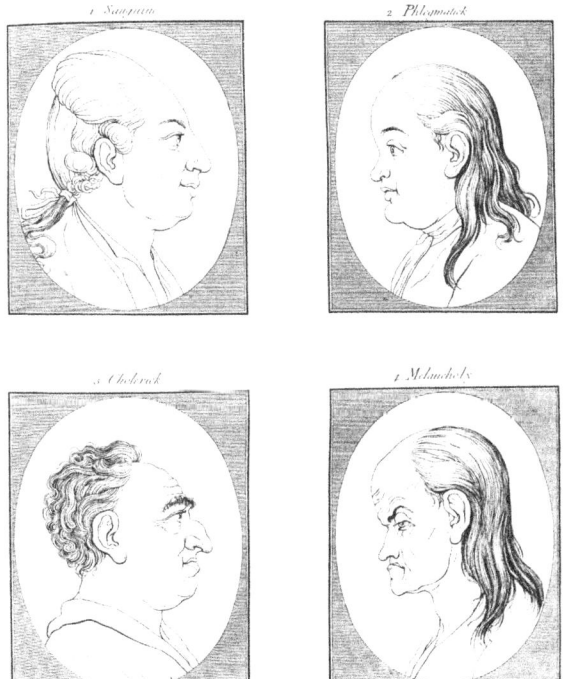

Figure 1.2 The Four Temperaments: Phlegmatic, Sanguine, Choleric, and Melancholic[3]

2   Wikimedia Commons, from an engraving of an ancient Greek coin by E. Hansen.

3   Lavater, J., *Essays on Physiognomy.* London: G.G.J. and J. Robinson, 1789.

Returning to the question of shared beliefs between the various styles of Oriental medicine, is there any historical data to substantiate an interrelationship between Hellenic, Unnani, Ayurvedic, and Chinese medicine? Both Chinese and Indian medical ideas have an oral tradition that probably predates any written record. Much Chinese medical lore is attributed to the Yellow Emperor, Huang Di (c. 2700 BCE), and there are corresponding fables concerning the origins of Ayurveda during the Neolithic and Bronze Age (c. 2300 BCE) along the Indus River in northwest India. The orthodox belief is that the four Vedas, or canons of wisdom, were originally revealed by the godhead, Brahma, creator of the universe, to a succession of divine entities including the god Indra, who passed this knowledge on until it was finally heard by a group of inspired sages, the Rishis, who in turn continued the teachings via an oral tradition maintained by the Brahmin or priestly caste. It was from this Vedic (Hindu) tradition that the Buddha (c. 563–483 BCE) initiated a new spiritual system, one that was as closely intertwined with Ayurvedic medical teachings as was its Hindu progenitor. Buddhism was much more widely disseminated than was Hinduism, and had a major impact on Chinese thought in all areas, including medicine. While the classics of Chinese medicine (*Neijing*, *Nanjing*, *Shanghanlun*, *Maijing*) were first written between 200 BCE and 200 CE, those of Indian medicine (*Charaka Samhita* and *Sushruta Samhita*) were more likely written between 760 and 660 BCE,[4] and thus possibly represent an earlier stratum of medical thought. These early texts already discuss the Humoral and Elemental theories that are to be found in most versions of Oriental medicine. Since there was undoubtedly a long period of oral transmission of these ideas prior to their being written down, it is impossible to know which is earliest. The question then becomes, was there any contact between these cultures prior to their first written texts? Certainly there are scholars who would answer in the affirmative. For example, the Chinese Yueh-chih tribes, the Kushans, coming from western China, occupied Benares (Varanisi) in northeast India. They are considered to have formed a bridge, the Silk Road,[5] between East and West. This trade route between the Mediterranean Sea and China was operative prior to 500 BCE, although it did not receive its name, or heavy traffic, until much later.[6] Likewise, the Burma Road (c. 115 BCE) to the south also opened the exchange of material goods and ideas to and from China.[7] There is no doubt of early contacts between Persia and Greece (c. 550 BCE, along the Silk Road) as related by the Greek historian Herodotus, and as both the Persians and the

---

4   Ninivaggi, F., *An Elementary Textbook of Ayurveda*. Madison, CT: Psychosocial Press, 2001, p.16.

5   Ibid., p.19.

6   www.livius.org/sh-si/silk_road/silk_road.html (accessed July 19, 2013).

7   Ninivaggi, 2001, p.19.

Vedic peoples in India were from the same Aryan stock, the likelihood that all these cultures exchanged ideas in the period prior to the writing down of medical texts seems inescapable.[8]

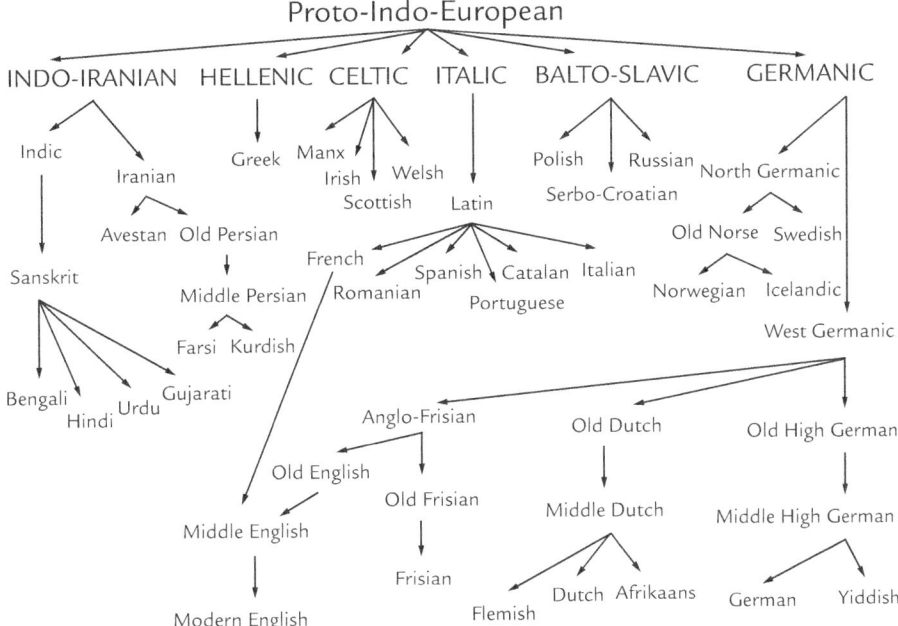

Figure 1.3 Indo-European language tree[9]

One final aspect of the attempt to reconstruct ancient medical history is worth mentioning. In almost every country of the ancient world, the great repositories of learning were destroyed, frequently by fires, from China (which supposedly spared medical texts), to the great library in Alexandria, whose destruction was begun by Caesar in 47 BCE and probably completed by the Muslims who

---

8   The two most thorough studies of which I am aware beg the question of whether these similarities are the result of convergence, diffusion from a common source, or some combination of the two. They both, however, document the enormous degree of concordance present: Filliozat, J., *The Classical Doctrine of Indian Medicine*. Delhi: Munshiram Manoharlal, 1964; Amber, R. and Babey-Brooke, A., *The Pulse in Occident and Orient*. New York: Dunshaw Press, 1966. On his pulse diagnosis listserve, Will Morris had this to say on January 27, 2013: "My new favorite…: *The Canon of Medicine Volume 2: Natural Pharmaceuticals*, Avicenna (Author), Laleh Bakhtiar (Editor). It reminds me of my trip to Italy in 1993 to review the pharmacies in the basilicas. There was not a single agent that did not occur in the Chinese pharmacopoeia. Early Persian medicine was essentially a melting pot of Greek, Ayurvedic and I believe also Chinese work."

9   Image: Adapted from http://soc-psych.wikispaces.com/file/view/Language_Tree.gif/323/9947/ Language_Tree.gif.

captured this Egyptian city c. 642 CE. The task of compiling a thorough history of medicine would undoubtedly have been much more revealing had these tragedies not occurred. My working hypothesis in this text will be that the primitive speculations about Elements and Humors can reasonably be supposed to have predated any written medical tradition, and might very well have been widely shared throughout the ancient world.

One implication of this historical hypothesis (a unitary conceptualization common to all of Oriental medicine) is that the various constitutional theories espoused by these distinct medical systems might appear contradictory at first glance but, being based on a common origin, could possibly be found to be reconcilable at a deeper level of understanding. This at least is the premise I have adopted, and in order to assess its validity, the various constitutional systems must be described in enough detail for the reader to be able to appreciate the hoped-for eventual synthesis. To facilitate the presentation, the systems will be briefly described using traditional numerology to order them, after which separate chapters will present each system that I use in greater detail. Following the presentation of constitutional theories, in Part Two I will devote several chapters to my approach to conditional pulse diagnosis, but for Part One, let us stay with the topic of constitutional analysis.

Therapeutic systems, of course, cannot distinguish constitutions until at least two possibilities are present, but the philosophical underpinnings are not constrained by this limitation. Let us begin with Zero. In both Chinese and Indian philosophy there is the notion that while all the manifestations of the phenomenal world are but expressions of One commonality (the Dao, Brahman), there is a way of looking at reality perhaps a step deeper. That would be the level of the absolutely unmanifested. In Chinese, this was called "Wu Ji" (without a pole) by the Neo-Confucian philosophers (see Figure 1.4) and corresponds to the Indian notion of "Avyakta," or pure unmanifested existence.[10] It is the great void (i.e. zero) out of which all of creation springs forth.

---

10   Ninivaggi, 2001, p.42, and Lad, V., *Secrets of the Pulse: The Ancient Art of Ayurvedic Pulse Diagnosis.* Albuquerque, NM: Ayurvedic Press, 1996, p.6.

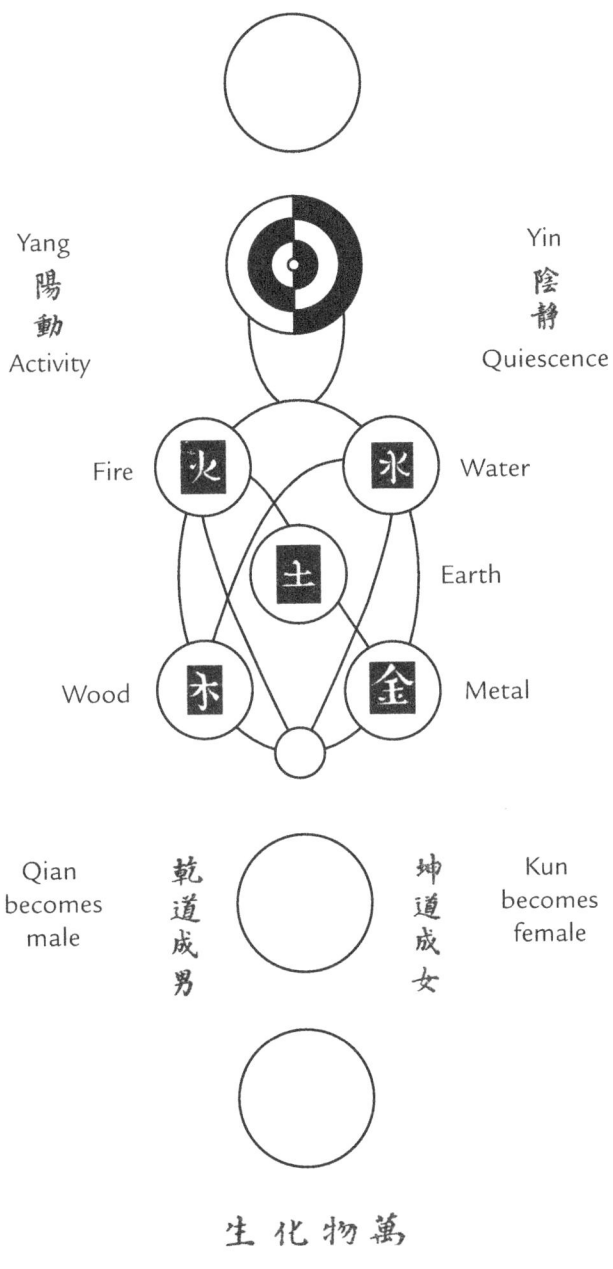

Figure 1.4 Diagram of the Supreme Ultimate[11]

---

11   Image: Chou Tun-I (1017–1073 CE).

This basic idea, the great void, which the Neo-Confucians elaborated, was already present in Lao Zi's *Daodejing*, where he says, "Ten thousand things under Heaven are born of being (Yu). Being is born of non-being (Wu)."[12] For those, like myself, who believe that the truths of Western science are fully compatible with (but not reducible to) those of Eastern medicine, this concept might be likened to that which preceded the "Big Bang," but Eastern medicine would not limit this idea to material reality; it would also include consciousness as a fundamental part of any description of "what is."

Keeping this analogy, we might think of One as the Big Bang itself, a singularity in which nature pours forth the whole of the universe, all of it sharing a common origin. In Chinese the term Tai Ji (Great Pole) is spoken of as the origin of the phenomenal world, and is thus an incarnation of the Dao, the One that everything comes from and to which it will return. Tai Ji, the ridgepole, is also translated as the "great primal beginning," and is introduced in the *Classic of Changes* or *Yijing*, one of the most ancient of Chinese texts, and the source of much of its medical conceptualization.[13] In a later interpretation of Tai Ji, Chu Xi described it as the Original Substance.[14] If we look for similar concepts in the Indian tradition, we may think of Purusha (Pure Consciousness, Spirit) as close to Wu Ji, and Prakriti (Primordial Nature) as close to Tai Ji.[15] The former is absolutely immaterial, while the latter is an unconscious kind of "Ur-matter." The former is limitless and has no discernible qualities, while the latter is capable of taking on qualities or properties (saguna).

We can think of the relationship of Purusha and Prakriti as descriptive of the transition out of the unmanifested state (Avyakta, zero) or as descriptive of the state of coming into being (Vyakta, one). In the Chinese tradition, the next transition, from one to two, was mentioned in both the *Yijing* and the *Daodejing*. There are many emblems in the Chinese tradition for representing the level Two, such as Heaven (Tian) and Earth (Di) or inner (Nei) and outer (Wai), but the archetypal pair is Yin and Yang. I must assume that the reader is reasonably familiar with these terms and, if not, there are numerous references to consult. Yin and Yang provide the first means for constructing a theory of constitutions. We can say, for example, that someone has either a predominantly Yin or a predominantly Yang constitution. What does this mean exactly? It is not as obvious as it may seem, because of the ambiguity in the term constitution itself. If we see someone of robust physique who is energetic and outgoing, we might say he has a Yang constitution, as compared to someone else who is

12   Chen, E., *The Tao Te Ching*. New York: Paragon House, 1989, chapter 40, p.152.

13   Wilhelm, R. and Baynes, C., trans., *The I Ching or Book of Changes*. Princeton, NJ: Princeton University Press, 1977, pp. lv and 318.

14   Needham, J., *Science and Civilization in China*, vol. 2. Cambridge: Cambridge University Press, 1956, p.462.

15   Ninivaggi, 2001, pp.43–44.

emaciated, frail, and withdrawn (having a Yin constitution by comparison). In this example, however, we are actually describing the person's condition or state, which might be quite different than their original natures.

There are terms for these different concepts in both Chinese and Indian medicine. In Chinese, the constitution is usually spoken of in reference to the Jing or Essence.[16] This same term, Jing, is used to describe both the inherited constitution (Xian Tian Zhi Jing), literally the "Before Heaven Essence," and the acquired constitution (Hou Tian Zhi Jing), literally the "After Heaven Essence." The former is said to be governed by the Kidney, while the latter is said to be governed by the Spleen. Often this distinction might be glossed over, with a person being referred to as one "type" or another, without regard to whether this "typology" is an inherited or an acquired issue. In Ayurvedic theory, this distinction is more commonly a subject of clinical importance and, as we shall see, it has led to an aspect of pulse diagnosis that provides a basis for distinguishing constitutions from conditions. The Indian term for constitution is Prakriti (Primordial Nature), which we have already encountered, while the term for (present) condition is Vikruti, with which it is contrasted.[17] Returning to the example of someone with either a Yin or a Yang "constitution," we can ask if there is a systematic approach to diagnosis and treatment based on this simple two part division and, if so, is it specifically identified with the inherited or acquired state?[18]

The best example I can think of, which is based on this simple differentiation of Yin and Yang, is Macrobiotics, a system of health care developed in Japan by Nyoitchi Sakurazawa, otherwise known as George Ohsawa. He did not come up with this system from scratch, but rather developed it based on an elaboration

---

16   There are references to constitutional types in the earliest strata of Chinese medical literature. Both the *Neijing* and the *Shanghanzabinglun* use the term Ti Zhi (Mathews, R. H., *Mathews' Chinese-English Dictionary*. Cambridge, MA: Harvard University Press, 1979, nos. 6246 and 1009) in this regard, but in both cases there is no implication that this constitutional typology refers to an inherited, as opposed to an acquired, attribute. I believe "body type" is the closest English translation of Ti Zhi (Wang Qi, personal communication, 2013).

17   The transliteration into English of these Indian terms is not standardized. Prakriti may also be rendered as Prakruti, and Vikruti may be rendered as Vikriti. These variants reflect differences in Northern and Southern Indian dialects. I have chosen Prakriti and Vikruti in order to make the terms more visually distinct.

18   After finishing the draft of this text, I did come across a reference to a two part constitutional typology by Zhang Zhongjing, author of the classical text *Shanghanlun*. Zhang discussed the differences between individuals with Zang constitutions versus those with Fu constitutions. Ti Zhi was the term Zhang used for constitution, which could refer to either an inherited or an acquired state. He thought Zang types were more delicate, but protected their health by careful lifestyles, while Fu types were hardier, but more prone to become ill due to reckless lifestyles. I am indebted to Wang Qi for this information in his publications (see Wang, J. *et al.*, "Cognition Research and Constitutional Classification in Chinese Medicine." *Am. J. Chin. Med.*, 39 (4), 2011, pp.651–660) and personal communications. Zhang's theory of Zang and Fu types is a prescient forerunner of Kuon's Eight Constitutions theory of the twentieth century, which also differentiates Zang and Fu constitutional types, to be discussed in Chapter 8.

of the clinical methodology (Shoku-Yo or Natural Food) of a Japanese army doctor, Sagen Ishizuka, who wrote several books in the late 1800s. Ohsawa adapted this primarily dietary modality by applying to it his understanding of the traditional Chinese concepts of Yin and Yang.[19] There are some differences between Ohsawa's understanding of Yin and Yang, and that which is shared by most Chinese sources, but these differences do not concern the question of whether or not Macrobiotics should be considered a "constitutional" system. While there is a minimal discussion of the factors that determine the differences individuals are born with, the thrust of Macrobiotics is aimed at achieving a harmonious balance of Yin and Yang, regardless of one's inherent nature. For example, one text states:

> Physical constitution is formed mainly during the fetal period and is most influenced by the mother's diet… A woman living in a cold climate will probably eat much animal and other Yang foods during her pregnancy, so her baby will tend to develop a husky physical body and a more aggressive character. Someone born in a warmer climate, and whose mother probably ate more fruits and Yin foods during pregnancy, will tend to acquire a more fragile body and a less outgoing personality. Constitution, environment, and stress greatly affect our health and happiness…[but] the most important factors contributing to health and happiness, or a normal healthy condition, are one's current diet and mental attitude—coupled with the understanding that the symptoms of an illness are only the signs of an unbalanced condition. If you balance your condition you can overcome any obstacles to health and happiness.[20]

I have quoted this passage at length because it illustrates what I believe to be two of the most fundamental questions in regard to constitutional treatment: How important is it to know someone's original constitutional makeup, and should the goal of treatment be to create some ideal state of balance that is a universal standard, or is the balanced state an individual variable that depends on the initial constitutional makeup? My understanding of the Macrobiotic literature is that the concept of a universal ideal balance of Yin and Yang is the fundamental factor in diagnosis and treatment, and that one's original constitution does not affect this ideal balanced state (that is, the goal of treatment is to treat Yin people with more Yang foods, and Yang people with more Yin foods, hoping to equalize Yin and Yang). As we shall see, various proponents of other constitutional systems have put forth quite different assumptions, the main one being that the very concept of balance is relative to the individual, and will vary widely from person to person. Systems with a belief in a universal standard of balance tend

---

19   Aihara, H., *Basic Macrobiotics*. New York: Japan Publications, 1985, pp.14–15.
20   Ibid., p.44.

to encourage the same treatment for anyone with a given condition (defined in Yin and Yang terms, for example), while systems with variable standards of balance tend to individualize treatment recommendations to a much greater degree. It is thus these latter types of systems that I would characterize as true constitutional approaches.[21] By this reasoning, Macrobiotics would not appear to qualify as a constitutional approach so much as a conditional one. There have undoubtedly been many amazing results from Macrobiotic treatment, but there are also many cases of people faring poorly on such a diet, rather than getting healthier.[22] Could it be that the reason for this disparity is the failure of Macrobiotics to take into account the fundamental differences in what it means to be balanced for people of different constitutional predispositions? I will not pursue this question further at the moment, nor will I delve any deeper into Macrobiotics as a constitutional system, since it has no direct connection to any constitutional acupuncture methodology, as far as I am aware. There have been other schools of thought regarding the use of acupuncture to directly affect the Yin/Yang balance, but none that I know of which treat this as a constitutional issue.[23]

It is surprising to me how little use is made of the systems that reflect the number Three in current acupuncture texts. There are, of course, several classical tripartite theories such as the division of energetics into Heaven, Man, and Earth levels, or the notion of the San Jiao or Triple Heater (see Figure 1.5), but neither of these was developed into a constitutional approach as far as I know.

One might also cite the "Three Treasures," Essence (Jing), Energy (Qi), and Spirit (Shen), which form an important theoretical basis for Daoist spiritual and health cultivation practices, and the Japanese style of practice based on differentiating syndromes of Qi, Blood, and Fluids, but here again we are not dealing with constitutional theories. Another, often forgotten, three part division found in classical acupuncture is the notion of three cycles in the Meridian system: Lung, Large Intestine, Stomach, and Spleen comprising the first circuit, Heart, Small Intestine, Bladder, and Kidney the second, and Pericardium, Triple Heater, Gall Bladder, and Liver the third (see Figure 1.6).

---

21 Even this distinction is not always clear-cut. Worsley's FEA approach teaches that, in health, all 12 pulses should be equal in volume and quality, but for reasons that I will elaborate, I consider his style constitutionally based. On the other hand, Kuon's KCA approach teaches that in a state of health, for each person, all 12 of the Organs are at different strengths, and that returning the patient to this individual "optimally unbalanced" condition is the goal of treatment. Lad's most recent text on Ayurveda appears to take an opposite position, in asserting that individuals whose Vikruti is the same as their Prakriti are the most difficult to treat (*Textbook of Ayurveda: General Principles of Management and Treatment*, vol. 3. Albuquerque, NM: Ayurvedic Press, 2012, p.10). These differing notions will be elaborated in the following chapters.

22 See *Footsteps*, p.180 and endnote 394.

23 See Niboyet, J., *Compléments d'acupuncture*. Paris: Editions Dominique Wapler, 1955.

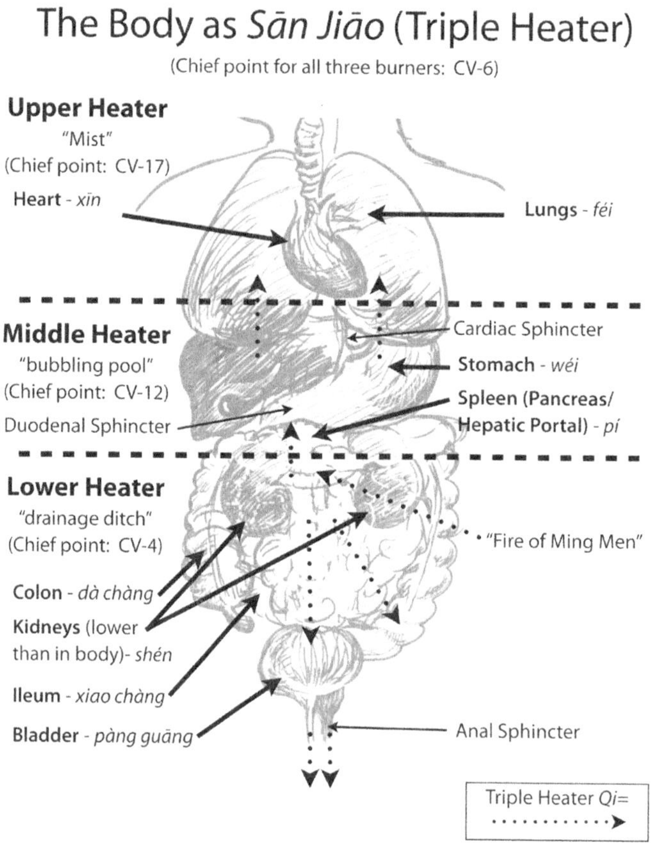

The Body as *Sān Jiāo* (Triple Heater)

(Chief point for all three burners: CV-6)

Upper Heater
"Mist"
(Chief point: CV-17)

Heart - *xīn*

Lungs - *féi*

Middle Heater
"bubbling pool"
(Chief point: CV-12)

Duodenal Sphincter

Cardiac Sphincter

Stomach - *wéi*

Spleen (Pancreas/
Hepatic Portal) - *pí*

Lower Heater
"drainage ditch"
(Chief point: CV-4)

"Fire of Ming Men"

Colon - *dà chàng*
Kidneys (lower
than in body)- *shén*
Ileum - *xiao chàng*
Bladder - *pàng guāng*

Anal Sphincter

Triple Heater *Qi*=
. . . . ▶

Figure 1.5 The Triple Heater or San Jiao[24]

The late French acupuncturist Jacques Lavier discussed the energetics of these three cycles in some depth, but did not attempt to tie them to a constitutional theory,[25] and they are also referenced by both H. B. Kim and Heiner Fruehauf, who point out that they resonantly reflect the Heaven, Earth, and Man trilogy.[26] Joseph Helms, based on the work of two French physician/acupuncturists, develops this model into what I might call the skeleton of a constitutional theory, which he refers to as the biopsychotypes; however, these constitutional types are not differentiated by pulse, color, odor, voice, or emotion. Because my own diagnostic approach, being described in this book, is almost entirely

---

24   Image: Neal White and Elisabeth Waller-White. The assignment of "Chief" Points is controversial. Most sources cite Ren 5 as the Mo Point of the Triple Heater, and Ren 7 as the Mo Point of the Lower Heater.

25   Lavier, J., *Histoire, doctrine et pratique de l'acupuncture chinoise*. Paris: Tchou, 1966, chapter 6.

26   Kim, H. B., *Minibook of Oriental Medicine*. Anaheim, CA: Qpuncture, 2009, p.367, and Fruehauf, H., "The Symbolism of the Organ Networks in Chinese Medicine," a class held in San Francisco, March 2013. For both Kim and Fruehauf, LU, LI, ST, and SP reflect Earth, HE, SI, UB, and KI reflect Heaven, and PE, TH, GB, and LV reflect Man.

dependent on pulse diagnosis, I will not present a detailed account of Helms' model, but highly encourage readers to avail themselves of his book.[27]

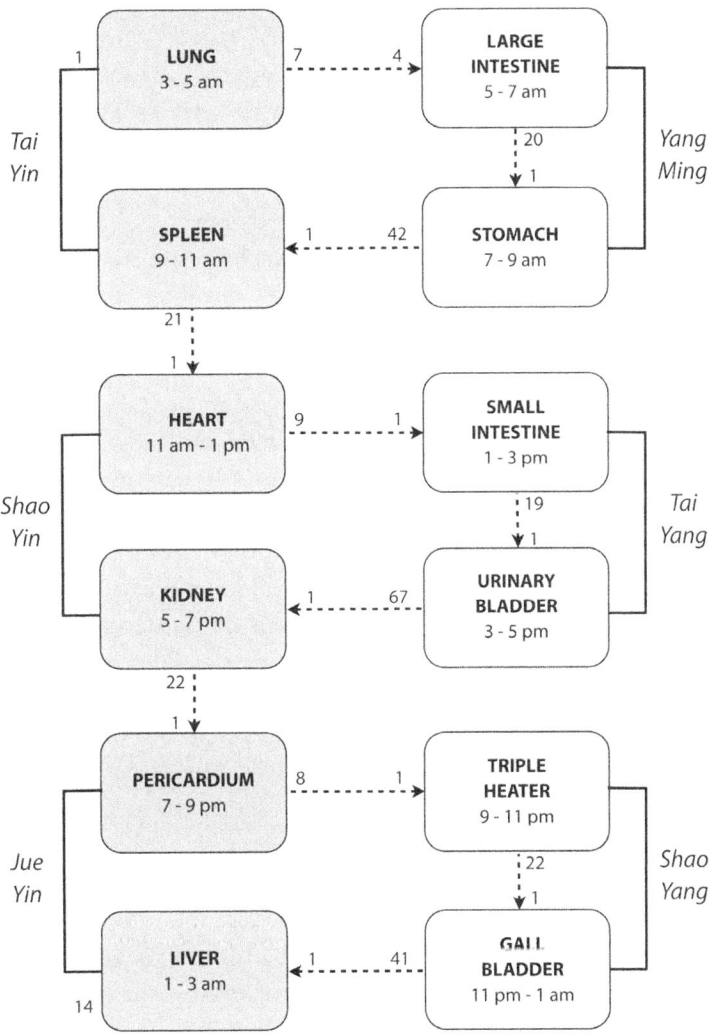

Figure 1.6 Three Cycles of the Meridians[28]

27   Helms, J., *Getting to Know You*. Berkeley, CA: Medical Acupuncture Publishers, 2007. The three types are: Vision/Action (Liver, Gall Bladder, Master of the Heart, Triple Heater), Nurture/Duty (Spleen, Stomach, Lung, Large Intestine), and Will/Spirit (Kidney, Bladder, Heart, Small Intestine).

28   Image: Neal White and Elisabeth Waller-White. The connections between the Meridians are indicated by the numbers of their Entry and Exit Points.

Perhaps because there has been some lack of focus on a threefold division of constitutional types, the contemporary teachings of Yoo Tae Woo, which form an important framework for his Korean Hand Acupuncture (KHA) methods, will seem strange to most acupuncturists. Several of his teachings are at odds with other widely held assumptions in Oriental medicine. He developed an empirical system of diagnosis which he called "Three Constitutions Theory," but which is really better translated as three "patterns" theory because the term Jeung in Korean is the same as Zheng in Chinese, which in turn is the same word as is found in the Eight Principal Patterns (Ba Gang Bian Zheng), the major diagnostic classification system of modern TCM. The Eight Patterns is clearly not meant to be a constitutional methodology.

Some of Yoo's possibly heterodox ideas include the notion that coupled Zang and Fu Organs/Meridians always reflect opposite energetic states (for example, if the Heart is Excess then the Small Intestine must be Deficient and vice versa)[29] and that the Kidney is commonly found to be in an Excess state and should be treated with Sedation or Dispersion in such a case.[30] Because Yoo's diagnostic and therapeutic systems formed the basis for uncovering a connection between the theoretical foundations of Indian medicine (Ayurveda) and those of acupuncture, and are also used in my own practice, I will devote a chapter to presenting the essential information on "constitutional" typology that he teaches, so the reader can understand and apply my methodology, and an appendix which will illustrate the locations of the Command Points on the hand (per KHA), which I use for pre-testing possible treatment protocols for feedback verification via the pulse or other sign and symptom responses. For now I will simply state that the three types that Yoo describes are called Yang Excess, Yin Excess, and Kidney Excess. It is interesting to note that Yang Excess and Yin Excess types are thought to derive from Kidney Deficiency conditions while Kidney Excess reflects the opposite. Although Yoo does not point this out explicitly, the situating of his "constitutional" analysis on the basis of Kidney energetics is quite consistent with the classical notion of the inherited constitution as being governed by the Kidney (Xian Tian Zhi Jing).

The discrimination of Yoo's three patterns is most easily made on the basis of his unique style of abdominal (Hara) palpation, but he also personally uses one of the oldest methods of pulse diagnosis, the comparison of the carotid and radial pulses, which was originally discussed in the *Neijing* and *Nanjing*. Yoo

---

29   This is contrary to the teachings in FEA, the Worsley Five Element style, where coupled Organs/Meridians are most often considered to share either an Excess or a Deficient state, and are both treated with either Tonification or Sedation in tandem. The exception is when the deep and superficial pulses at any position are discordant. However, Chapter 9 of the *Lingshu* explicitly advocates treating the coupled Organs/Meridians of the same Element in opposite polarity, in accordance with the findings from carotid/radial pulse diagnosis.

30   This idea is counter to teachings of TCM that state there are no Excess patterns of the Kidney, and it should never be Sedated.

teaches this pulse diagnostic method of distinguishing the "Three Constitutions" only to his more advanced students, but he also uses carotid/radial pulse diagnosis to evaluate the Eight Extraordinary Meridians, and teaches this in his more elementary classes. Based on my experience, I have questions about the reliability of conclusions drawn from carotid/radial pulse diagnosis regarding the Six Levels, as taught by Yoo, but do not discount the possibility that my own understanding and skill in this regard may be insufficient. At present, I do not use the carotid/radial pulse for Six Level diagnosis, but do use it in combination with other findings for Extra Meridian diagnosis. I think it is important to present Yoo's teachings in this regard, but will relegate them to Part Two, which discusses conditional pulse diagnosis, as Yoo uses pulses to evaluate the Six Levels and the Eight Extra Meridians as part of a conditional assessment.

Following my description of KHA, I will discuss some aspects of Ayurveda, which seem to me to share striking conceptual parallels with KHA. Ayurveda is above all a system based on the three Humors: Vata (Wind), Pitta (Bile), and Kapha (Phlegm). These Humors are called "Doshas," which literally denote faults or impurities, but only carry this connotation when describing pathology. In usage as a physiological concept, the Doshas are the means by which homeostasis is maintained in the body, mind, and spirit. For now, the most important aspect of Ayurveda to mention is its own unique method of pulse diagnosis. I should really say methods, because just as in Chinese medical traditions there are numerous ways to examine and interpret the pulse, such is also the case in Indian medicine. In fact, if one were to simply rely on the material about Ayurvedic pulse diagnosis published in the English literature, one would hardly encounter the methods that I have learned and used, methods that have been transmitted by oral rather than literary traditions. Perhaps the most interesting thing about Ayurvedic pulse diagnosis is its ideas about the way the pulse reflects different layers of information with respect to depth of pressure of the palpating finger. The deepest level at which the pulse can be felt is said to reflect the person's Prakriti or constitution, while the more superficial level of the pulse is said to reflect the current condition, or Vikruti. As far as I know, there is no similar concept in Chinese pulse diagnosis, although there are references to the deepest pulse as corresponding to the Kidney, guardian of the constitutional energy or Jing.[31] The position for examining the radial pulse in Ayurveda is approximately two to three fingerbreadths more proximal than in Chinese medicine.

---

31 *Nanjing*, Chapter 5.

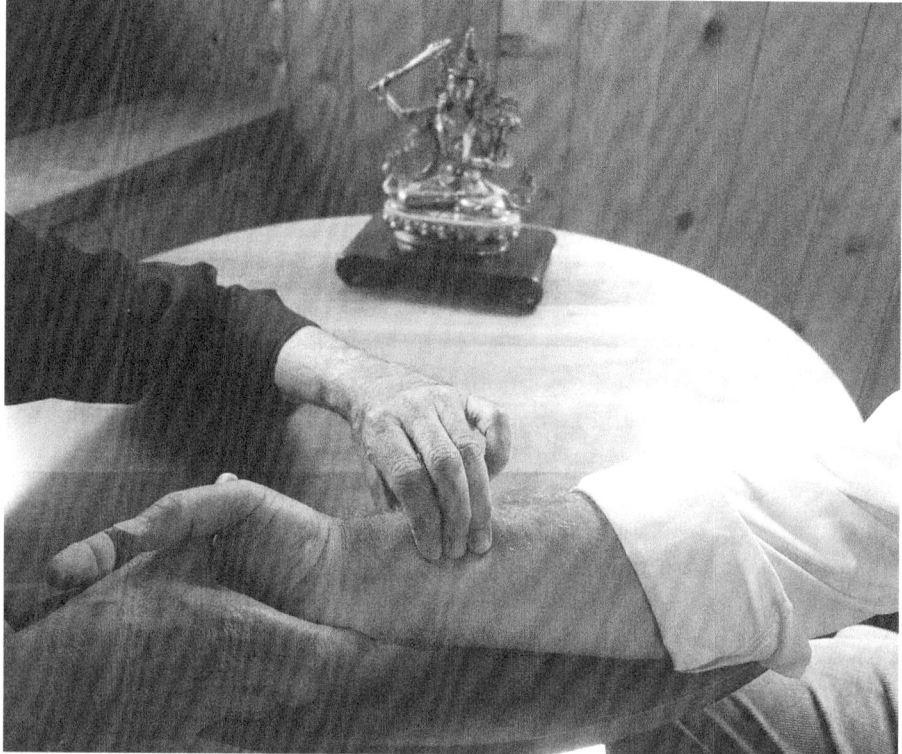

Figure 1.7 The more proximal location for examining the Ayurvedic pulses[32]

I will presently introduce two other methods of constitutional pulse diagnosis, both from Korea, and both of which use this more proximal location and deepest aspect of the pulse. I do not know if this similarity is coincidental, or if there was a borrowing of methods involved, but it is possible that the Chinese did not evolve a similar method of constitutional pulse diagnosis simply because they were feeling around in the "wrong" place.

About the same time that Sagen Ishizuka was using nutritional therapy to lay the groundwork for the birth of Macrobiotics in Japan (late 1800s), a Korean doctor, Lee Jeh-ma, was developing a new approach to herbal therapy, called Sasang (Four Images) Constitutional Medicine or SCM.[33] The Four Images is a term from the *Yijing*, where Yin and Yang are each subdivided further into Greater and Lesser types. Thus the Four Images are Greater Yang, Lesser Yang, Greater Yin, and Lesser Yin. They have also been referred to as Yang in Yang, Yin in Yang, Yin in Yin, and Yang in Yin.

---

32   Image: Marina Chentsova Eckman.
33   The Korean word Sang is the same as the Chinese word Xiang (Mathews 1979, no. 2568).

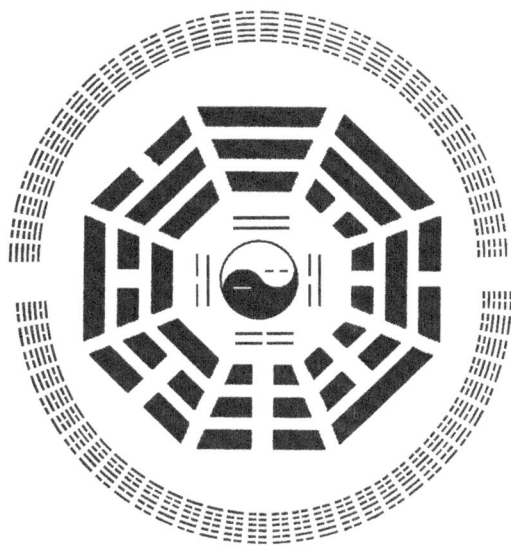

Figure 1.8 The Four Images from the Yijing[34]

Lee's original idea was that people vary in both physical and psychological characteristics, and as a result will respond differently to herbs even if their signs and symptoms when ill are the same. A staunch Neo-Confucian, Lee believed that the virtues or lack thereof in an individual's personality was the most reliable guide to understanding which of the four types they belonged to, and thus served as his discriminator for choosing herbal remedies. Sasang medicine (SCM) has since become widespread in Korea, but is not very well known elsewhere. The biggest hindrance to the development of SCM has been its lack of uniform and reliable diagnostic methods to classify people. Although Lee used herbal medicine as his therapeutic modality, he predicted that, in the future, someone would figure out how to use acupuncture according to Sasang principles. His prediction came true in the twentieth century, following the discovery of a method of constitutional pulse diagnosis by Kuon Dowon. I will

---

34   Image: Neal White and Elisabeth Waller-White. Based on Legge's 1899 translation of the *Yijing*. The central circle shows Yang (white) rising on the left and Yin (black) falling on the right. Solid lines are Yang and broken lines are Yin, so one can see that there is Yin in the middle of Yang (usually depicted as a black circle) and Yang in the middle of Yin (usually depicted as a white circle). Around the central Yin/Yang symbol are the Four Images, or bigrams, of two lines each. Greater Yang is at the top, Lesser Yang is on the left, Greater Yin is at the bottom, and Lesser Yin is on the right. The bottom line of each image is the one closest to the center of the picture. Surrounding the Four Images are the Eight Trigrams and, further out, the 64 Hexagrams.

devote a chapter to Dr. Kuon's method of Eight Constitutions Medicine (ECM, which I have previously referred to as Korean Constitutional Acupuncture, or KCA), but I will first include a chapter on Sasang theory itself. Following Kuon's lead, another Korean doctor, Puramo Chong, developed a method of constitutional pulse diagnosis that conforms more closely to Lee's teachings, and is based on four rather than eight types. I learned this method of pulse taking at Chong's clinic, and have developed my own variation, which I use in its place.[35]

The acupuncture style taught by J. R. Worsley, a style which I have previously called Leamington Acupuncture (LA), is often called classical Five Element Acupuncture (FEA) by its practitioners. Worsley did not use the word constitution in his teachings, to my knowledge, and I believe there is a simple explanation for that. His central concept—one of the Elements as the Causative Factor (CF) in each individual's presentation—did not insist that everyone was already born with a CF established. While he left open the possibility that the CF could be congenital in some cases, he also seemed to think that it might be established by one's early childhood experiences in others. I do not know if his opinion on this issue changed in the years after I had studied with him, but some of his students clearly saw the CF as a constitutional matter. The texts *Nourishing Destiny* and *Five Element Constitutional Acupuncture*,[36] as well as *Footsteps* and the several publications by Worsley himself, can be consulted for extended discussions of FEA, but I will include a chapter here giving enough of the essentials of this style of practice so that the material I present later in the clinical applications of my own synthetic approach will be more readily understood. It is my hope that Five Element practitioners in particular will find the new perspectives that I introduce helpful in both diagnosis and treatment planning. Of all the teachers with whom I have studied, Worsley was perhaps the most insistent that acupuncture treatment should not be based on the symptoms, but rather on the root cause in every case. For this reason I feel

---

35   It might be argued that the four "Root" types in Japanese Meridian Therapy (Liver Deficiency, Kidney Deficiency, Lung Deficiency, and Spleen Deficiency) represent a constitutional approach to acupuncture. While this system is based on pulse diagnosis, I believe that there is no dogma stating that these Root imbalances are inherent or fixed in nature. My understanding is that individuals may present with different Root imbalances on sequential examinations. Thus I do not consider Meridian Therapy to be a constitutional system, although at the same time it is not primarily a conditional system either, as the Root imbalance is not discernible via the symptomatic presentation. How to classify Meridian Therapy is a topic that merits further consideration.

36   Jarrett, L., *Nourishing Destiny*. Stockbridge: Spirit Path Press, 1999, and Hicks, A., Hicks, J., and Mole, P., *Five Element Constitutional Acupuncture*. Edinburgh: Churchill Livingstone, 2004.

quite comfortable treating FEA as representing the constitutional approach at the level of Five.[37]

There is one obvious candidate for using Six as the foundation of a constitutional methodology, the six levels of Yin and Yang. This model is present in both the *Neijing*, where it is used to name and organize the Meridians, and in the *Shanghanlun*, where it forms the basis for the herbal treatment of illnesses due to pathogenic cold invasion. The six levels are Taiyang, Shaoyang, Yangming, Taiyin, Shaoyin, and Jueyin.[38] Several teachers from France, notably Maurice Mussat and Yves Requena, have taught material that can be thought of as a constitutional system based on this sixfold model. Mussat's approach is based on identifying the trigrams of the *Yijing* with the various levels of Yin and Yang. He teaches several treatment methods to address symptomatology arising from each of these constitutional levels, such as triangular equilibration. That material is beyond the scope of this text (although I do find it clinically useful), but can be accessed through the American Academy of Medical Acupuncture (AAMA) or the book by Joe Helms.[39] Requena also has published a number of books that describe his conceptualization of the six levels as constitutional indicators.[40] I should also mention a text in German by the late Heribert Schmidt,[41] which uses the herbal six level tradition to propose a constitutional acupuncture system, but not reading German, I'm unable to say to what degree it might contribute to this general presentation of constitutional systems. The main reason I've not incorporated these teachers' views on the Six Levels of Yin and Yang into my personal method of constitutional diagnosis is that they are not associated with a method of pulse diagnosis, unlike the other components of my synthetic approach.[42]

---

37 Worsley's main teachers were French, Chinese, and Japanese, but he was subsequently influenced by Korean notions, including the idea of constitutional diagnosis, which I believe preceded his development of the concept of the CF. There is also a five part Korean approach to pulse diagnosis called "Hwa Chim," developed by Song Jae-Hoon, and written about by him in 2001, although not available in English. Unlike the Japanese Meridian Therapy approach, which is based on Deficiency patterns of four Zang Organs, Hwa Chim is based on Excess patterns of five Zang Organs. Like Meridian Therapy, however, it is not presented as a reflection of an individual's constitution, but must be assessed anew at each treatment session. See Kim, 2009, p.363.

38 One English translation of these terms is Greater Yang, Lesser Yang, Bright Yang, Greater Yin, Lesser Yin, and Fading Yin. I have used the single word transcriptions for these terms to distinguish them from their usage in the Sasang approach (e.g. Taiyang vs. Tai Yang). The actual Chinese characters are the same in both systems, but using different styles of transcription allows for less confusion regarding the model being discussed. For a hypothesis about the origin of these terms, see Eckman, P., *The Book of Changes in Traditional Oriental Medicine*. Columbia, MD: Traditional Acupuncture Institute, 1988.

39 Helms, J., *Acupuncture Energetics*. Berkeley, CA: Medical Acupuncture Publishers, 1995.

40 Requena, Y., *Terrains and Pathology in Acupuncture*, vol. 1. Brookline, MA: Paradigm, 1986.

41 Schmidt, H., *Konstitutionelle Akupunktur*. Stuttgart: Hippokrates Verlag, 1988.

42 Mussat has actually stated (class notes) that he does not take pulses, being unconvinced that they are a meaningful diagnostic parameter.

My initial approach to constitutional diagnosis at the level of six was based on an expansion of the Ayurvedic pulse findings, taking into account that the Doshas may be present either singly, or in combination. If the imbalance is occurring in either one or two Doshas at the same time (a quite common finding), then there are exactly six possibilities: Vata, Pitta, Kapha, Vata/Pitta, Vata/Kapha, and Pitta/Kapha.[43] Since these imbalances can be perceived by pulse diagnosis, this turns out to be a very useful constitutional model, and will be explained in detail.

At present, however, I find that there is an additional, complementary, method of Six Level constitutional pulse diagnosis, harking back again to the Six Energetic Levels of Yin and Yang (SEL). The method I will discuss was first enunciated by Wang Shu-he in the *Maijing*, and its clinical application is very similar to one described by Will Morris in 2004.[44] Morris has found this methodology to be particularly effective in treating Sinew Channel pathology involving the Wei Qi (Defensive Energy), but he views the *Maijing* map as the basic approach for dealing with issues of Six Level energetics, including internal medicine problems of the Organ systems, and their Principal and Divergent Meridians.[45] What I am adding to the understanding of the *Maijing* map is its additional use in constitutional diagnosis, which specifically involves the Yuan Qi (Original Energy). I learned the practical skills of Six Level palpation that Morris teaches from his student Joseph Adams, who emphasized its use in diagnosing Sinew Channel pathology. After reviewing the original text of the *Maijing*, I realized that its author did not stipulate whether he was discussing Wei Qi or Yuan Qi. My clinical experience has led me to believe that the *Maijing* Six Levels model is the easiest and most reliable pulse method for constitutional diagnosis at the level of six, and narrows to two the possible Elemental candidates for the CF. It is imperative, however, that this pulse assessment be done in a specific manner, so I will explain how this examination is carried out in some detail.

There isn't any theoretical model of constitution that I'm aware of which uses Seven for its typology.[46] On a theoretical level, however, the possibility

---

43   In this text, I am using the nomenclature of dual Doshas as reversible terms. Thus Vata/Pitta is equivalent to Pitta/Vata. This is a simplification I'm adopting in order to present the theoretical underpinnings of constitutional classification as clearly as possible. In fact, some of these dual Dosha individuals may be Pitta dominant and others Vata dominant, but such a difference does not change their constitutional classification.

44   Wang Shu-he, *The Pulse Classic: A Translation of the Mai Jing* (Yang Shou-zhong, trans.). Boulder, CO: Blue Poppy Press, 1997, Book Ten, pp.351–354; Morris, W. R., "Chinese Pulse Diagnosis: Epistemology, Practice, and Tradition." Dissertation. California Institute of Integral Studies, San Francisco, CA, 2009.

45   Will Morris, personal communication, 2013.

46   Will Morris (in a personal communication) has pointed out that the Seven Planetary types might provide the basis for a constitutional model, and indeed Kuon's KCA theory does use the Roman terminology for four of the planets in a truncated version of the seven. The seven planet system is the basis for the naming of the seven days of the week.

exists of using the Ayurvedic system of the Seven Chakras to discover one. There is at least one way to gather information about the Chakras from the pulse, but it seems to reflect the current issues in a person's life rather than those at a constitutional level.[47] John Cross has recently published another way to use the pulses to evaluate the Chakras,[48] and it appears to me to also deal with the present condition rather than the constitution. I have myself devised a way to glean information about the Chakras, using Ayurvedic pulse information, again focusing on the condition as reflected in the superficial part of the pulse. I have used Cross' protocols for treating the Chakras with some good results based on my diagnostic method, and will present my ideas in Parts Two and Three. I do not mean to exclude the possibility that constitutional information related to the Chakras might be inscribed in some other way on the pulse, but given their apparent connection to the present condition, I am inclined to doubt that such a connection will be found. Since my synthetic model of constitutions involves 24 types, and 24 is not divisible by 7 (it is divisible by 2, 3, 4, 6, 8, and 12), it is possible that seven is simply not a basis for constitutional differentiation. Thea Elijah has proposed an interesting explanation for this finding in discussing the difference between "fiveness" and "sevenness" in TOM theory, in the context of the emotions.[49] She notes that, when speaking of the five emotions, the focus is on the healthy or physiological manifestations of the organism, whereas the seven emotions are invoked when discussing pathology, which would certainly not belong in a constitutional model. This does raise the question of why 24 is not divisible by 5, if the Five Elements are operative at the constitutional level. While I cannot provide a definitive answer, I believe that the Fire Element, being double (having four Officials rather than the two of each of the other Elements), must be treated as providing a sixth Element for the purpose of constitutional analysis. Thus in using Five Element diagnosis (for example via color, sound, odor, and emotion), one may not be able to distinguish Imperial (Heart/Small Intestine) from Ministerial (Pericardium/Triple Heater) Fire; nevertheless these represent, in an important way, quite different constitutions, and should therefore be classified as Six, numerologically.

Eight Constitutions Medicine (ECM) is the name currently used by Kuon to describe what I have called Korean Constitutional Acupuncture (KCA) in the past. In my own training as an acupuncturist, this was the first constitutional system I was exposed to, and I am very grateful to have had the rare opportunity to study it in person with its originator, Kuon Dowon, in Seoul. Although Kuon's methodology has evolved over time, the one aspect

---

47 My teacher, Mary Jo Cravatta, uses this technique. She reserves teaching it until one has mastered the more elementary aspects of Ayurvedic pulse diagnosis, which I am still working on. My observation, however, is that the Chakra she finds on the pulse often changes over time in a given individual, and therefore cannot be a constitutional reflection.

48 Cross, J., *Acupuncture and the Chakra Energy System*. Berkeley, CA: North Atlantic Books, 2008.

49 T. Elijah, personal communication.

that has remained unchanged is his discovery of eight unique pulse types which are unvarying throughout the life of any individual, reflecting only their constitutional tendencies, and being unaffected by any changes in the individual's state of health. My interpretation of the meaning of this unique pulse represents a somewhat different viewpoint than Kuon's, but I believe he has correctly stated that there are only eight patterns of presentation of this pulse, and my interpretation of their meaning is merely an extension of his own, rather than a fundamental disagreement. Kuon's theoretical model and treatment style are so unique and powerful that I will devote a chapter to describing them, limited only by my promise to share solely those aspects that he has already publicly disclosed.[50]

While on the subject of eightfold analysis, I should at least mention the system of Eight Extraordinary Meridians, especially as they have been associated with at least two different methods of pulse diagnosis (Morris' Neoclassical version, and Yoo's KHA version), besides which they are spoken of as being precursors of the 12 Regular Meridians in embryological development on the one hand, and are believed to transmit Jing (Essence) and Yuan Qi (Original Energy) on the other, both factors making them ideal candidates for involvement in constitutional issues. While this is certainly true on a theoretical level, in practice I have never seen any reference to a constitutional acupuncture system based on them. Perhaps it is well to remember that the Extraordinary Meridians also transmit Wei Qi (Defensive Energy), and as such are involved in adapting to the current condition. In fact, the major clinical teaching about these eight Meridians, as described in the *Nanjing*, sees them as receptacles for the overflow of Xie Qi (Perverse Energy) when the Regular Meridians are unable to contain this pathological intrusion.[51] Clinically, the Eight Extraordinary Meridians are often chosen on the basis of symptomatology alone. My opinion is that while these eight are instrumental in creating a new individual (embryogenesis), the

---

50   In addition to Kuon's published work, detailed in the bibliography, there is also quite a lot of information about KCA available on the website of his son, Wujon Kuon: Eight-Constitution Medicine (www.ecmed.org). In addition, one of Kuon's main disciples, Bae Cholwan, published several articles on KCA in Korean, which were approved at the time by Kuon Dowon; however, Kuon and Bae have since diverged in their approaches (personal communication from Puramo Chong). Although Bae's articles have not been translated into English, I have incorporated material from them that I learned from both Puramo and H. B. Kim.

51   I have found it to be surprising that many of my patients with serious chronic illnesses, such as "chronic fatigue syndrome," or even cancer, do not necessarily display Extraordinary Meridian pulse patterns, while patients with more superficial problems, such as frozen shoulders, may often display Extraordinary Meridian pulses. If this finding proves to be generally applicable, it may indicate that perhaps some of these "serious" illnesses could reflect a failure of the Extraordinary Meridian system to operate in such a way as to cope with Perverse Energy (Xie Qi) that has overwhelmed the capacity of the Regular Meridians. The Perverse Energy would thus be able to directly disrupt the functioning of the Organs (Zang/Fu) themselves. I believe such an interpretation fits the understanding of the Extraordinary Meridians' role as explained in the *Nanjing*, by attributing the failure of this "overflow" mechanism as a significant cause of serious chronic illnesses.

CF or constitution does not arise until the Organs/Officials/Meridians have been created and take over responsibility for this new life.

Once we get to Nine and above, the constitutional theories tend to be based more on traditional biorhythmic theory than on pulse diagnosis. The Nine Stars,[52] Ten Stems, and Twelve Branches are all examples of what might be called astrological constitutional systems. These methods are actually all applications of the Heavenly Stems and Terrestrial Branches, an ancient system of cyclical dating shared by the Chinese, Japanese, and Koreans, among others, and which has been used in various ways in traditional acupuncture.[53] The system of hourly open points is one well-known example (although certainly not a constitutional method). There is an entirely different system of Vedic astrology from India, that has its own complex method of constitutional analysis, but these astrological systems are outside the scope of this presentation, and are mentioned simply as a point of reference. For the reason already stated, I would not expect the constitution to reflect sets of 9, 10, or 11, but, as 24 is divisible by 12, there should be a 12 part constitutional analysis, and I think it is readily apparent that these 12 constitutions correspond to the 12 Organs/Officials/Meridians which organize and maintain our lives.

There are many possibilities for constitutional theories based on more than 12 types, but the only one that has influenced my own thinking was a doubling of Kuon's Eight types into 16, which was proposed by Lee Dong Woong in Korea, and is the method used in clinic by Puramo Chong, whose practice I observed. Sixteen is not divisible into 24, nor is it divisible by three itself, so such a model would seem to me to be incomplete on theoretical grounds, but because it provided a key insight that led to the development of my own understanding of the relationship of the various constitutional theories, I will explain his approach. My own method of constitutional diagnosis involving 24 types was arrived at using the 16 types as an intermediate stepping stone, and then integrating it with all the preceding systems. For the moment, I should say that this number of constitutional types may seem large, complex, and unwieldy, but in fact is rather simple. It is based on the idea that the constitution is fundamentally a reflection of the inherent strengths and weaknesses of the 12 Organs/Officials/Meridians, and that the predominant tendency towards Excess or Deficiency (hyperfunctioning or hypofunctioning) in one of them is the underlying determinant of the constitution in each

52   Kushi, M., *Nine Star Ki*. Becket, MA: One Peaceful World Press, 1991.

53   The general name for this aspect of Chinese energetic theory is Zi Wu Liu Zhu Fa. Many of the chapters in the *Neijing* are based on this approach, but there is scholarly debate as to whether they were part of the original text, or were later additions. Zi and Wu are the Branches corresponding to midnight and noon, so it is easy to see the well-known "Law of Midday/Midnight" as one example of the application of the teachings of this methodology.

individual, producing exactly 24 possibilities.[54] Of course each of these 24 constitutions may be composed of various subtypes (similar to the concept of Element within Element, in Five Element theory, and I do actually use this deeper level of analysis clinically at times), but that is a subject best left for future discussion. I should also mention that the *Neijing* does mention a system of 25 constitutional types, but this appears to me to be a purely theoretical exposition of Yin/Yang and Five Element speculation, and is not presented with the necessary diagnostic criteria (especially pulse indicators) that would make it clinically useful.[55] It may, however, have been the impetus for Worsley to have routinely employed the concept of Element within Element in the diagnostic schema he employed from the middle of his career onwards. Using the Element within Element model yields exactly 25 constitutional types,[56] while adding another level of Element within the first two increases the count to 125 types. During the period of my study with Worsley, he never discussed how knowing the Elements "within" was clinically useful, so I believe that FEA practitioners need have no fear that adopting a 24 type constitutional model will diminish the range of therapeutic possibilities to be considered, but should, on the contrary, increase it. Finally, I would be remiss not to emphasize that constitutional theory is just that, a theory. When faced with a real person as a client, theories are like maps that help us orient ourselves, but we must never mistake the map for the territory. Each individual is unique, and not merely a constitutional type.

---

54   The Japanese author Honma Shohaku, one of the most influential teachers of the Meridian Therapy school (Keiraku Chiryo), mentioned this idea in his writings, but did not elaborate on the methodology for identifying the various types, at least in English reports of his work. None of his writings have been translated into English, to my knowledge.

55   *Lingshu* 64.

56   These, however, are not the same 25 types described in *Lingshu* 64.

Chapter 2

AN OVERVIEW OF CONSTITUTIONAL PULSE DIAGNOSIS

There are several basic methods of pulse examination whose combined findings should allow one to uniquely define the 24 distinct constitutions. Only one of these methods involves taking the traditional "Chinese" pulses at the Inch (Cun), Bar (Guan), and Cubit (Chi) positions along the radial artery, and I will suggest an adaptation to even this aspect of pulse examination in order to make it even more reliable regarding constitutional information. There are other methods of constitutional pulse diagnosis which I will describe below, but all methods of constitutional pulse diagnosis share one common feature: since the constitution does not vary throughout the life of the individual, neither do their constitutional pulses. Thus, once the constitution has been determined and confirmed by clinical feedback, there is no need to continue to take the constitutional pulses on subsequent visits, other than to use repetition to solidify one's skill in this regard. The other types of pulse examination, which I find to be tremendously informative at every patient visit, relate to the present condition, which is continually subject to change. These include the carotid/radial pulse (for Extra Meridian diagnosis), the Vikruti evaluation of the Ayurvedic pulse (primarily at the Dosha and Subdosha levels), and the standard Cun, Guan, and Chi pulses in two separate locations. To reiterate, in my understanding, one does not treat the constitution (it is unchanging and unchangeable), but rather the present condition with respect to the constitution. This distinction will be illustrated in all of the case histories to be presented.

The different methods of pulse examination that I use to determine the constitution are borrowed (with adaptations) from Ayurveda, Korean Constitutional Acupuncture (KCA), the Sasang pulse method of Puramo (SCM), and the variant of orthodox Chinese pulse examination of the Six Levels (SEL) which I adapted from Morris' "neoclassical pulse diagnosis." All four are methods of examining the radial pulse along a segment that is more proximal than the location used in "Chinese" pulse diagnosis. As mentioned in Chapter 1, the use of this proximal location in Indian medicine is possibly as old as, or older than, "Chinese" pulse diagnosis, but the accuracy of this claim is a moot point. The fourth method is derived from a version of the standard "Chinese" finger placement (in both TCM and FEA, for example) and bases its interpretation on the *Maijing* as per Morris' neoclassical pulse teachings; however, I have discovered that the constitutional findings embedded in the Cun, Guan, and Chi positions are more clearly displayed at the more proximal location just mentioned.[1] I interpret this particular proximal location as one "wavelength" away from the standard location (Yang) for Chinese pulse examination (see Figure 2.1). These relationships, confirmed by clinical feedback, support my view that the pulses are resonant phenomena, and should display aspects of waveform behavior, a topic that is common to the history of both Eastern and Western science. The congruence of all these various methods of pulse examination, with some aspects exhibiting locations one "wavelength" apart, is an example of what has been described as the holographic representation of information in the human body. The holographic hypothesis is in turn a natural implication of resonance theory, to which I have made allusion. In summary, my synthetic approach to constitutional diagnosis, using this panoply of pulse examination techniques, can be thought of as being simultaneously ancient and modern.

Before describing in detail these components of constitutional (and later, conditional) pulse diagnosis, I will briefly summarize the steps I most commonly use in clinical practice. In actuality, I switch back and forth between palpating the constitutional and conditional pulses, so I will briefly mention the techniques I also use for feeling the conditional pulses, but I will not describe them in detail here, nor explain them until Part Two of this book. One order in which I might (and often do) perform these examinations in clinic is presented below, but I do not have a fixed ritual about the ordering of these steps. In fact, the first step I will describe is not really used in determining the constitution

---

1   The reason, I believe, for some degree of unclarity regarding the constitutional information at Cun, Guan, and Chi is that these positions also simultaneously reflect Eight Extraordinary Meridian information, and the overlap of these two informational inputs can distort the constitutional picture. Fortunately, the Extraordinary Meridian mapping does not appear to be projected at the more proximal pulse location, so that the constitutional information there is clearer.

but, as it is given such importance in the *Neijing*, I like to check it in each patient, and use it to evaluate the general state of Yin/Yang balance.

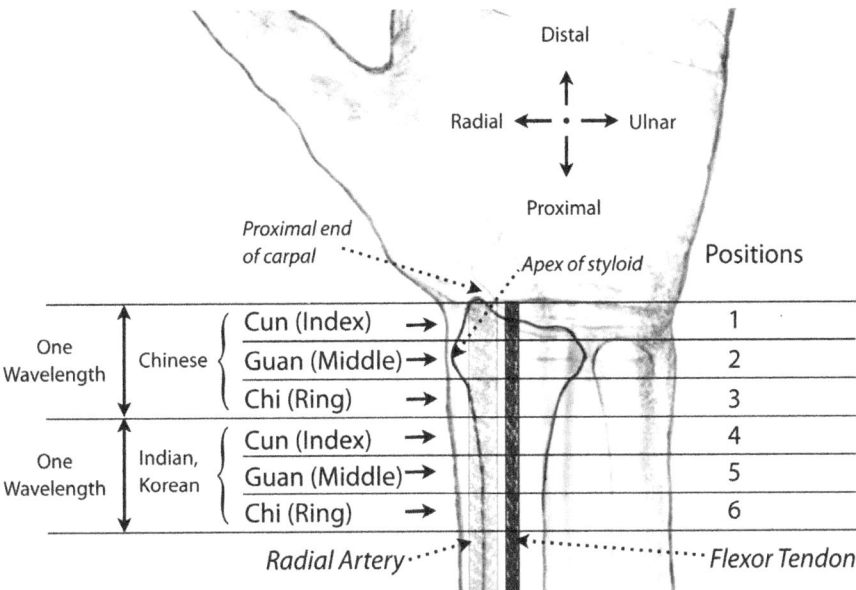

Figure 2.1 Distal and proximal locations for radial pulses[2]

The order of the steps presented below has been chosen for the sake of clarity of presentation, but is not the same order that I will follow in the subsequent textual exegesis. The text will proceed in a more systematic way through the hierarchy of constitutional theories, while the actual clinical protocol that I most often use is a synthesized route to an accurate constitutional (and conditional) diagnosis based on conclusions drawn from each of these theoretical models.

1. I often start the pulse examination, with the patient sitting on the exam table, by comparing the radial and carotid pulses on each side of the body, remembering that this was the most clearly described method of pulse diagnosis in the *Neijing*. My Korean Hand Acupuncture teacher, Yoo Tae Woo, used this method in a similar manner as described in the *Neijing*, that is, to evaluate the Six Great Meridians, but he also described a way to apply it to diagnosis of the Eight Extraordinary Meridians. I do not use this examination to evaluate the Six Great Meridians,

---

2   Image: Neal White and Elisabeth Waller-White. The distal pulse positions shown are what I call the Yang locations of Cun, Guan, and Chi.

having found that the results are not sufficiently reliable in my hands;[3] however, I do use it in evaluating the Extraordinary Meridians, but add other diagnostic indicators to improve its reliability. What seems to be an additional reliable finding is that an imbalance in the caliber of the radial and carotid pulses often indicates the side of the body which is most out of balance energetically (usually opposite to the side that is out of balance materially and symptomatically), and which could be treated unilaterally with acupuncture; however, I often opt to treat bilaterally in order to strengthen the treatment. This exam is carried out as follows: With the client seated on the exam table, I check the ratios of the *sizes* of the radial and carotid pulses, first on their left side, then on their right. In many cases this will only take a few seconds, as it is not unusual for individuals to have marked differences. In other cases this can take quite a while, as individual variations in anatomy can lead to confusion, as can pulses which are close to balance. Yoo Tae Woo has proposed an explanation for why this pulse ratio is such an important diagnostic indicator, basing his interpretation on the idea that these two arteries reflect the blood flow to the posterior (radial artery, serving as a surrogate for the vertebral artery—these two arteries share a common origin) and anterior (carotid artery) parts of the brain on that side of the body. He sees the brain as being involved in the functional control of all the Organs via the Meridians and their reflected Micromeridians on the hand. My own thinking is an extension of this hypothesis: If one treats the energetically imbalanced side of the body, the blood flow to the brain on that side will change in the direction of normalization. However, the affected side of the brain has its biggest impact on the contralateral side of the body, due to the crossing or decussation of nerve fibers in the central nervous system. Thus the impact will be observed on the opposite side of the body. Now it is well known that classical references recommend treating the side opposite to the symptoms, and this is done in many styles of acupuncture including Korean Constitutional Acupuncture, Sa Am Korean Acupuncture as taught by Byoung Kim,[4] and in the balance method taught by Richard Tan, based on the system developed by Master Tong in Taiwan. My speculation at least provides

---

3   In fact, I believe that the Six Level interpretation of carotid/radial pulses, as presented in both the *Neijing* and by Yoo, is invalid. I have treated many cases where this theory posits that the Yang Meridians should be Sedated and the Yin Meridians Tonified, but my patients fared extremely well by doing exactly the opposite!

4   Kim, B., *The Silver Bullet, KOSA.* Buena Park: KOSA of the Americas, 2012.

a rationale for this method of opposite side needling, as it is usually the case that the carotid/radial imbalance is most pronounced on the side opposite (contralateral) to the main symptoms; however, this is not always the case, and each treatment session should be based on the actual pulse findings combined with the presenting symptomatology.[5] With regard to carotid/radial pulse examination, the details of how to carry out this procedure will be more fully described in Part Two, as it is an aspect of the conditional diagnosis relating to the Six Levels and the Eight Extraordinary Meridians.

2.   Now it is time for the first part of the constitutional analysis, which I do with the patient lying face up on the exam table. To discuss the constitutional pulse exam itself, I need to first establish what I call the Yin and Yang locations of the Cun, Guan, and Chi positions. For the Yang location (see Figure 2.1), I start by placing my middle finger just over the high point of the radial styloid process, and then let my index and ring fingers come to rest adjacently, with my index finger just distal to the styloid process. In checking one's own pulse, the index finger will be found to lie just proximal to the bone at the base of the thenar eminence, close to or right over the deepest depression at the wrist crease, which is the location of Point LU 9 (Tai Yuan).[6] In contrast to the Yang location of Cun, Guan, and Chi, I will just mention here the Yin location of Cun, Guan, and Chi, which are all located about one half Cun proximally. The Yin locations are found by placing the index and middle fingers on either side of the crest of the styloid process, and with the ring finger placed adjacent to the middle finger, the three fingers keeping exactly the same relationships as just described for the Yang locations.

---

5   There are many connections in the central nervous system that allow for a transmission of information between the left and right sides. The corpus callosum is an obvious example, but there are many others in the brain itself, as well as at the spinal cord level. Thus symptoms and signs do not have an inherently fixed localizing relationship. It is also possible that the degree to which these findings appear contralaterally versus ipsilaterally may reflect the chronicity of the condition. It is to be hoped that future studies will be able to shed light on this matter.

6   Theoretically, if the patient's fingers are wider than the examiner's, then the fingers would need to be spread out very slightly, and scrunched closer together for children or those with smaller fingers. While this holds true for children's pulses, my experience is that the adjustment necessary in taking the pulses of adults is quite small, to the point of virtual insignificance in almost all cases. I believe that this finding is a result of the rather small difference in the length of people's arms from wrist to elbow, which serves as the standard for proportional measurement along the arm. If there is even a 10 percent difference in arm length, this would result in needing to adjust the fingers taking the pulse by only 10 percent, which is barely noticeable.

Returning to a discussion of the Yang location, it is a preliminary step for carrying out the first part of the constitutional examination. With one's fingers in this Yang location, if the examiner now puts his or her little finger adjacent to their ring finger, and then replaces their little finger with their index finger (now located in what I call the "fourth position"; see Figure 2.1 again), this new location is the correct place to carry out all of the methods of constitutional diagnosis, starting with Kuon's KCA determination. An alternate way to arrive at this finger position is to slide one's index finger distally along the radius until it is naturally stopped by the beginning of the bulging of the styloid process.[7] It often seems to me that there is a palpable depression in the soft tissues in this location, and I have come to think of it as a unique location that I designate as the "Constitutional Point." I like to start the constitutional exam with the KCA step because it was the first method of constitutional pulse taking that I learned, both from reading Kuon's publications, from studying with his students, and finally by observing Kuon himself in his clinic in Seoul. I should mention that I have slightly adapted Kuon's technique following years of experimentation concerning the method that gives the most accurate and reproducible results. I will describe KCA pulse taking in detail in Chapter 8 but, as a quick overview, I take the KCA pulse on first the patient's left wrist and then on their right wrist. The pattern felt on the two sides is not necessarily the same. There are only eight patterns that may be found, just as Kuon has discovered, but my interpretation of the meaning of these patterns entails an expansion of Kuon's theories. For each of Kuon's original eight types, I believe there are three possible constitutional variants (two of which always share the same Great Meridian of the Six Levels), the rationale for which will be presented in Chapters 8, 9, and 10. Kuon's eight pulse types represent four patterns that deal with constitutions based on the Fu Organs, and four patterns that deal with constitutions based on the Zang Organs.[8] Kuon discovered dietary guidelines for each of the eight types, and when patients are found to have constitutions that fit Kuon's original types, I have found these recommendations to be very helpful.

---

7   The beginning of the proximal end of the bulging out of the styloid process is more proximal than the apex of the styloid process. The two methods of arriving at the location for taking the constitutional pulses should give identical results.

8   These correspond to the Greater Yang, Lesser Yang, Greater Yin, and Lesser Yin patterns of SCM.

3. After taking the KCA pulses, keeping my fingers in the same locations, I usually take the SCM or Puramo pulse, named after the Korean practitioner who devised this method, and taught it to me in his clinic. Although the location of the fingers along the radial artery is the same as in KCA, the SCM pulses are felt with different parts of the practitioner's fingers. For KCA one presses down with the fingers' pads, while for SCM one presses down with the fingertips. The details of these differences will be explained in Chapters 4 and 8. The SCM pulse is intended to identify which of the Four Sang the client represents (Greater Yang, Lesser Yang, Greater Yin, or Lesser Yin). As was the case with KCA and Kuon, I also perform the SCM examination and interpret its results slightly differently than Puramo does, but I will explain this in detail in Chapter 4. Puramo used only the patient's left wrist to examine the SCM pulse, but I find that the results are the same on both sides, and they can be used to verify each other. When possible, I like to confirm the SCM pulse bilaterally for maximum reliability. This constitutional classification system also provides a more general set of dietary recommendations than does KCA, and I have found them to be helpful. By itself, the Sasang classification does not indicate which Element, Organ, Official, or Meridian is the constitutional locus, but in conjunction with the other constitutional steps, it guides one towards a correct diagnosis. The SCM and KCA pulse findings should corroborate each other, as they developed from the same original theory. If there is a contradiction between these two methods' findings, then a mistake has been made, and the examination should start anew.

4. Next, I often proceed to a Six Level pulse evaluation, keeping my fingers at this proximal location, and employing the map described in the *Maijing*. Later, I will repeat this Six Level exam at the traditional distal Cun, Guan, and Chi locations for comparison, using the same *Maijing* map. If there is a difference between the findings at these two locations, I suspect the presence of an Extraordinary Meridian imbalance. The *Maijing* map depicts the medial to lateral locations where the impulses of the Six Levels (Taiyang, Yangming, Shaoyang, Jueyin, Taiyin, or Shaoyin) can be felt, and explains, in my opinion, how the orientation of the Cun, Guan, and Chi pulses reflect which of the Six Levels of Yin/Yang is constitutionally dominant. The *Maijing* also describes the effects of Extraordinary Meridian activity on the locations of the impulses at Cun, Guan, and Chi, so there is the possibility that the constitutional pulse pattern may not be clearly displayed in the more distal standard

location for Chinese pulse examination. This is the reason I evaluate the Six Levels first in the more proximal location, where it is apparently not distorted by Extraordinary Meridian imbalances. If an Extraordinary Meridian imbalance is suspected, it can be interpreted according to the standards described in the *Maijing*, or by other methods to be explained in Part Two. The Six Level diagnosis should once again agree with the previous constitutional assessment. If not, these steps need to be rechecked.

5. With my fingers still at the proximal locations, I usually proceed to checking the Ayurvedic pulses, both at the constitutional (Prakriti) and conditional (Vikruti) levels. The deeper pulse determines if the constitution is Vata, Pitta, Kapha, Vata/Pitta, Vata/Kapha, or Pitta/Kappa in type, and is the same on both wrists. Each of these Doshic types corresponds to only one or two of the (Chinese) Five Elements. This correlation of Doshas with Elements is central to the coherence of constitutional pulse diagnosis, and as such will be fully elaborated in Chapter 3. The Prakriti pulse type can be difficult to clearly discriminate, but I will indicate two variations of pulse technique that can help arrive at a more reliable conclusion (one is described by Lad in his textbook, and the other is the method I learned from my teacher of Raju's tradition). Only certain Prakriti pulses are possible for each SCM and KCA pulse type, so once again, if there is not agreement, a mistake has been made, and the pulse diagnosis should start over again.[9] The Vikruti pulses include Superficial, Dosha, and Subdosha determinations, all of which relate to the conditional state, but which can also contribute to a better understanding of the constitution, as will be discussed in Chapter 12.

    In summary, at this point in the constitutional pulse analysis one should be able to form a hypothesis about the Great Meridian connected to the CF (Six Levels), whether it tends towards Excess or Deficiency, and whether it represents either the Hand or Foot branch of the Great Meridian. Furthermore, having carried out all these steps, the practitioner should be able to identify each of the following aspects of the constitution: Ayurvedic diagnosis, Sasang diagnosis, Five Element CF diagnosis, Eight Constitutions typology, and, finally, which of the 12 Officials is at the root of the constitutional predisposition, and whether it will tend towards Excess (hyperfunctioning) or Deficiency

---

9   One of my discoveries is that the Subdosha level of the Vikruti pulse can help to clarify, confirm, or reject one's conclusions about the constitution. This involves a more advanced and more subtle aspect of Ayurvedic pulse diagnosis, together with my own speculations on concordances between the Subdoshas and the Chinese Elements. This material will be presented later in the text.

(hypofunctioning) according to the schema in Table 2.1, which I have likened to a Rosetta Stone, as it serves to correlate findings across the various medical systems which developed in unique ways in different parts of Asia.[10]

6. Having completed the four constitutional examinations, I return my fingers to the Yang locations of Cun, Guan, and Chi to continue the conditional pulse examination. This Yang position is used to ascertain the (conditional) state of the Yang aspect of each of the 12 Organs/ Meridians as is specified in both the *Maijing* and *Nanjing*. I call this finger position the Yang location because I believe it reflects the state of the Yang of each of the Organs. In a similar fashion, I then move my fingers one half Cun proximally, to the Yin locations of Cun, Guan, and Chi to assess the Yin of each of the Organs. I also use both the Yin and Yang locations of Cun, Guan, and Chi to help clarify the abnormality within the constitutional Meridian by using the pulse image theory of Adams (based on the *Nanjing*), also discussed in Chapter 6. Adams' and Morris' teachings are the starting point for this step in the evaluation, but I have come to somewhat different conclusions from them about the interpretation of these pulses, and will present both their ideas and my own for comparison.

Before leaving this introduction to pulse diagnosis, I'd like to say just a few words about diagnosing the current condition, which after all is the target of treatment. As I indicated previously, the constitution cannot be changed by treatment; only the condition is subject to change.

I use several pulse exams, as I've briefly indicated, to analyze the current condition. One is the carotid/radial pulse comparison; another is evaluation of the superficial Ayurvedic pulse known as the Vikruti (at three levels: Superficial, Dosha, and Subdosha); and, lastly, the combined examination of the Yin and Yang locations of the Cun, Guan, and Chi pulses. I use both pulse quality and pulse volume in the assessment at each of these positions, differing in this regard from the FEA tradition transmitted by Worsley, who used only pulse volume.[11] I have found that transferring Qi from Meridians that are Excess to Meridians

---

10 The methods described so far do not distinguish constitutions of the Water and Fire Elements, which represent the two branches of the Taiyang and Shaoyin Meridians. Currently my main method for making this distinction is on the basis of the Subdosha Vikruti pulses, to be described in Chapter 12. I have indicated this component in Table 2.1 using the symbols ▼ for the Water Element and ▲ for the Fire Element in the Subdosha pulse.

11 Clearly there are occasions when Excess pulses are small in volume, but very hard in qualitative terms. Also, at times Deficient pulses might be bigger in size, but almost totally lacking in force. These exceptions must be considered diagnostically.

that are Deficient, using the Creative (Sheng) and Control (Ke) Cycles of the Five Elements, is one of the most reliable and powerful ways to use acupuncture to restore balance to the individual, but it is necessary to understand the relative Yin and Yang effects of the different Command Points to carry out this strategy, and here I am guided by Thambirajah's excellent text as well as by Worsley's teachings in this regard, although, as I have indicated, there is a slight disparity between their teachings about the Control Cycle (Xiang Ke). Usually the constitutional Official/Organ/Element will be either the most Excess or the most Deficient by pulse volume (in either the Yin or Yang location), but not always. In any case, if the CF tends towards Deficiency by the above diagnosis, I will usually transfer Qi into it from the most Excess location. Contrariwise, if the CF tends to Excess, I will transfer Qi out of it towards the most Deficient pulse felt, or Disperse the Excess Qi using Points of the CF itself. I commonly (although not always) use only "Command" Points[12] for treatment, an approach that was characteristic of the esteemed Japanese practitioner Mme. Hashimoto, who was one of the first Asians to teach acupuncture clinically in the West,[13] and is also characteristic of many practitioners of Japanese Meridian therapy and Korean Constitutional and other Korean styles of acupuncture.[14] This is just an initial suggestion, however. In many instances, I choose to treat using KCA or other approaches. The use of distal Command Points is a popular response to trying to practice acupuncture in the spirit of the *Nanjing*. Other acupuncture styles, which emphasize the use of Points on the whole body, are more reflective of the spirit of the *Neijing*.[15] I am not saying either approach is superior to the other. They are different, but both are valid and effective when used properly. The chapters on treatment and on case histories will give more specific details on using the pulses to devise treatments based on these and other clinical strategies. Finally I would like to add one more comment about acupuncture treatment in general. The reader will undoubtedly become aware at some point that I do not discuss the different Meridian systems consisting of Primary, Sinew, Connecting, or Divergent Channels, nor do I differentiate treatment by Wei, Ying, and Yuan Qi, nor by the six Exogenous Pathogenic

---

12   The Command Points were so named by Soulié de Morant, and include the Five Transport Points (Five Element Points), the Source and Connecting Points (Yuan and Luo), and the Front Mu and Back Associated Shu Points. Additional Points that I include in Command Point treatments are the Group Luo Points, the Xi (Cleft) Points, and the Key Points of the Extraordinary Meridians.

13   See my publication *Footsteps*, pp.109–119, for a discussion of the contributions of Soulié de Morant and Hashimoto to the transmission of acupuncture from Asia to the West.

14   See Kim, 2012, for a presentation of Korean Sa Am style acupuncture, which only uses Command Points in its treatment protocols.

15   J. Kespi's *Acupuncture: From Symbol to Clinical Practice*. Seattle: Eastland Press, 2012, is a good example of a modern adaptation of this *Neijing* inspired usage of all the body Points. It is based on a deep understanding of the "Spirits of the Points."

Factors. The reason for this is quite simple: My conviction is that the basis of health is the normal functioning of the 12 Zang Fu and their Meridians (reflecting healthy Zheng Qi). If these 12 are doing their jobs, the organism will do its best to heal itself. By diagnosing the current imbalances in these 12, and adjusting them with respect to their constitutionally proper state, a movement towards healing should occur. I do not disagree with any traditions that use the different Meridian systems in other ways, but only offer a simple approach that has proven useful in my own practice. As a preview, I would like to suggest here that one of the goals of acupuncture treatment should be to return the conditional pulse pattern (Vikruti) to the original pattern found in the constitutional pulse (Prakriti), recognizing that all the Organs and their Meridians are not equally strong in a state of health, but display a pattern characteristic of that individual.[16]

Table 2.1 will doubtlessly seem overwhelmingly complex at first sight, and is not meant to be memorized. It is like a map, shown on the frontispiece of a novel, to illustrate the stage upon which the action will take place, and to serve as a handy guide if the reader wants to check back and see the bigger picture at any later point in this presentation.

---

16 For now, I am leaving open the possibility that, in a state of health, the Vikruti might reflect either the Doshas of the Prakriti or their exact opposite! The reason for this is that both possibilities can reflect the same order of Elemental balance. The difference is that one state might represent dominance of the Zang Organ of that Element, while the opposite state would reflect dominance of the Fu Organ of the same Element. These two possibilities might reflect equally appropriate homeostatic responses to keeping Elemental balance, while allowing more flexibility of the organism to adapt to its environment. I present this possibility based on my clinical experiences with changes in Vikruti brought about by treatment.

Table 2.1 The "Rosetta Stone" for Oriental medicine

Sasang	KCA	Ayur	6L	Constitution	5E
1. Lesser Yang	Saturno	PK ▼	Shaoyin	Kidney Deficiency	Water
2. Lesser Yang	Saturno	PK ▲	Shaoyin	Heart Excess	Fire
3. Lesser Yang	Saturno	P	Taiyin	Lung Deficiency	Metal
4. Lesser Yang	Saturna	PV	Yangming	Stomach Excess	Earth
5. Lesser Yang	Saturna	PV	Shaoyang	Gall Deficiency	Wood
6. Lesser Yang	Saturna	PK	Shaoyang	Triple Heater Deficiency	Fire
7. Lesser Yin	Mercurio	V ▼	Shaoyin	Kidney Excess	Water
8. Lesser Yin	Mercurio	V ▲	Shaoyin	Heart Deficiency	Fire
9. Lesser Yin	Mercurio	VK	Taiyin	Lung Excess	Metal
10. Lesser Yin	Mercuria	K	Yangming	Stomach Deficiency	Earth
11. Lesser Yin	Mercuria	K	Shaoyang	Gall Excess	Wood
12. Lesser Yin	Mercuria	PK	Shaoyang	Triple Heater Excess	Fire
13. Greater Yin	Jupito	VP	Jueyin	Liver Excess	Wood

14. Greater Yin	Jupito	VP	Taiyin	Spleen Deficiency	Earth
15. Greater Yin	Jupito	V	Jueyin	Pericardium Deficiency	Fire
16. Greater Yin	Jupita	VK	Yangming	Large Intestine Deficiency	Metal
17. Greater Yin	Jupita	V ▲	Taiyang	Small Intestine Excess	Fire
18. Greater Yin	Jupita	V ▼	Taiyang	Bladder Deficiency	Water
19. Greater Yang	Hespero	K	Jueyin	Liver Deficiency	Wood
20. Greater Yang	Hespero	K	Taiyin	Spleen Excess	Earth
21. Greater Yang	Hespero	PK	Jueyin	Pericardium Excess	Fire
22. Greater Yang	Hespera	P	Yangming	Large Intestine Excess	Metal
23. Greater Yang	Hespera	PK ▲	Taiyang	Small Intestine Deficiency	Fire
24. Greater Yang	Hespera	PK ▼	Taiyang	Bladder Excess	Water

Key: ▲ = Fire Subdosha present in the Vikruti pulse
▼ = Water Subdosha present in the Vikruti pulse

CHAPTER 3

KOREAN HAND ACUPUNCTURE (KHA)[1] AND AYURVEDIC MEDICINE

KHA is a therapeutic system that uses points exclusively on the hands for treatment (with needles, moxa, magnets, metallic pellets, etc.), but its diagnostic system embraces examination of the whole body. The hand is seen as a microcosm of the body but, unlike other treatment styles that work via microsystems, KHA includes the full range of Meridians and Points that are present in whole body acupuncture. Thus virtually any treatment that can be formulated for traditional acupuncture can be performed via the hand microsystem. Its advantages include accessibility, safety (there are no organs that can be inadvertently injured), and responsiveness to minimal stimulation, making it appealing to those who are averse to the discomfort of conventional needling.[2]

1　Originally named such as a direct translation of Koryo Sooji Chim, it has subsequently been styled as Korean Hand Therapy (KHT), ostensibly to emphasize the non-invasive and self-treatment opportunities that it advocates. I will stick to the original nomenclature.

2　I often use gold and silver colored press pellets on the KHA Points to "pre-test" a constitutional treatment, and verify that this produces a change in the signs and symptoms, especially the abdominal sensitivity and the pulse. I will describe the location of the KHA Points necessary for this pre-test in Appendix 1. To reiterate, the goal of this chapter is to present, as clearly as possible, the three "constitutional" patterns, and to show the tendencies towards Excess or Deficiency of each of the 12 Organs/Meridians that are specific to each of these patterns.

A

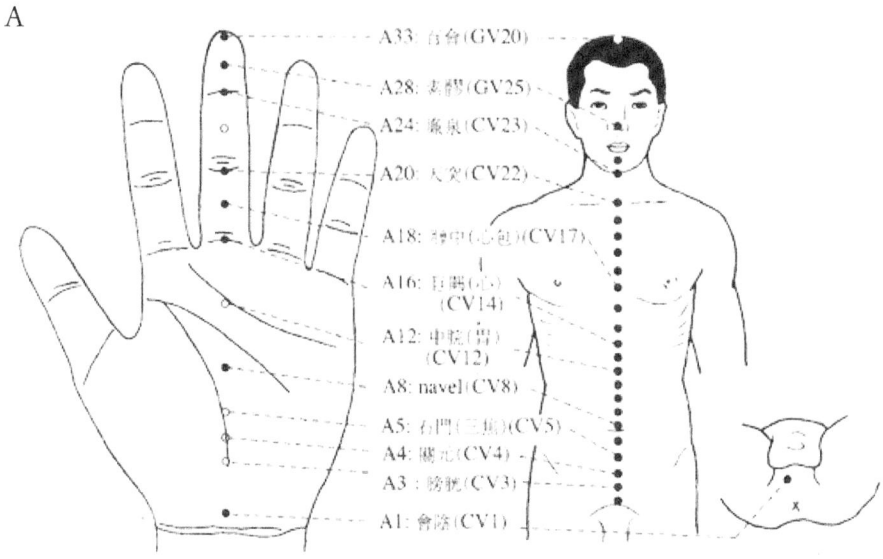

B

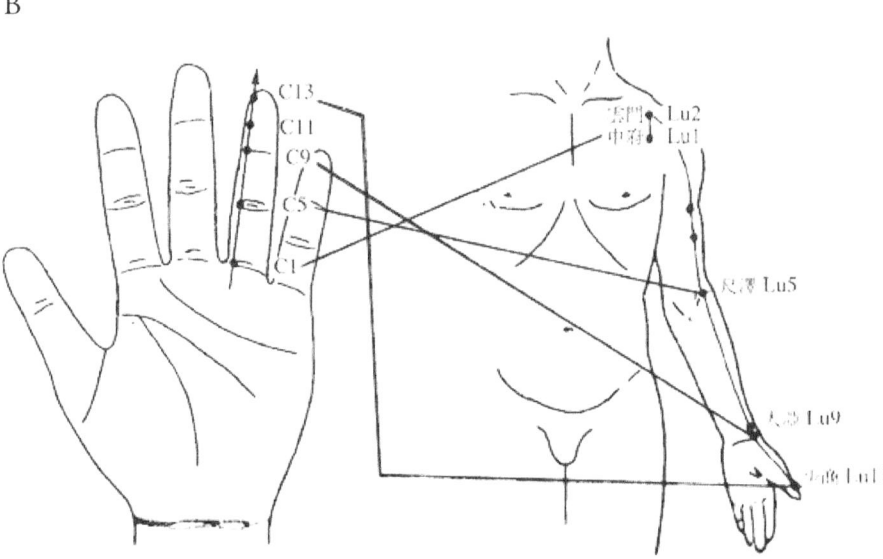

Figure 3.1 Correspondences between KHA and Body Acupoints of the Conception Vessel (A) and Lung Meridian (B)[3]

3   Image: Yoo Tae Woo, *Koryo Hand Therapy*, Vol. 1 (second edition). Seoul: Eum Yang Mek Jin, 2001.

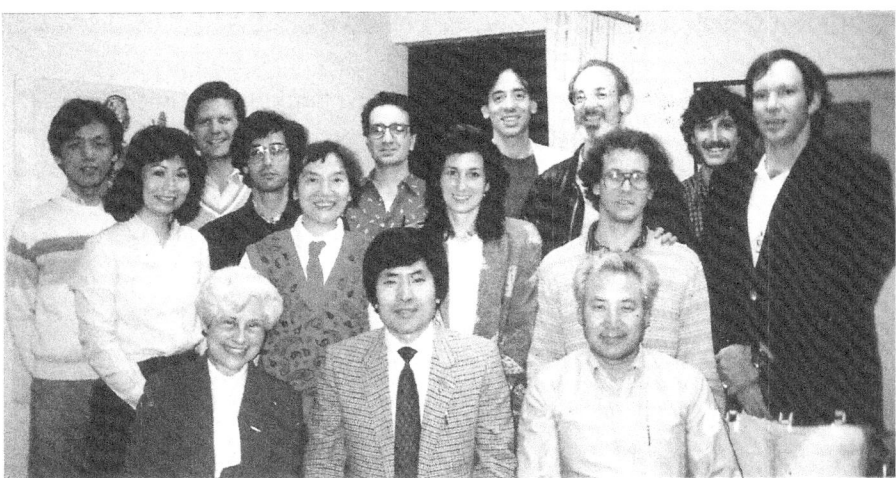

*Figure 3.2 Yoo Tae Woo (front row, center), originator of Korean
Hand Acupuncture, teaching in San Francisco*[4]

Korean Hand Acupuncture (KHA), developed by Yoo Tae Woo starting in 1971, employs a threefold analysis of constitutions or, more accurately, patterns.[5] This "constitutional" theory is based on the clinical observation by Yoo that there are three locations on the abdomen (site of the Hara or Dan Tian), which become tender as an early indicator that one's Organ/Meridian system is out of balance. These sites are at the acupuncture points Stomach 25 for what he calls the Yang Excess pattern, Spleen 15 for what he calls the Yin Excess pattern, and the region from Conception Vessel 4 to 5 for what he calls the Kidney Excess pattern (see Figure 3.3). I will give a brief overview of these three patterns, so that the reader can appreciate their apparent congruence with the patterns of the three Doshas of Ayurveda, but for a more complete presentation, the reader is referred to Yoo's basic text.[6]

Yang Excess types sweat easily, dislike heat, are mesomorphic in body shape, are prone to spasms and pain in general, are athletic, and tend to form purulent discharges (pus). They feel worse in the Summer and Spring, while being ameliorated in the Winter and Fall.

Yin Excess types are prone to edema, dislike cold (but are usually well insulated by fat), are endomorphic in shape, usually healthy, but tend towards profuse bodily discharges and a sedentary lifestyle. They feel worse in the Fall and better in the Spring.

---

4   Image: From the author's private collection (the author is in the back row, third from the right).
5   This is called "Sam il che jil" in Korean. See Yoo Tae Woo, *Koryo Hand Acupuncture*, vol. 1 (ed. P. Eckman). Seoul: Eum Yang Mek Jin, 1988, for more detailed descriptions.
6   Ibid.

Kidney Excess types tend towards constipation and the production of stones of various sorts, and dislike cold the most, are ectomorphic in shape, have scanty discharges, and are prone to forming hard lumps rather than fat or muscle spasm, leading to conditions that are more frequently difficult to treat. They feel worst in the Winter and best in the Summer.

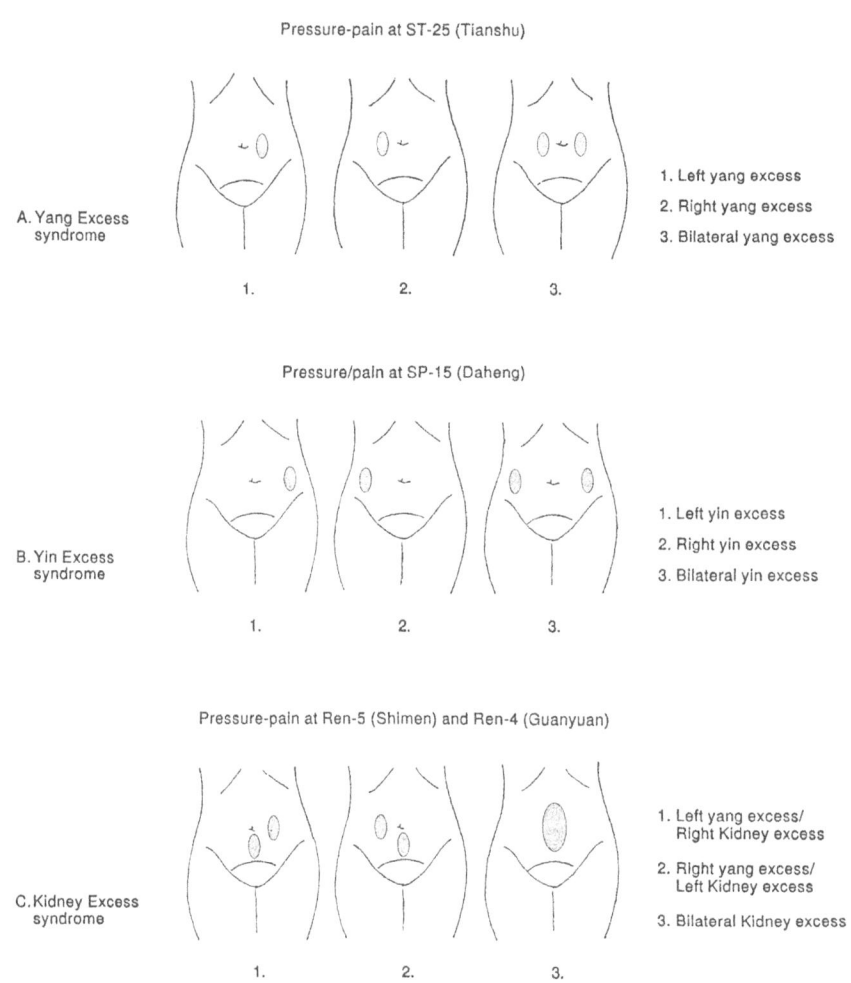

Figure 3.3 Pressure sensitivity patterns of the three syndromes in KHA[7]

In KHA, the diagnosis of these three types is mostly made on the basis of abdominal palpation rather than by pulse examination. Yang Excess typically presents with tenderness due to underlying muscle spasm at the Acupoint

---

7   Eckman, P., "Ayurveda and Korean Hand Acupuncture: A Brief Introduction to Some Similarities between Constitutional Typologies." *Amer. J. Acup.*, 23 (2), 1995, p.154.

ST 25 (Tianshu). Yin Excess typically presents with more diffuse sensitivity to pressure at SP 15 (Daheng), but without palpable muscle spasm. The obesity often accompanying this presentation may make the abdominal sensitivity difficult to elicit. Kidney Excess typically presents with both tenderness and hardness along the Conception Vessel, primarily at Ren 4 (Guanyuan) and Ren 5 (Shiguan). As the condition worsens, this sensitivity will spread up and down the midline, both anteriorly and posteriorly, but also laterally, so that the whole abdomen may become extremely tender.

We can begin to think about each of these patterns from the perspective of the Kidney, which is in charge of storing the Original Yin (Water) and Original Yang (Fire) of the body. In a state of health, Yang should go down and Yin should go up,[8] leading to warm extremities and a cool head. What would happen, though, if the Kidney Water were relatively weak? Then the Kidney Fire would overpower it, and start to rise, leading to a hot head and cold extremities. This is a very common pattern, and is frequently seen in skinny, hyperactive people.[9] Yoo called this the Yang Excess pattern, because it presents with fiery symptoms such as acute and severe pains, hypertension, nervousness, insomnia, hot flashes, infections, and a rapid pulse. This is commonly taught in many schools of Oriental medicine as the pattern of "Water weak, Fire active."

What Yoo noticed is that patients with this pattern invariably demonstrated tenderness and muscle spasm at Stomach 25, the Alarm or Mo Point of the Large Intestine, which he interpreted as indicating an Excess state of the Large Intestine. He speculated that even though the origin is Deficient Kidney Water (Yin), the expression is Excess Yang, and will show up first in a Yang Organ, but why that particular one? By the Law of Midday/Midnight, the Large Intestine is the Organ directly opposite the Kidney, and it is interesting to note that Stomach 25, the Large Intestine Mo Point which becomes tender, is physically more or less directly opposite the Back Shu Point of the Kidney, Bladder 23.[10] From this beginning, Yoo speculated that the Large Intestine was thus the first Organ to become imbalanced in the Yang Excess state, and determines the relative Excesses and Deficiencies of the other Organs. By applying the axioms of Five Element and Yin/Yang theory, we can predict the tendencies for all the other Organs. If the Large Intestine is Excess, then its Mother and Son Organs (Stomach and Urinary Bladder) will also tend to become Excess via the Creative Cycle (Xiang Sheng), while the Grandmother and Grandson Organs (Small Intestine/Triple Heater and Gall Bladder) will tend to become Deficient via the Control Cycle (Xiang Ke). In Yoo's experience, the basic

---

8   These directions are indicators of healthy biological function. Inorganic matter follows the opposite direction, with Yang rising and Yin descending.

9   This is the pattern of Kidney Yin Deficiency in TCM.

10   We will see in Chapter 4 that, in Sasang theory, the Large Intestine is considered part of the Kidney system.

opposition of Yin and Yang results in their coupled Organs tending to have inverse states; therefore the Lung, Spleen, and Kidney will become Deficient and the Heart, Pericardium, and Liver will become Excess in their functions. These relationships are summarized in Figure 3.4. We can see that the Organs that most typically have Fire patterns in TCM, the Heart, Liver, and Stomach, are all Excess in the Yang Excess pattern. This pattern is more often found to appear (via both symptoms and signs) on the left (Yang) side of the body, to be most symptomatic around noon (peak of Yang), and in the Spring and Summer (Yang seasons). It is usually found in people who are symptomatically better in the Fall and Winter (Yin seasons). In TCM terms, it is quite similar to the pattern of Kidney Yin Deficiency.

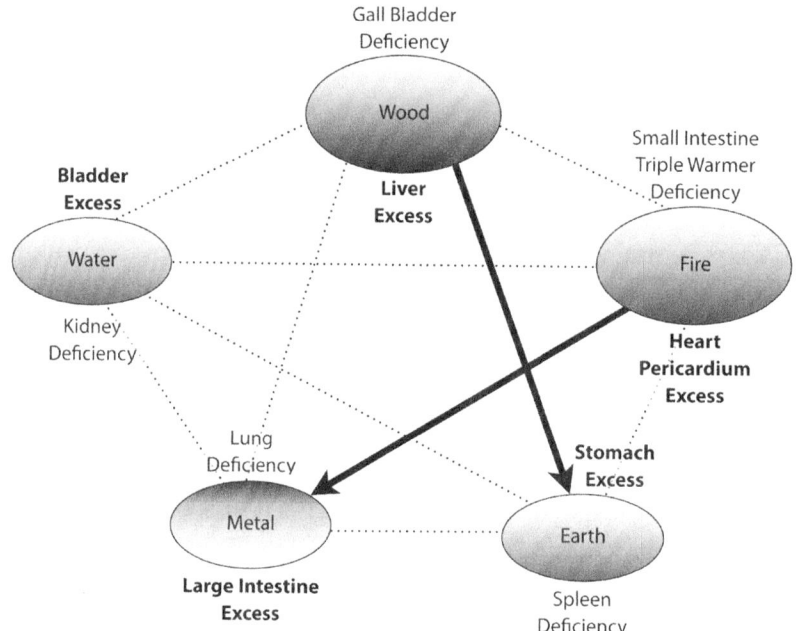

Figure 3.4 Organ states in Yang Excess syndrome[11]

Suppose that instead of the Kidney Water being relatively weak, it was the Kidney Fire (Yang) that had a relative Deficiency. This would lead to an accumulation of Dampness, so people with this situation would typically be overweight and sluggish, rather than skinny and hyperactive. Yoo noted that many people with this body type are sensitive at Spleen 15, which is again at the same horizontal level as Stomach 25 and Bladder 23. He called this pattern Yin Excess. Dampness is associated with the Earth Element, and

---

11   Image: Neal White and Elisabeth Waller-White. Based on Yoo Tae Woo, 1988, p.395.

Yoo's conclusion was that the Yin Organ of the Earth Element, the Spleen, was the first to develop Excess manifestations in this situation. He found that Spleen 15 was more commonly sensitive than the classical Mo Point of the Spleen, which is Liver 13. Again, it is interesting to note that Spleen 15 is more or less opposite in location to Bladder 52, the outer line which also reflects the state of the Kidney. The feeling at Spleen 15 is not usually one of muscle spasm (Yang), but of diffuse pressure (Yin). There is an obscure passage in the *Neijing*, which may make sense in the context of this analysis. It says the Kidney is "the Yin in the Yin," but that "the Spleen is the Absolute Yin in the Yin."[12] This may reflect a recognition that the Spleen is the first Organ to develop signs of Excess in the Yin Excess pattern. We can use the same method as above to determine the states of the other Organs. The Spleen's Mother and Son will both tend towards Excess, so the Heart, Pericardium, and Lung will all exhibit this polarity, while the Grandmother and Grandson, the Liver and Kidney, will tend towards Deficiency. Using the opposition of coupled Organs rule, the Small Intestine, Triple Heater, Stomach, and Large Intestine will tend towards Deficiency, while the Gall Bladder and Bladder will tend towards Excess, as illustrated in Figure 3.5.

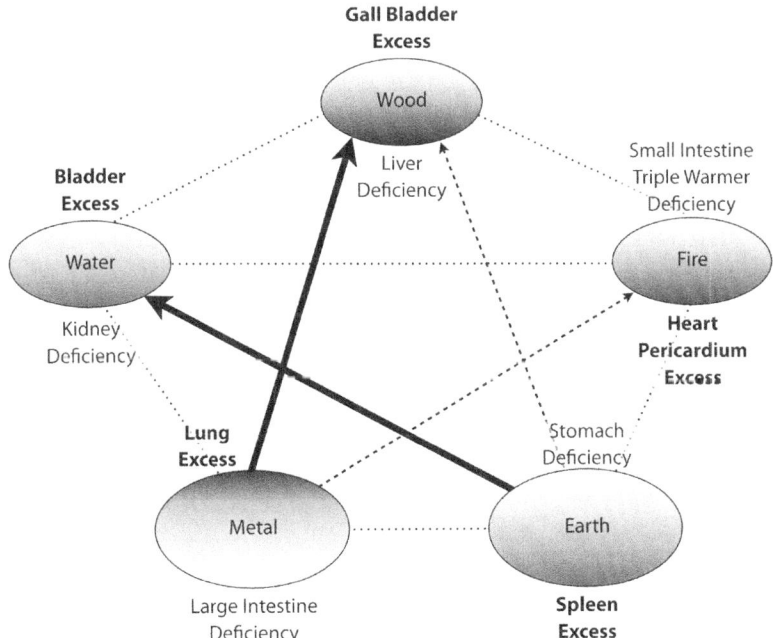

Figure 3.5 Organ states in Yin Excess syndrome[13]

---

12   *Suwen* 4.

13   Image: Neal White and Elisabeth Waller-White. Based on Yoo Tae Woo, 1988, p.411.

As mentioned, the sensitivity at Spleen 15 is generally not accompanied by muscle spasm, and may actually display a laxity (Yin) of the musculature. People with this pattern are more commonly afflicted on the right (Yin) side of the body, but often have painful complaints that are difficult to localize. In fact, the tenderness at Spleen 15 may be quite subtle, and it may seem as if there is no particular place in the abdomen that is reactive to pressure (Yin). There is often a marked coldness (Yin) around Conception Vessel 12, and a tendency towards kyphosis of the spine. The tendency is for such patients to get worse at night (Yin) and in the Fall (Yin). In TCM terms, this pattern is very similar to that of Kidney Yang Deficiency. Although this is the least common of the three "constitutions" statistically, it is often found in individuals who have had adverse reactions to acupuncture, especially treatment at Large Intestine 4 or 11, Stomach 36, or Liver 3, which are all very commonly used Points.

Finally we have the controversial "Kidney Excess" pattern. Clinically it is more commonly found than the Yin Excess pattern, but not as often as the Yang Excess pattern. The hallmark of this pattern is sensitivity in the region between Ren 4 and 5, which are the Mo Points of the Small Intestine and Triple Heater, but there is also sensitivity at Kidney 16, again on the same horizontal level as the test points for the other patterns, and directly indicating an imbalance of the Kidney. The sensitivity in this area is neither one of muscle spasm nor laxity, but rather has the feeling of a congelation or lump. The Kidney is responsible for storage of the Jing, but if pathogenic energies invade the Kidney (leading to the Excess state) they will also be stored in the Dan Tian, which is what the congealed sensation represents. This can be thought of as a kind of Yin condition (worst in Winter and best in Summer), so it should show up first in a Yin Organ, which it does at Kidney 16, but this is not a clinically useful discriminator since the periumbilical area is sensitive in almost everyone. The lump is usually most readily felt between the Mo Points of the Small Intestine and Triple Heater, so the Excess state of these Organs is taken as the indicator of this pattern, but the Kidney is still taken as the starting point for determining the situations of the other Organs. Its Mother and Son Organs, namely the Lung and Liver, will also tend towards Excess, while the Grandmother and Grandson, the Spleen, Heart, and Pericardium, will tend towards Deficiency. The coupled Organs have inverse tendencies, so the Large Intestine, Bladder, and Gall Bladder will be Deficient and the Small Intestine, Triple Heater, and Stomach will be Excess, as shown in Figure 3.6.

The Kidney Excess pattern is more commonly found in women (Yin) and on the right side (Yin), although the most predominant symptoms tend to be in midline organs. Thus most uterine and other gynecological problems show this pattern, as do most cases of spinal scoliosis. Because the test points are on the midline, it is not obvious which side of the body is imbalanced. Yoo's basic rule for deciding this question is that if either of the other two patterns is present, then the Kidney Excess is on the side opposite to it. If neither of the other two patterns is present, the Kidney Excess is interpreted as being bilateral. In my experience, this rule does not always appear to be clinically accurate.[14]

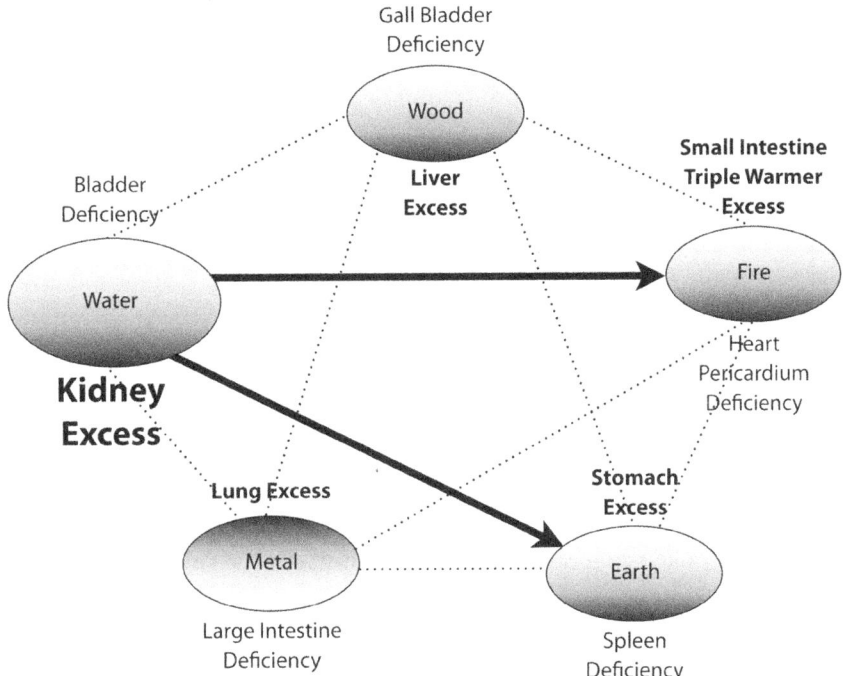

Figure 3.6 Organ states in Kidney Excess syndrome[15]

The Kidney Excess pattern starts out with tenderness, but as it aggravates, it begins to show congelation. This "lump" begins on the midline below the navel, but gradually spreads in all directions as the imbalance becomes worse. The Kidney Excess pattern is frequently seen in chronic and recalcitrant diseases. If treated early, it responds as well as the others, but if the congelation has progressed, it becomes more difficult to treat. Such patients often have abdominal tenderness anywhere they are palpated, so this may be the key diagnostic finding. I'm not sure if there is really a satisfactory TCM analog of the Kidney Excess pattern, but stagnation (Excess) of Qi, Blood, and/or Fluids is probably the closest.

---

14   I believe that an individual can manifest sensitivity on both ST 25 and Ren 5 as a result of an imbalance of either the Stomach or Liver, for example, on one side of the body alone. Further clinical experience with correlating the Ayurvedic Vikruti pulse and the abdominal exam should clarify this issue. See Chapters 11 and 12 for further discussion of this topic.

15   Image: Neal White and Elisabeth Waller-White. Based on Yoo Tae Woo, 1988, p.405.

Although these three patterns are not truly constitutions in the strict sense (their manifestation can change from day to day, reflecting changes in the person's condition, as opposed to their constitution), by recognizing their analogy to the constitutional types in Ayurveda, it becomes possible to hypothesize about the Excess or Deficient states of the Organs in a system which does have true constitutional types. Further information on KHA will be found in Appendix 1, which will provide the necessary basic knowledge to use KHA Points for "feedback" pre-testing of possible acupuncture treatments on the Regular Meridian Points.

To build a bridge from syndromic thinking to constitutional thinking, I will now discuss Ayurvedic medicine, which as I indicated earlier provided my initial insight in the search for a method of constitutional pulse determination of the Causative Factor (CF). As most readers will probably be relatively unfamiliar with Ayurveda, the traditional medicine of India, I will start by introducing one of its basic concepts: the three Doshas (Humors). These are Vata (Wind), Pitta (Bile), and Kapha (Phlegm), using the customary English translations to emphasize that the concept of Doshas is usually applied to pathology, although in fact these categories are simultaneously at play in normal physiological circumstances as well. The Doshas have the following characteristics:

> Vata is dry, cold, light, irregular, mobile, thin, rough, and is aggravated in the Fall and early Winter, while being ameliorated in the Summer. These characteristics correspond closely to those of the Kidney Excess pattern in KHA.

> Pitta is oily, hot, light, intense, fluid, malodorous, and is aggravated in the Summer and late Spring, while being ameliorated in the Winter and Fall. These characteristics correspond closely to the Yang Excess pattern in KHA.

> Kapha is oily, cold, heavy, stable, viscous, thick, smooth, and is aggravated in the late Winter and early Spring, while being ameliorated in the late Spring and Summer. These characteristics correspond closely to the Yin Excess pattern in KHA.

These three Doshas, either alone or in combinations, are invoked as the pathological imbalances that need to be addressed in Ayurvedic medicine, at both the symptomatic and constitutional levels. Imbalances that are creating the current symptomatology are called the Vikruti, while those present in an individual's constitution are called the Prakriti. The contributions of these three Doshas to a person's Vikruti and Prakriti can be diagnosed from the pulse, but since the focus of Part One of this text is on the constitution, I will be referring to the Prakriti pulse unless specified otherwise.

Let me start out by warning the reader about a major source of confusion in comparing Ayurveda to Chinese medicine. Each system has what it calls a "Five Element" theory, but they are not equivalent, nor can one transpose the Elements from one to the other system. In the Indian tradition, the Elements are Aether, Air, Fire, Water, and Earth. Three of these (Fire, Water, and Earth) also appear in Chinese medicine but, even with these three, there are significant differences between how they are understood in the two traditions, so it is imperative that if the Five Element model is being discussed, the relevant tradition is clear. In this treatise, unless stated otherwise, the Chinese system is being referred to when I mention Five Elements, with the exception being this chapter, where the Ayurvedic Elements are the basis of discussion.

In Ayurveda, each of the three Doshas is composed of two of the Elements, so it would be best to give a description of the Ayurvedic Elements. I think the easiest way to understand these Elements is in the context of their progression from least to most "material" in character, which is classically their order of appearance from the void, or Avyakta.

Aether is like the space in which events occur. It has no "physical" manifestation of its own.

Air is like the gaseous state. It represents existence without form, and is manifested in all instances of movement.

Fire is like the transformation between states, such as solid to liquid to gas in water, changing from ice to liquid to vapor. It represents form without substance, and is manifested in all metabolic processes.

Water is like the state of substance without stability. Its essential character is fluidity, and is manifested in all bodily secretions, juices, and liquids.

Earth is like the solid state of matter, and represents stability of structure.

The makeup of the Doshas is as follows:

Vata is composed of the Aether and Air Elements.

Pitta is composed of the Fire and Water Elements.

Kapha is composed of the Water and Earth Elements.

In Ayurvedic pulse diagnosis, the Elements are not perceived as such, only through their manifestation via the Doshas. Ayurvedic medicine is obviously much too complex a field to cover completely in this text, but I wanted to demonstrate how it has a way of reconciling the orders of five and six,[16] just as I have proposed for Chinese medicine.

There are many traditions of Ayurvedic pulse diagnosis, just as there are in Chinese medicine. Regardless of tradition, however, all seem to agree that the location for examining the radial pulse is approximately two to three fingerbreadths more proximally than the position used in Chinese pulse diagnosis (see Figure 1.7). Thus the index finger is situated proximal to the styloid process of the radius, which appears to me to be most accurately placed just proximal to the "Chi" or "Cubit" position in Chinese pulse taking, using what I have named the Yang location. Cravatta, my Ayurvedic teacher, used the method of sliding her fingers distally along the radius until they naturally stopped due to the beginning of the styloid prominence ("fourth position"), in order to locate the place for her index finger. The middle and ring fingers are placed adjacently. The various styles of Prakriti diagnosis with which I am familiar all depend on the same principle: that Vata, being most mobile, will show up most distally (from the heart); Pitta, being of average mobility will be in the middle; and Kapha, being the most static, will show up most proximally. The Prakriti pulse is felt at a deep level, and most traditions teach that the pulse should be completely compressed, and then, as the pressure is released, the first impulses perceived denote the Prakriti, but I sometimes find it more useful to start with the Vikruti pulses at the superficial level, and gradually increase the pressure of the palpating fingers until there is a distinct change felt somewhere deeper than halfway to the bone (radius). Both of these methods are "correct," and it is probably a good idea to employ the one that gives the clearest information.

Published English references to Ayurvedic pulse diagnosis (other than Lad's)[17] typically do not refer to the Prakriti level, and mostly present a totally different methodology than the one I am describing, a methodology which simply compares the pulse images to various animals: snake, frog, and swan being the most common.[18]

---

16   The six are Vata, Pitta, Kapha, Vatta/Pitta, Vata/Kapha, and Pitta/Kapha.

17   Lad, V., *Secrets of the Pulse: The Ancient Art of Ayurvedic Pulse Diagnosis*. Albuquerque, NM: Ayurvedic Press, 1996.

18   Gupta, K., *Science of Sphygmica or Sage Kanad on Pulse*. Delhi: Sri Satguru, 1891; Upadhyay, S., *Nadi Vijnana*. Delhi: Chaukhamba, 1986; Upadhyay, G., *The Science of Pulse Examination in Ayurveda*. Delhi: Sri Satguru, 1997; Athavale, V., *Pulse*. Delhi: Chaukhamba, 2000.

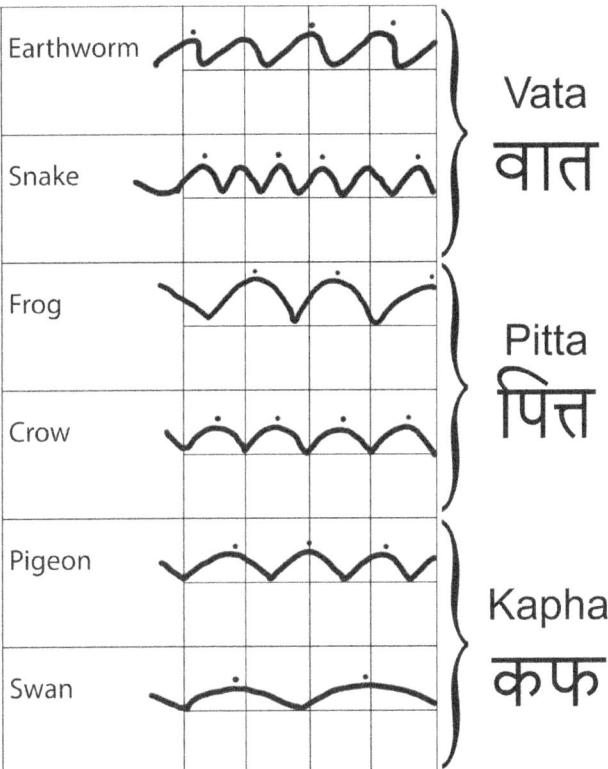

Figure 3.7 Animal images in the Ayurvedic pulse[19]

According to my training and experience, this animal image refers only to the utmost superficial aspect of the pulse, which in turn reflects the most fleeting aspect of the current condition or Vikruti, rather than the Prakriti. Since treating the current energetic state (Vikruti) is the routine approach in Ayurvedic practice (although always with regard to the underlying constitutional make-up), I will present an explanation of this part of Ayurvedic pulse diagnosis, and show how the Vikruti pulses are used clinically in the case history chapter. There are also several levels in between the most superficial and the deep pulses, which are very important in Ayurvedic pulse diagnosis (specifically, the Dosha level, which includes the Subdosha level, and the Dhatu or tissue level) (see Figure 3.8). The Dhatu level of diagnosis is beyond the scope of this text, and it does not provide information about the constitution, as far as I can

---

19   Image: Neal White and Elisabeth Waller-White. Based on image by Dr. V. Mittal, www.mittalayurveda. com. As Figure 3.7 illustrates, the animal iconography is not limited to snake, frog, and swan; however, these are the most common choices for Vata, Pitta, and Kapha respectively.

determine. I mention this degree of complexity in evaluating the Ayurvedic pulses simply as a warning that, absent a good mentor, the written tradition of Ayurvedic pulse diagnosis can be both incomplete at best and frankly misleading at worst.

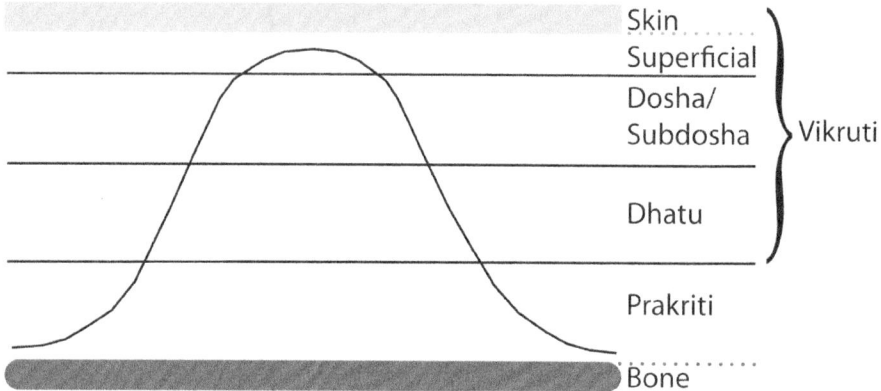

Figure 3.8 Layers of the Ayurvedic pulse[20]

To reiterate, the Ayurvedic concept of the pulse, although varying somewhat by tradition, always includes the notion that the levels felt, from superficial to deep, reflect different aspects of energetic functioning. The most superficial level represents the present physiopathologic state, and thus varies with the individual's recent meals, urinary and bowel functions, activities, emotional experiences, etc.[21] This level changes quickly, and also reflects diurnal and seasonal changes. It is not always easy to decide if what one feels in the superficial pulse is an expression of these normal physiological fluctuations, or is rather the first indication that a pathological imbalance in the Doshas has begun. Normally, at the most superficial level, the index finger feels a pulse that is described as moving in a "snakelike" manner, which I experience as narrow, undulant, and vibratory, all at the same time. These are all Vata characteristics, and the index finger resonates with Vata, being the furthest from the heart along the radial artery. Normally, the middle finger feels a pulse that is described as moving in a "froglike" manner, which I experience as bounding or jumping in quality. This is a Pitta characteristic, and the middle finger resonates with Pitta Dosha. Normally, the ring finger feels a pulse that is described as moving

---

20   Image: Neal White and Elisabeth Waller-White.

21   This is the pulse that is most properly described as feeling like a snake, frog, or swan.

in a "swanlike" manner, which I experience as wider, smoother, and gentler or less vibratory than the other two images. These are Kapha characteristics, and the ring finger resonates with Kapha Dosha. In a healthy individual, the "animals" should be in their correct locations, so, if they are not, one can begin to interpret the Vikruti. The animal images are not always iconic, however, and one may feel pulses that are mixtures of several animal types blended together. This is also an indication of imbalance. Finally, and most importantly in my experience, the relative strengths of these three pulse positions, felt by the three fingers, needs to be assessed. The Vikruti may be determined from an unusually strong animal image, even if it is in the correct location, but first one must be sure to rule out the normal physiological increases and decreases in the Doshas resulting from time, season, climate, and behavior (e.g. eating, urinating, defecating, etc.). Even more important than the animal image, in determining the Vikruti, is the strength of the pulse under each finger as the palpating pressure is gradually increased. If a Dosha is significantly imbalanced at the Vikruti level, the pulse under the corresponding finger will maintain its resistance despite increased pressure, while healthy Doshas will feel more like a thin membrane of the superficial pulse has been pushed through without further resistance. There are six possible imbalanced Vikruti findings using this methodology, which are: Vata, Pitta, Kapha, Vata/Pitta, Vata/Kapha, and Pitta/Kapha.

Slightly deeper than where the animal images are felt, and taking up the biggest part of the pulse volume, is the Dosha/Subdosha level, which indicates the imbalances that have been present for some time. Each of the Doshas has five Subdoshas, which allow the practitioner to more accurately ascertain the location and nature of the energetic perturbation. There are textual explanations of the physiological differences associated with each of the Subdoshas that present them in a manner similar to the syndromes in TCM, but do not give any information about the constitution. As in TCM, the Subdosha pattern can be a crucial factor in deciding on the initial treatment strategy. If one or more Subdoshas are clearly exaggerated, this may be a better guide to the Vikruti than the animal image in the superficial pulse.

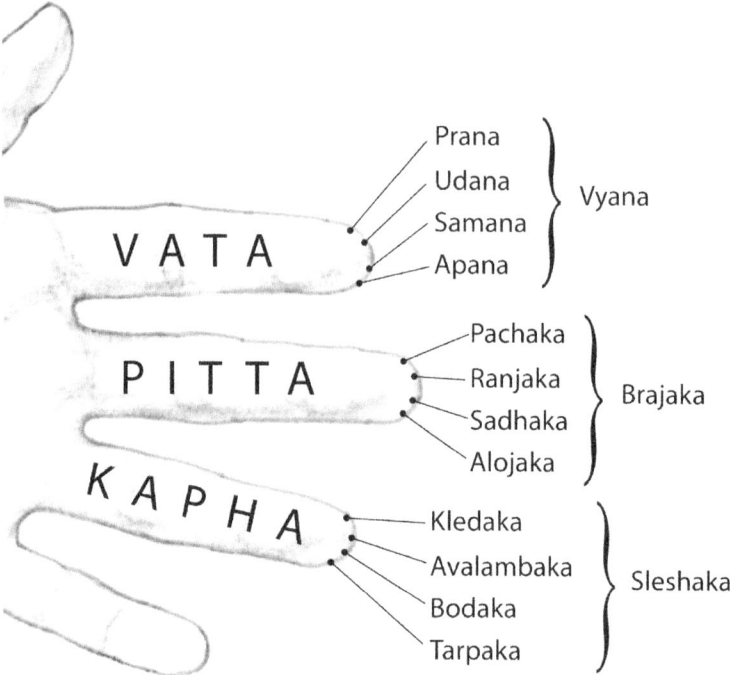

Figure 3.9 The Subdoshas[22]

If perturbations penetrate even deeper energetically, they will show up on the next deeper level of the pulse, which reflects the seven Dhatus, or tissues. This level is affected in all chronic and serious illnesses; however, none of these levels reflect the constitution (Prakriti). The constitution is revealed only at an even deeper level of the pulse, although this may not be the deepest level just above the bone.[23] To some degree, what is felt in the pulse is affected by the expectations of the examiner. In order to capitalize on this phenomenon, I recommend following an abridged Ayurvedic pulse taking protocol, which I use myself at the current time. I first place my index, middle, and ring fingers on the radial pulse and gently increase the pressure one finger at a time. When a Dosha is perturbed, the finger will continue to perceive resistance even as the pressure and depth increase. This reveals the Vikruti on the side of the body being examined. A Dosha that is not contributing to the Vikruti pulse will only show a thin membrane of resistance when the pressure is increased on

---

22   Image: Neal White and Elisabeth Waller-White. The Subdosha pulses are felt at the indicated locations on their associated finger. If two Subdoshas are felt equally strongly on the same finger, then it indicates the Subdosha designated by the bracket on the right.

23   According to Cravatta, this deepest pulse reflects the mother's energetics during fetal life (personal communication).

each finger. If a distinct Vikruti pulse is detected, then I will feel to identify which part of the examining finger feels the greatest impulse, in order to identify the relevant Excess Subdosha. There is controversy between different teachers about this interpretation, but I follow Cravatta in attending to four locations on each examining finger, which I will call 1st, 2nd, 3rd, and 4th positions, going from distal to proximal with respect to the patient's heart. If any of these four positions feels as if it is hollow. or sucking your finger into a vacuum, then the corresponding Subdosha is Deficient. Finally, if any two positions on the same finger are felt simultaneously and equally strongly, that becomes a "5th position." Figure 3.9 shows the Subdoshas for each of the five positions on the index, middle, and ring fingers.[24] I have discovered that the Subdosha patterns on the three fingers together can illuminate the possible choices for the person's Prakriti and Vikruti, but as the Subdoshas are really part of the conditional pulse assessment, I will discuss this finding in Part Two. After assessing the Vikruti pulse, I next slowly increase the pressure on all three fingers until the pattern changes to a new stable one. This new pattern, felt at a relatively deep level, is the Prakriti.[25] While the Vikruti may be totally different on the two sides of the body, the Prakriti is always the same. I cannot stress too highly that, in my experience, the only reliable method of assessing the Ayurvedic constitution is via the pulse. There are many sources that claim to diagnose Ayurvedic constitution via a survey of physical, mental, and physiological or pathological characteristics, but these typically reflect a combination of constitutional and conditional influences (Prakriti and Vikruti). In many cases, the condition (Vikruti) has an opposite Doshic make-up from the constitution (Prakriti). This is not so surprising when one notices that opposite Doshic patterns are always consonant with the same Elemental imbalance; it is just that the coupled Organ is more strongly imbalanced. For example, in the Metal Element, if Excess in the Large Intestine creates a Pitta pulse (equivalent to Yang Excess in KHA), Excess in the Lung creates a Vata/Kapha pulse (equivalent to combined Kidney Excess and Yin Excess in KHA). This finding may be a manifestation of the same phenomenon that Yoo teaches in KHA, i.e. that Zang and Fu coupled Organs show opposite energetic states (if Yang is Excess, then Yin is Deficient and vice versa). In any case, in applying the constitutional diagnostic recommendations in this text, the pulse is the only acceptable method of Ayurvedic diagnosis. However, when it comes to treatment, the present condition (Vikruti) may be the main factor in guiding

---

24 In order, the Vata Subdoshas are: Prana, Udana, Samana, Apana, and Vyana. The Pitta Subdoshas are: Pachaka, Ranjaka, Sadhaka, Alojaka, and Brajaka. The Kapha Subdoshas are: Kledaka, Avalambaka, Bodaka, Tarpaka, and Sleshaka.

25 The Dhatu, or tissue, level is felt between the Subdosha and Prakriti levels, but manifests in a totally different way, by continuously fluctuating pulse impressions, so that finding a stable pulse pattern deeper than the Subdosha level can be considered as having already passed through the Dhatu level.

the specifics of treatment, rather than the Prakriti. This is the style of practice of my principal Ayurvedic teacher.[26]

Having introduced the general approach, I'll now describe the specifics of Prakriti pulse determination. The first method of Prakriti pulse determination is the one I learned from Cravatta, and represents Raju's tradition. It is simple in principle, and consists of ascribing percentages to the strengths of the impulses (at the Prakriti depth) under the index, middle, and ring fingers, corresponding to Vata, Pitta, and Kapha respectively. Thus a Prakriti might be described as 40 percent Vata, 40 percent Pitta, and 20 percent Kapha. This would be called a Vata/Pitta or Pitta/Vata constitution. For the purpose of the methodology I am introducing, as a way to correlate Ayurvedic diagnoses with KHA patterns, I consider any Prakriti pulse that has 50 percent or more of one Dosha to be classified as reflecting that Dosha alone. Thus a pulse that is 60 percent Pitta, 30 percent Vata, and 10 percent Kapha is called a Pitta pulse.

The second method of Prakriti pulse determination is a variation of Lad's method as follows. Under each finger (index, middle, and ring), the practitioner searches for pulse spikes (at the Prakriti depth) that are either on the distal, middle, or proximal portion of the finger, using the client's heart as the point of reference. Distal spikes are Vata, middle spikes are Pitta, and proximal spikes are Kapha. Experience and mathematical possibility indicate that, again, only six varieties are encountered in the vast majority of cases: Vata, Pitta, Kapha, Vata/Pitta, Vata/Kapha, and Pitta/Kapha.

There is a rational way of accounting for both these methods of pulse diagnosis. One might think of the palpating fingers as acting somewhat like a prism, which diffracts light energy into a spectrum, except in this case the fingers are diffracting the energy of the pulse wave according to the properties of the Doshas. Vata (shortest wavelength, highest frequency), being the most mobile, travels the furthest and shows up on the index finger and the distal edges of the fingers in general. Pitta, being moderate, shows up on the middle finger and in the center of the fingers in general. Kapha (longest wavelength, lowest frequency), being the most static, shows up on the ring finger and on the proximal edges of the fingers in general. Both these methods can be thought

---

26   In his book on Ayurvedic pulses, Lad teaches that the aim of treatment is to return the Vikruti pulse to the same pattern, or state of Doshic balance, as the Prakriti pulse (Lad, 1996, p.33). Interestingly, this is quite similar to Kuon's understanding of constitutional dynamics, to be presented in Chapter 8. Contrariwise, in his most recent text, Lad states that individuals whose Vikruti is the same as their Prakriti are the most difficult to treat successfully (Lad, V., *Textbook of Ayurveda: General Principles of Management and Treatment*, vol. 3. Albuquerque, NM: Ayurvedic Press, 2012, p.10). These assertions appear to me to be contradictory. It is my own observation that the most effective acupuncture treatments do often result in pulses that have identical Vikruti and Prakriti patterns; however, they may also result in a Vikruti showing the opposite Doshas, which always correspond to the same Element. In such cases it is the coupled Organ that is showing the greater imbalance. Another pattern I have seen following successful acupuncture treatment is that the Vikruti may be in a state where no Doshas are manifesting. This topic certainly needs further study.

of as holographic, and theoretically could be applied to pulses anywhere in the body. I have on occasion used this principle to make a Prakriti determination on clients with aberrant radial arteries on both wrists, and it should be equally helpful in the case of amputees. These two methods can be practiced until they clearly confirm each other, or the practitioner may alternatively decide that they are much more skilled at using one of these methods, and stay with that one alone. We are now ready to return to the correlation between the Ayurvedic (Prakriti) findings, KHA patterns, and the Five Element CF.

Table 3.1 shows the correlations I previously reported between the KHA and Ayurvedic categories. A comparison of the Ayurvedic and KHA typologies reveals a significant similarity between Yang Excess and Pitta, Yin Excess and Kapha, and Kidney Excess and Vata. If this association is accurate, then Ayurvedic pulse diagnosis could be used to identify the KHA types at a truly constitutional level. While Yoo did not speculate on constitutional pulse characteristics of the three types he described, it is easy to see that the Ayurvedic Prakriti pulse can provide just such information. The potential value of this correlation is that, by using the additional material from KHA theory, each of these types is known to correspond to only a fixed set of possible Zang/Fu or Meridian imbalances, as has already been described. This approach could therefore lead to a first step in diagnosing which Organ/Official/Meridian is at the root of an individual's constitution, and also the polarity of imbalance (Excess or Deficiency) they will express. To review, the corresponding KHA imbalances are as follows:

> Yang Excess (Pitta) includes Excess tendencies in the Large Intestine, Stomach, Bladder, Liver, Heart, and Pericardium, and inversely, Deficiency tendencies in the Lung, Spleen, Kidney, Gall Bladder, Small Intestine, and Triple Heater.

> Yin Excess (Kapha) includes Excess tendencies in the Spleen, Heart, Pericardium, Lung, Bladder, and Gall Bladder, and inversely, Deficiency tendencies in the Stomach, Small Intestine, Triple Heater, Large Intestine, Kidney, and Liver.

> Kidney Excess (Vata) includes Excess tendencies in the Kidney, Lung, Liver, Stomach, Small Intestine, and Triple Heater, and inversely, Deficiency tendencies in the Bladder, Large Intestine, Gall Bladder, Spleen, Heart, and Pericardium.

Table 3.1 Comparison of the constitutional typologies between Ayurveda and Korean Hand Acupuncture[a]

Parameters		Ayurveda Vata	KHA Kidney Excess	Ayurveda Pitta	KHA Yang Excess	Ayurveda Kapha	KHA Yin Excess
Moisture		Dry*	Stone-forming, constipation	Oily	Sweat easily	Oily	Prone to edema
Temperature		Cold	Dislikes cold most	Hot*	Dislikes heat	Cold	Dislikes cold, but insulated
Density		Light	Thin, ectomorph	Light	Balanced, mesomorph	Heavy*	Obese, endomorph
Patterns		Irregular	Hard to treat	Intense	Severe spasms/pain	Stable	Usually healthy
Motion		Mobile	Ethereal	Fluid	Athletic	Viscous	Sedentary
Excretions		Thin (gassy)	Scanty	Malodorous (bilious)	Purulent	Thick (mucoid)	Profuse
Texture		Rough	Lump forming	Liquid	Spasm forming	Smooth	Fat forming
Climates	Best	Heat	Heat	Cold	Cold	Warm (wind, sun)	Warm
	Worst	Cold (wind, dry)	Cold (fire, damp)	Heat (cold)	Heat	Damp	Damp

Season	**Best**	Summer	Summer	Winter (fall)	Winter (fall)	Late spring/summer	Spring/winter
	Worst	Fall, early winter	Winter	Late spring, summer	Summer (spring)	Later winter, early spring	Fall, late summer
Times	**Best**	Noon	Noon	Morning	Morning	Afternoon	Afternoon
	Worst	Dusk (and dawn)	Evening	Noon and midnight	Early afternoon	Morning/night	Morning (night)

*   indicates the most characteristic findings for each Ayurvedic type

a   Eckman, 1995, p.156.

Combining the Ayurvedic and KHA findings into the six possibilities created by imbalances in either one or two Doshas together leads to the following conclusions about the relationship of the Doshas to the Organs/Officials/ Meridians:

Pitta (Yang Excess) by itself indicates either Large Intestine Excess or Lung Deficiency.

Kapha (Yin Excess) by itself indicates either Spleen Excess, Gall Bladder Excess, Stomach Deficiency, or Liver Deficiency.

Vata (Kidney Excess) by itself indicates either Kidney Excess, Small Intestine Excess, Triple Heater Excess, Bladder Deficiency, Heart Deficiency, or Pericardium Deficiency.

Vata and Kapha combined (Kidney Excess and Yin Excess) indicates either Lung Excess or Large Intestine Deficiency.

Vata and Pitta combined (Kidney Excess and Yang Excess) indicates either Liver Excess, Stomach Excess, Gall Bladder Deficiency, or Spleen Deficiency.

Pitta and Kapha combined (Yang Excess and Yin Excess) indicates either Heart Excess, Pericardium Excess, Bladder Excess, Small Intestine Deficiency, Triple Heater Deficiency, or Kidney Deficiency.

Thus we can see that making an Ayurvedic diagnosis of the constitution (Prakriti) can potentially narrow the possibilities for the CF in a Five Element (Chinese from here on) perspective, to one or two Elements at most. In summary, these are: Metal CFs will be either Pitta or Kapha/Vata. Fire and Water CFs will be either Vata or Pitta/Kapha. Wood and Earth CFs will be either Kapha or Vata/Pitta.

For example, a pure Pitta Prakriti pulse can be thought of as a Yang Excess type indicator *at the constitutional level*. In KHA, the only Organs that will reflect only the Yang Excess state are the Large Intestine, when it is in Excess, and the Lungs, when they are Deficient. Thus an individual with a pure Pitta Prakriti pulse is already identified as having a Metal Element CF. The other Ayurvedic pulse findings are not so simple in their indications of the CF, but they narrow it down to two possible Elements. Because this material is somewhat complex and most likely new to the reader, I will review these associations in more detail. Vata pulses, when found alone, reflect Kidney Excess syndrome tendencies, and might be expected in constitutions with Excess tendencies in the Small Intestine, Triple Heater or Kidney, or Deficient tendencies in the Heart, Pericardium, or Bladder. Thus individuals with pure Vata Prakriti pulses will have either a Fire or a Water Element CF. Kapha pulses, when found alone, reflect Yin Excess syndrome tendencies, and might be expected in constitutions with Excess tendencies in the Spleen or Gall Bladder, or Deficient tendencies in the Stomach or Liver. Thus individuals with pure Kapha Prakriti pulses will have either an Earth or a Wood Element CF. However, we know that in both KHA and Ayurveda, there are individuals with more complex situations. In KHA, an individual may have Yang Excess syndrome on the left side and Kidney Excess syndrome on the right side. This is actually a very common finding. If we project these tendencies onto the constitutional level, we would expect combined Pitta and Vata Prakriti pulses. The only Organ imbalances that can produce these combined findings are Excess tendencies in the Liver or Stomach, or Deficient tendencies in the Gall Bladder or Spleen. Thus, once again, we have identified individuals with either a Wood or an Earth Element CF. Likewise, Yang Excess tendencies on one side and Yin Excess tendencies on the other would correspond to Pitta/Kapha constitutions, which would be expected in cases of Excess in the Heart, Pericardium, or Bladder, or in Deficiencies in the Small Intestine, Triple Heater, or Kidney. Here we have again identified individuals with either a Fire or a Water Element CF. Finally, the combination of Yin Excess tendencies together with Kidney Excess tendencies would produce a Kapha/Vata Prakriti pulse, and would be expected in individuals of either an Excess Lung or Deficient Large Intestine nature. These individuals can have only a Metal Element CF. The correspondences of Zang/Fu and the Doshas can be summarized as follows:

Lung Excess = Vata/Kapha

Lung Deficiency = Pitta

Large Intestine Excess = Pitta

Large Intestine Deficiency = Vata/Kapha

Stomach Excess = Pitta/Vata

Stomach Deficiency = Kapha

Spleen Excess = Kapha

Spleen Deficiency = Pitta/Vata

Heart Excess = Pitta/Kapha

Heart Deficiency = Vata

Small Intestine Excess = Vata

Small Intestine Deficiency = Pitta/Kapha

Bladder Excess = Pitta/Kapha

Bladder Deficiency = Vata

Kidney Excess = Vata

Kidney Deficiency = Pitta/Kapha

Pericardium Excess = Pitta/Kapha

Pericardium Deficiency = Vata

Triple Heater Excess = Vata

Triple Heater Deficiency = Pitta/Kapha

Gall Bladder Excess = Kapha

Gall Bladder Deficiency = Pitta/Vata

Liver Excess = Pitta/Vata

Liver Deficiency = Kapha

In Part Two of this treatise (Chapter 12) I will revisit the Vikruti pulses, which should theoretically correlate better with the abdominal diagnosis, and I will elaborate both on their interpretation, and on the ways of using them in treatment planning, but for now we will stay with the discussion of constitutional pulse diagnosis.

CHAPTER 4

SASANG CONSTITUTIONAL MEDICINE (SCM)

Throughout the history of Oriental medicine, various teachers have adopted opposite points of view regarding the wisdom of treating oneself with herbs or acupuncture. Professor Worsley, in a homily against self-treatment, recounted the case of one of his senior protégés, who died at an early age from cancer, following a prolonged period of self-treatment.[1] On the other hand, the literature is replete with accounts of famous individuals who began their study of Oriental medicine by successfully treating themselves after experiencing a failure to be helped by the practitioners of their era. I have always felt inspired by such stories, and am pleased to introduce a dramatic example here.

---

1 J. Worsley, personal communication.

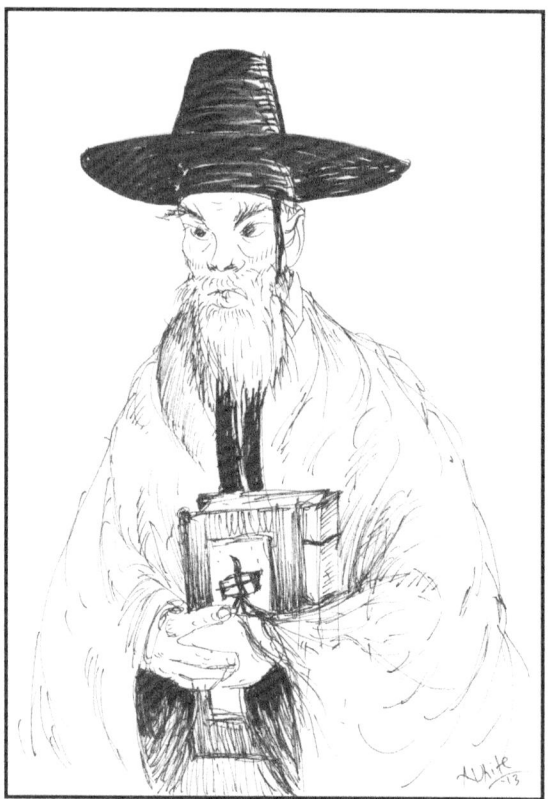

Figure 4.1 Lee Je-Ma, originator of Sasang Constitutional Medicine[2]

Lee Je-Ma (1836–1900) was a Korean Neo-Confucian philosopher who was plagued by health problems throughout his life. As a child, he began to suffer from episodes of vomiting and difficulty swallowing, together with lower body weakness resulting in difficulty walking. Over the years, these symptoms intensified despite treatment by the most famous doctors, shamans, and other healers that Lee could find. It was at this point that he began to study the classics of Oriental medicine, and to experiment with novel herbal strategies, which ultimately led to a cure.[3] The principle that guided his self-treatment was the recognition that people fall into four different constitutional types, and that the herbs which work for one type are often counter-productive for the same symptoms in individuals of other constitutions. Lee's bases for this four constitutions theory, apart from his observation of its clinical efficacy, were the philosophical principles codified in the Confucian and medical classics.

---

2   Image: Neal White. Based on Lee Je-Ma, *Longevity and Life Preservation in Oriental Medicine*. Seoul: Kyung Hee University Press, 1996.

3   Kim, J., *Compass of Health*. Franklin Lakes, NJ: Career Press, 2001, pp.16–17. The editor in the Lee, 1996, text cites the *Lingshu*, *Shanghanlun*, and *Zhongyong* as Lee's main sources, although obviously the *Yijing* is an even deeper root.

Beginning from the energetics described in the *Yijing* (*Classic of Changes*), Lee called his method Sasang (Four Images)[4] medicine, following the model presented there of the division of Yin and Yang into four subtypes, which Lee characterized as follows: Greater Yin (strong Liver and weak Lung), Lesser Yin (strong Kidney and weak Spleen), Greater Yang (strong Lung and weak Liver), and Lesser Yang (strong Spleen and weak Kidney).[5] It is important to note that Lee's concept of these "Organs" was radically different than the classical Chinese concept, and did not include the standard coupling of Zang and Fu paired Organs. In fact, while Lee associated the Stomach with the Spleen, he associated the Small Intestine with the Liver, the Large Intestine with the Kidney, and the Esophagus with the Lung.[6] The following list elaborates on these new groupings:

Spleen system: Stomach, breasts, eyes, midback, and tendons.

Liver system: Small Intestine, navel, nose, and muscles.

Kidney system: Large Intestine, urethral opening, mouth, Bladder, and bones.

Lung system: Esophagus, tongue, ears, brain, and skin.

It is readily apparent that the Heart does not appear in Lee's constitutional theory at all, and this reflects the approach many practitioners of Oriental medicine have taken in regard to the "Emperor" Organ.[7] This missing Organ is one reason that I was not satisfied with Lee's original strictures, and found myself attracted to modern interpreters of Sasang theory who incorporate the Heart into their models for both acupuncture and herbal treatment. I will reprise this topic in Chapter 9.

Lee did not think that these four constitutions were equally distributed among the population, but estimated that about 50 percent of people were of

---

4   Si Xiang, in Chinese.

5   There are few references in English to Sasang medicine. In addition to Kim, 2001, there are the following: Song, I., *An Introduction to Sasang Constitutional Medicine*. Seoul: Jimoondang International, 2005; and Lee Je-Ma, 1996.

6   In trying to reconcile Lee's Organ theory with the energetics of the *Yijing*, one proposal is that Lee's essential teaching is that the Qi in Greater Yang types tends to ascend straight up, in Lesser Yang types it ascends obliquely, in Greater Yin types it descends obliquely, and in Lesser Yin types it descends straight down. This theory, while giving a physiological basis for the differences between the constitutions, also allows for an expansion of the model such as will be presented in Chapters 8, 9, and 10. Also, Yang types are seen as energy dominant, whereas Yin types are seen as matter dominant, perhaps leading to differences in their reactivity, or inertia, to energetic treatment. The unique Organ pairing does not follow a universal rule, but tends to follow the Midday–Midnight relationships of Yin and Yang, rather than their Elemental Yin–Yang relationships.

7   The Heart is not included in this model, as Lee regarded it as the mind, rather than as one of the Organs.

Greater Yin type, 30 percent of Lesser Yang type, 20 percent of Lesser Yin type, and only about one in a thousand were of Greater Yang type. It is interesting that Lee classified himself as having a Greater Yang constitution. Not all practitioners of SCM find these same proportions, but that is to be expected based on my observation that the diagnostic criteria are quite uncertain. My own conviction is that the true proportions are quite different, but my understanding of the Four Sang deviates from Lee's teachings for reasons that I will explain in Chapter 10, so that probably explains the different frequencies we encountered.

Lee divided the trunk into four Jiao instead of three: Upper (seat of the Lung), Upper Middle (seat of the Spleen), Lower Middle (seat of the Liver), and Lower (seat of the Kidney).

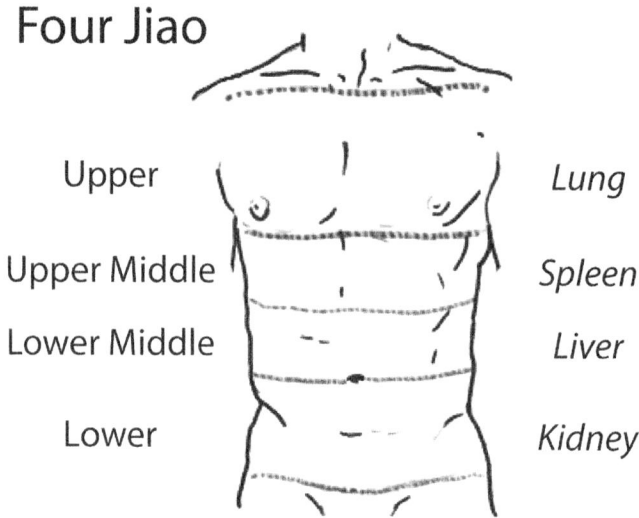

Figure 4.2 The four Jiao[8]

Although Lee devised effective herbal treatments for each constitutional type, as noted he was never able to develop a definitive method for classifying individual typology. He did use body type and other physical characteristics as suggestive guidelines, but he placed more emphasis on a person's emotional reactions and moral character, following the teachings of Mencius in this

---

8   Image: Neal White and Elisabeth Waller-White. These are energetic, as opposed to anatomical, correspondences, as the kidneys are physically in the Lower Middle Jiao and the Liver is physically in the Upper Middle Jiao.

regard.[9] While he may have been quite adept at using this form of diagnosis (one that is very similar to the Five Element practitioners' use of emotion testing), his followers have found the lack of clear diagnostic criteria to be the greatest challenge in practicing Sasang medicine. Lee made a few casual remarks about the differences in the pulse in the four types, but these are unreliable guides to constitutional diagnosis. Thus the situation for Sasang practitioners is very similar to that of contemporary Five Element acupuncturists to which I alluded in the Prologue: the lack of a definitive method of pulse diagnosis for determining the constitution or CF. As I mentioned, Kuon Dowon did discover a method of constitutional pulse diagnosis that was inspired by Sasang theory, but it is not accepted by most Sasang practitioners because Kuon's theories and practices deviated from strict Sasang tradition in many ways. I will elaborate on Kuon's approach in Chapter 8, but at least one strictly traditional Sasang practitioner used Kuon's breakthrough to develop his own method of Sasang pulse diagnosis.

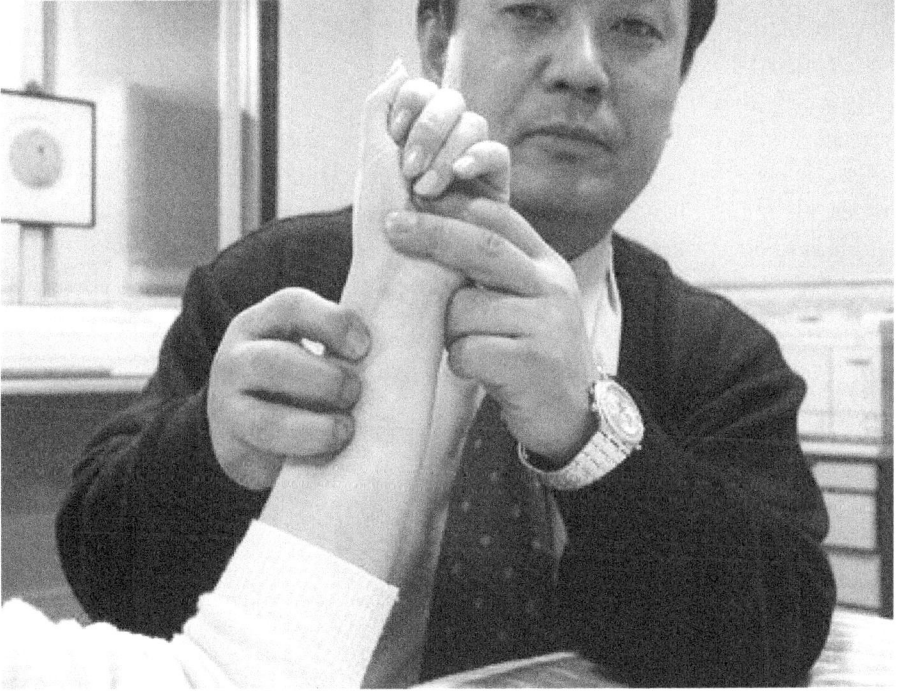

Figure 4.3 Puramo Chong, demonstrating SCM pulse examination[10]

---

9   The four emotions discussed are sorrow, anger, joy, and pleasure. The four virtues discussed are benevolence, righteousness, propriety, and wisdom.

10   Image: www.koreanmedicine.org/english.

Puramo Chong is a strict follower of SCM, and uses a form of constitutional pulse diagnosis he developed as his main indicator of constitutional typology. His methodology is described in detail on his website, www.puramo.com, but when I spent time observing in his clinic, I learned some of the subtleties in applying his technique which need explaining. Puramo only uses the subject's left wrist for constitutional diagnosis and, like other forms of constitutional pulse taking, he uses the more proximal location on the radial artery. The practitioner's fingers are placed over the flexor tendon in such a way as to pull it towards the radius, while pressing down hard enough with the fingertips of the index, middle, and ring fingers to completely obliterate the radial pulse. As the pressure is released, he notes which finger is the first to perceive the pulse. The index indicates Lesser Yang, the middle indicates Greater Yin, and the ring indicates Lesser Yin. Puramo, like Lee, believes that Greater Yang types are exceedingly rare, and will not be identified by this method. His website article presents a hypothetical rationale for these findings but, interestingly, they are based on Chinese medical principles, and not on anything unique to SCM. While in his clinic, I tried to duplicate his findings, and discovered that actually he felt the Greater Yin pulse between the middle and ring fingers, and he felt the Lesser Yang pulse between the index and middle fingers. This led me to speculate that these pulses were reflecting the anatomical order of the strong Organs in the four constitutions, and that individuals of Greater Yang type might be expected to manifest a pulse on the middle of the practitioner's index finger. He is currently testing this hypothesis in his practice, but I have already had abundant confirmation of this personal interpretation of the SCM pulse in my own clinic, and can report that this method identifies a substantially larger group of individuals as having a Greater Yang constitution than Lee originally reported.

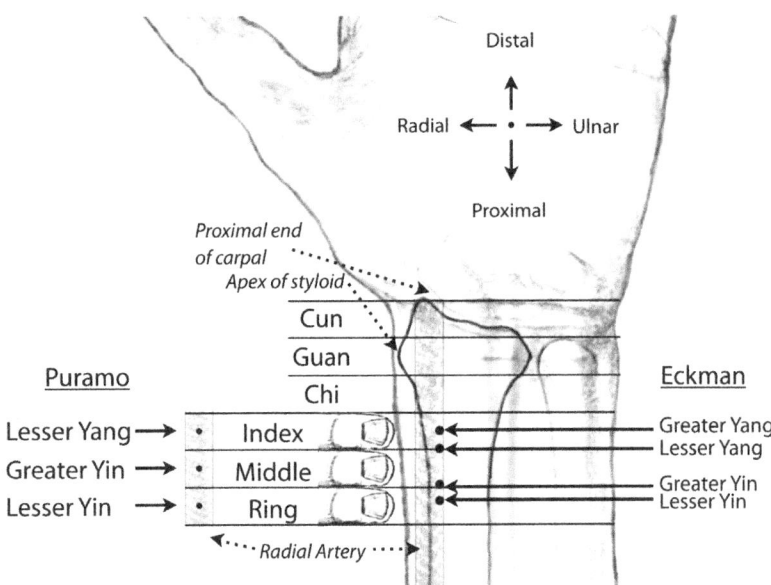

Figure 4.4 SCM pulse diagnosis per Puramo (left) and Eckman (right)[11]

Because this method of pulse examination can be uncomfortable, I have experimented with variations of technique that give accurate results with less discomfort. Here are my recommendations: First, line the palpating fingertips just above the flexor tendons on the radial side of the wrist, using the fingertips, and press straight down onto the radius so as to obliterate the pulse, if the artery runs close enough to the tendons. It is important to locate the index finger by sliding it distally along the radius until it naturally stops due to the beginning of the prominence of the styloid process. If the pulse is not felt with the fingertips right next to the tendons, try moving the fingers radially in a parallel manner until the pulse is felt, but try to keep the palpating fingers as close to the flexor tendons as possible, while still feeling a radial pulse. I find the ulnar edge of the radial pulse to give the most clear and accurate results. As the pressure is released, the pulse will emerge first at one of four locations, as shown in Figure 4.4. My method of Sasang pulse diagnosis gives the same results whether taken on the left or right wrists. The symmetrical nature of this pulse is supportive of its identification as a constitutional indicator of the Sasang diagnosis.

---

11   Image: Neal White and Elisabeth Waller-White.

Although Lee's treatments were herbal in nature,[12] he did predict that in the future someone was bound to discover a way to apply acupuncture according to Sasang theory. In this vision Lee was quite prophetic, for, as I indicated, Kuon Dowon discovered both a method of constitutional pulse diagnosis and a method of formulating appropriate acupuncture treatments, which will be described in Chapter 8. I have included this chapter on SCM because it is important in understanding the evolution of constitutional theory. In this regard, I'd like to return briefly to the question of treating only the constitution, versus treating the condition in the context of knowing the constitution. In actuality, Lee proposed different herbal treatments for each constitution, depending on the symptomatology. His analysis of different symptom presentations was based on concepts that would have been familiar to his contemporary practitioners of Chinese medicine: Hot/Cold, Exterior/Interior, and Zang/Fu manifestations. As this text is not about herbal medicine, the interested reader is referred to the works of Lee and Song in the bibliography for further details.

---

12   The herbal prescriptions were specifically indicated for dealing with disease manifestations. Lee's recommendations for preventive health maintenance and self cultivation had more to do with proper diet and emotional/spiritual practices respectively. In the healthy condition Greater Yang types have no difficulty with urination, Lesser Yang types have no difficulty with bowel movements, Greater Yin types have no difficulty sweating, while Lesser Yin types have no digestive difficulties. If these conditions are not fulfilled, it is an indication that more aggressive treatment is indicated.

FIVE ELEMENT ACUPUNCTURE (FEA)

Since its earliest days, the Five Element theory in both acupuncture and Chinese philosophy in general has been periodically criticized as being unreliable, unscientific, and generally a remnant of superstitious beliefs. For example, Mo Zi, writing about the same time as the demise of Zou Yan, the putative founder of the Five Element philosophical tradition (c. 170 BCE), said, "The Five Elements do not perpetually overcome one another… Quite apart [from any cycle] fire naturally melts metal, if there is enough fire; or metal may pulverize a burning fire to cinders, if there is enough metal."[1] Wang Chong, in the first century CE, wrote that "the cock is connected with [Metal], and the hare with [Wood]. If metal really conquers wood, why do cocks not devour hares?"[2] Although it is admirable, in my opinion, to distinguish superstition from knowledge, it is also necessary to base one's judgment on sufficient practical experience, so as not to "throw the baby out with the bathwater." The true contribution of Five Element theory to the practice of acupuncture is undeniable to anyone who carefully studies its history and has experience in applying it. The Five Shu Points on each Meridian are individually associated with the Five Elements, and many styles of acupuncture (Chinese, Japanese, Korean, Vietnamese, and English, to cite a few) are derived from, and totally dependent upon, their use and their specific interrelationships according to Five Element theory.

Whether or not there was a traditional Five Element style of acupuncture in ancient China, which has been passed down to the present time by oral

---

1 Needham, J., *Science and Civilization in China*, vol. 2. Cambridge: Cambridge University Press, 1956, pp.259–260.

2 Ibid., p.266, from *Lun Heng* (*Discourses Weighed in the Balance*).

transmission, is open to debate, but as I have argued in *Footsteps*, the contemporary methodology taught as classical Five Element Acupuncture (FEA)[3] is actually a modern synthesis of various "traditional" teachings, compiled by the late J. R. Worsley in England. In brief, I conjecture that this style is mostly derived from Japanese and Chinese sources (agreeing in this regard with Worsley's named teachers), although filtered through the experience of other European teachers. In this chapter I will only touch on enough of the principles of FEA to pique the interest of those trained in other traditions. For a more thorough exposition of FEA, the reader is referred to *Footsteps* or *Five Element Constitutional Acupuncture*.[4] As I have already stated, there is as yet no method of pulse diagnosis in this tradition, for identifying the constitution or CF as it is called, a situation which this text is attempting to redress.

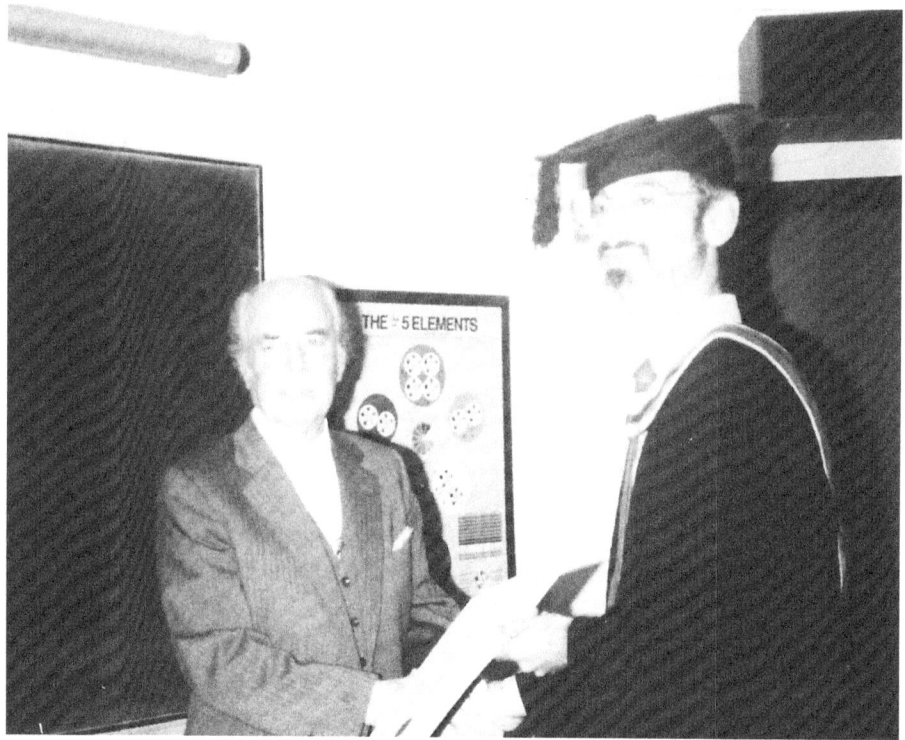

Figure 5.1 J. R. Worsley in front of his Five Element Chart at the author's M.Ac. graduation

---

3   I referred to this style as Leamington Acupuncture (LA) in *Footsteps* as a way of emphasizing its syncretic nature, but that designation has not been adopted as normative, and I am referring to it as Five Element Acupuncture (FEA) in the present work.

4   Hicks, A., Hicks, J., and Mole, P., *Five Element Constitutional Acupuncture*. Edinburgh: Churchill Livingstone, 2004.

Perhaps the best way to characterize FEA is to note that it follows the direction of thinking that can be traced from *Suwen* to *Lingshu* to *Nanjing*, and adopts the radial pulse position interpretations common to the latter text and the *Maijing*.[5] This trajectory is specifically focused on the practice of acupuncture, in contrast to the seminal texts that are more particularly about herbal medicine, such as *Shanghanlun*, *Jingguiyaolue*, and the later works by Liu Wan-su, Li Dong-yuan, Zhang Cong-zheng, Zhu Zhen-heng, Zhang Jie-bin, Li Shi-zhen, and Ye Tian-shi. These latter authors followed the revised interpretation of the radial pulse in the Ming dynasty text *Leijing*. The acupunctural teachings of modern TCM are mostly based on the ideas of this more herbally focused tradition, and so these two styles of practice (FEA and TCM) are quite dissimilar in many ways. Readers who are primarily trained in TCM (currently the dominant style of acupuncture in the USA as well as in China) may find the following list of attributes of FEA rather "foreign."

1. The primacy of the Spirit (Shen). I have already indicated that Oriental medicine recognizes the hierarchical organization of living beings, and in this regard, the Spirit is considered to be of a higher nature, and thus more important in terms of treatment, than the mind or body.

2. An imbalance in one of the Five Elements is characteristic of all individuals, and is called the Causative Factor (CF). It manifests in specific colors, sounds, odors, and emotions. Successful acupuncture treatment depends on giving attention to restoring this Element to balance, although it is not limited to that sole objective.

3. The mechanism for adjusting the balance among the Elements is primarily through use of the Creative Cycle (Xiang Sheng) and the Control Cycle (Xiang Ke) of the Elements. Additionally, the Source (Yuan) Points, Horary (Ben) Points, Connecting (Luo) Points, Front Assembly (Mo) and Back Associated (Shu) Points, and Entry/Exit Points are similarly employed, as are all other Acupoints, based on their individual potential as codified in their traditional names (Spirits of the Points).

4. Several kinds of energetic states act as "blocks" to the efficacy of Five Element treatment, and must be dealt with initially. These include Aggressive Energy, Husband/Wife Imbalances, and Demonic Possession. It is also possible for blocks to occur between sequential Meridians according to the 24 hourly tides in the flow of Qi. These latter blocks are cleared by using Entry/Exit Point treatments. Blocks can also occur between the different levels of body, mind, and spirit, and between the left

---

5   Wang Shu-he, *The Pulse Classic* (Yang Shou-zhong, trans.). Boulder, CO: Blue Poppy Press, 1997, Book 1, Ch. 7, pp.12–13.

and right branches of any Meridian (Akabane imbalances). The meaning of these terms and their historical lineage in traditional acupuncture are all discussed in *Footsteps*.[6]

Before leaving the topic of FEA, I would like to reiterate the way in which the constitutional pulse determination that I am introducing in this text can be integrated into FEA practice. Essentially the practitioner has two options. Either one can simply use constitutional pulse diagnosis to make or confirm a decision about the CF, or one can expand one's therapeutic options by making use of the additional information that such a diagnosis provides. Specifically one can incorporate diet, lifestyle, and herbal recommendations based on the Ayurvedic constitution (although it would be best to develop skill in diagnosing the Vikruti as well), and the same can be said for using Sasang recommendations. In terms of acupuncture, there is a whole range of new treatment strategies that can be employed based on the Ayurvedic, KCA, and KHA diagnoses. But even if the practitioner prefers not to mix in any of these other treatment strategies, there is a definite benefit in simply reassuring oneself about the accuracy of the CF. Of course, there is a whole separate range of treatment options that arise from an understanding of the current conditional pulse examination, but that discussion must wait until Parts Two and Three.

Finally, there is a European system of therapy that was developed by a French physician who was familiar with the Chinese Five Element theory, which fits nicely in this chapter, as it is specifically "constitutional" in approach. I am referring to oligotherapy, also known as functional diathetic medicine, originated by Jacques Menetrier (c. 1954).[7] He identified the following five pathological tendencies as characteristic of individuals with comparable Elemental imbalances at the constitutional level:

Allergic/arthritic corresponding to Wood, treated by Manganese (and/or Sulfur)

Dystonic corresponding to Fire, treated by Manganese-Cobalt (together)

Disadaptive corresponding to Earth, in two forms:

Pituitary/Gonadal, treated by Zinc-Copper

Pituitary/Pancreatic, treated by Zinc-Nickel-Cobalt

---

6   In my opinion, patterns of Extraordinary Meridian activation should be included in the list of "blocks." In Part Two I will discuss a reinterpretation of the concept of Demonic Possession. Lonny Jarrett gives an excellent presentation on blocks to Five Element treatment in *The Clinical Practice of Chinese Medicine*. Stockbridge: Spirit Path Press, 2006.

7   Menetrier's work is difficult to track down, even in French, this overview being based on two books in English by Requena, Y., *Character and Health*. Brookline, MA: Paradigm, 1989, pp.35–39; and *Terrains and Pathology in Acupuncture*, vol. 1. Brookline, MA: Paradigm, 1986.

Hyposthenic corresponding to Metal, treated by Manganese-Copper

Anergic corresponding to Water, treated by Copper-Gold-Silver

This approach is called oligotherapy because the dosage of these trace elements is about one millionth of a gram! These supplements can be helpful in supporting Five Element acupuncture, taken intermittently between treatments.[8] As with all other modalities, treatment with oligoelements must be individualized, as some people are much more sensitive to their effects than others, who hardly notice any changes. It is the author's preliminary sense that knowing the Sasang diagnosis might be helpful in choosing dosage recommendations here. Greater Yang types (which may have their CF in any of the Elements) tend to be the most energetically sensitive, and might respond to one dose of the oligoelement per week, or less. By contrast, Greater Yin types (also of any CF) seem to need higher dosages, and perhaps they are the best responders to the manufacturer's suggestion of daily dosage. The appropriate dosages for Lesser Yang and Lesser Yin types would be somewhere in between. Further study is needed to determine if the oligoelements corresponding to Officials which are not part of the CF can be used intermittently, to better coordinate their relationship with the CF. The information I have presented on oligotherapy is only an introductory overview, and there are both many other oligoelements that can be used, and many other areas of theoretical unknowns to be explored.

---

8   Oligoelements can be ordered in the USA from I & E Organics in San Diego, CA. Their website is www.iandeorganics.com. The author has no connection with this company or the products it sells.

CHAPTER 6

THE SIX WARPS OR SIX ENERGETIC LEVELS (SEL)

I am not the only contemporary acupuncturist who has been trying to grapple with more than 2000 years of Oriental medical lore concerning the pulse, and its relationship to the various energetic levels and systems in the human organism. Many, many years ago, when Leon Hammer was only thinking about writing a book on Chinese pulse diagnosis, he had the idea that I was already working on such a text, when in reality it was the furthest thing from my mind, and I so informed him. Hammer went on to write an 800-page book on the subject,[1] defining what has become known as the Shen/Hammer system of pulse diagnosis, referring to his main teacher, the late John Shen. I personally have not incorporated much of his methodology in my own, more constitutional approach, but I'd like to thank him for at least putting the idea of such a book in the back of my mind to incubate. Many American practitioners have studied the Shen/Hammer system and been influenced by it, and several of them have in turn contributed greatly to my thinking. The first is Will Morris, who has published a number of papers about pulse diagnosis,[2] and with whom I have corresponded online. One of Morris' students, Joseph Adams, taught a series of classes at a nearby acupuncture school, which I was fortunate enough to have been able to attend, and Adams came up with a

---

1   Hammer, L., *Chinese Pulse Diagnosis*. Seattle, WA: Eastland Press, 2001.
2   Available at www.pulsediagnosis.com.

methodological interpretation of one of the passages in the *Nanjing*,[3] which I have found to be helpful in constitutional pulse diagnosis, and so I'd like to acknowledge my debt to them both.

As the aim of this chapter is to present a methodology for gleaning constitutional information from the pulse using a six part model, let me start with Morris' teachings,[4] which are based on passages in the *Maijing*, or *Pulse Classic*, by Wang Shu-he, written in the second century CE.[5] In Book 10 of this text, Wang describes the location of various pulses on the radial artery according to their Six Energetic Level (SEL) designation, viz. Taiyang, Shaoyang, Yangming, Taiyin, Shaoyin, and Jueyin.

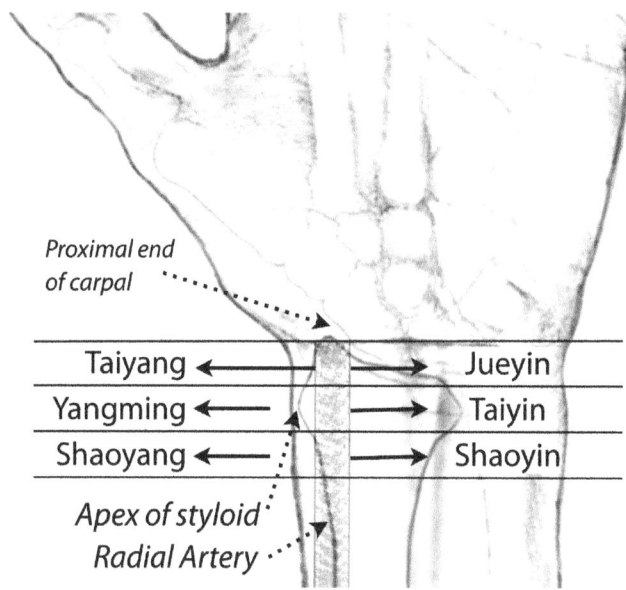

Figure 6.1 SEL pulses per the Maijing[6]

Morris has proposed that this model is describing sensations felt in the most superficial aspect of the pulse,[7] and furthermore that these locations disclose deviations in the architecture (radial or lateral deviation) of the pulse in these locales. It is logical to associate the most superficial aspect of the pulse with the

---

3   *Nanjing*, Chapter 5.

4   Morris, W. R., "Chinese Pulse Diagnosis: Epistemology, Practice, and Tradition." Dissertation. California Institute of Integral Studies. San Francisco, CA, 2009.

5   Wang Shu-he, *The Pulse Classic* (Yang Shou-zhong, trans.). Boulder, CO: Blue Poppy Press, 1997, Book 10, p.352.

6   Image: Neal White and Elisabeth Waller-White.

7   Morris has stated that he uses the most superficial aspect of the pulse because pressing deeper into the pulse allows for distortion of the artery's natural shape, leading to inaccurate readings of the SEL architecture (personal communication, 2013).

Sinew Channels (TMs)[8] and the Wei Qi (Defensive Energy) that they transport, which would account for their efficacy in treating TM problems. This deviation in the alignment of the radial pulse is not only reflective of Wei Qi and the TMs, however. In the *Maijing* passage being discussed, there is no mention of TMs or Wei Qi. Rather, the text seems to simply state where the pulses of the various energetic levels can be felt beating. Thus the *Maijing* map may be applied to other applications of SEL phenomena, such as internal medical conditional diagnosis, and I am in turn applying it to constitutional diagnosis. Here is the schema, simplified for my purposes by leaving out additional information that I have yet to verify in my clinical experience:

> At the radial side of the Cun (distal) position beats the (foot) Taiyang pulse.
>
> At the radial side of the Guan (middle) position beats the (foot) Yangming pulse.
>
> At the radial side of the Chi (proximal) position beats the (foot) Shaoyang pulse.
>
> At the ulnar side of the Cun position beats the (foot) Jueyin pulse.
>
> At the ulnar side of the Guan position beats the (foot) Taiyin pulse.
>
> At the ulnar side of the Chi position beats the (foot) Shaoyin pulse.

It is of interest that, in this very same passage, Wang describes the pulses of five of the Extraordinary Meridians as follows:

> Striking forcefully, both radial and ulnar, at the Cun...the Yangqiao pulse.
>
> Striking forcefully, both radial and ulnar, at the Guan...the Dai pulse.
>
> Striking forcefully, both radial and ulnar, at the Chi...the Yinqiao pulse.
>
> From the (foot) Shaoyang to the (foot) Jueyin...the Yinwei pulse.[9]
>
> From the (foot) Shaoyin to the (foot) Taiyang...the Yangwei pulse.

From these descriptions, it is possible to envision the existence of an actual deviation in the architecture of the radial artery, depicting a chronic (constitutional?) pattern of energetic imbalance. There are three locations, Cun, Guan, and Chi. There are only a limited number of ways that the artery's shape can be deformed. If it deviates radially at Cun, it indicates Taiyang; radially at

---

8   "TMs" stands for Tendinomuscular Meridians, an alternate translation for Sinew Channels.

9   The editor of the English translation of *Maijing*, Yang Shou-zhong, adds a footnote that these last two descriptions of trajectory can be identified in an ulnar/radial orientation, by reference to the SEL locations given immediately above (Wang Shu-he, 1997, p.352).

Guan, it indicates Yangming; radially at Chi, it indicates Shaoyang; ulnarly at Cun, it indicates Jueyin; ulnarly at Guan, it indicates Taiyin; ulnarly at Chi, it indicates Shaoyin; running obliquely from radial to ulnar as it goes from Chi to Cun, it indicates Yinwei; and running obliquely from ulnar to radial as it goes from Chi to Cun, it indicates Yangwei. These are the only possible simple variations of this basic topography, and it has been my experience that these are reliable indicators of the constitutional imbalance in SEL terms, as long as the pulses are examined in the locations that I will explain. In order to get reliable and reproducible pulse readings, it is also important that the methodology for taking the pulse conform to a standard. The particular standard that I use (a variation of that taught by Morris and Adams) is to take the pulse with the patient lying face up, with their wrist resting on its ulnar surface, or cupped in my other hand. I support their wrist from below with my non-palpating hand, which I either allow to rest on the exam table, or hold at a comfortable elevation. Alternatively, I have found comparable results by using the "hand-holding" approach taught by Worsley, as long as the ulnar side of the wrist is facing downwards.[10] Another crucial factor is the positioning of one's fingers at the Cun, Guan, and Chi positions. Morris uses the Yang locations of Cun, Guan, and Chi for the SEL determination, following the tradition shared by Wang Shu-he and John Shen, whereas Adams recommended the slightly more proximal Yin locations in the class I took with him. The difficulty in this exam is twofold: first, the Extraordinary Meridian pulse patterns are also reflected at this same location, so if an Extraordinary Meridian has been activated, the SEL pattern might not be discernible here, and second, the Yang Cun pulses are frequently deceptively difficult to clearly discern due to the natural narrowing of the radial artery as it reaches the wrist flexure. For these reasons I have found a more accurate alternate procedure: taking the "SEL pulse" first at the "constitutional" location one "wavelength" proximally (fourth position), and then checking the Yang locations of Cun, Guan, and Chi for either corroboration, or possible Extraordinary Meridian patterns (see Figure 6.2).

The most important aspect of this examination, in either place it is studied, is to start with all three fingers parallel to the flexor tendon, which is the standard for judging deviations in the radial or ulnar directions. It is also helpful to use two methods of palpation: first with the pads of the fingers and then with the tips of the fingers, to best evaluate the pulse architecture. Additionally, one can use any part of the fingers to palpate these pulses by rolling them lightly or more forcefully over the artery in order to find the center of the pulse at each position, so as to confirm the pattern and avoid erroneous results. If these steps are followed, the practitioner should come up with one of the above

---

10   The patient's wrist may be perpendicular, or alternatively slightly rotated radially outwards, so as to be comfortable for both patient and practitioner. This is quite different than the standard practice in TCM, where the patient's wrist is positioned palm upwards, resting on a pillow or cushion.

patterns. To reiterate, I'm hypothesizing that one reason this pattern does not always appear at Cun, Guan, and Chi might be the presence of an imbalance of one of the Extraordinary Meridians.[11] These include the patterns already indicated (per the *Maijing*) for the Yinqiao, Yangqiao, Yinwei, Yangwei, or Dai Vessels, but also includes the patterns of the three other Extra Meridians whose pulse I have not yet described. These last three pulses are as follows: If all three positions are beating strongly at the superficial (Qi level) depth, it reflects a Du imbalance. If all three positions are beating strongly at the middle (Xue or Blood) depth, it reflects a Ren imbalance. And if all three positions are beating strongly at the deep (Jing or Essence) level, it represents a Chong imbalance. These correlations have also been described by Morris and Adams, again following the *Maijing*.

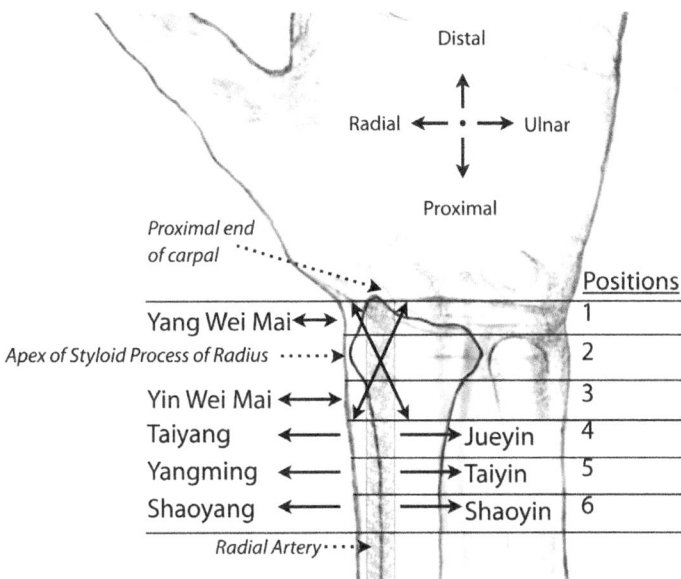

Figure 6.2 SEL transposed proximally and Extraordinary Meridians shown distally[12]

To summarize, in diagnosing the constitution, feel for the deviation of the radial pulse in either the Cun, Guan, or Chi position at the proximal "constitutional" location, and note if it is radial or ulnar. This should tell you which of the Six Warps (SEL) is constitutionally imbalanced. The *Maijing* attributed all of these imbalances to the foot branch of the Great Meridian, but my experience is that it might be either the foot or the arm branch that is constitutionally imbalanced in each case, and one must use additional methods to differentiate these two possibilities.

---

11   See Case 33 in Chapter 19.

12   Image: Neal White and Elisabeth Waller-White.

One method that I have found to be helpful in confirming or refining the SEL constitutional diagnosis is the pulse shape approach, taught by Adams, based on the *Nanjing*.[13] As usual, I have a slight difference in interpretation from Adams, but it is quite minor. The *Nanjing* describes the pulses of the Five Elements in terms of their depth (measured in the number of beans of pressure one needs to apply to feel the pulse most clearly). Going from superficial to deep, the sequence is Metal, Fire, Earth, Wood, and Water. Ideally, a healthy Element should have its widest and clearest pulse at its "natural" depth. In discriminating which half of a Great Meridian is the constitutional one indicated by the radial pulse, I use the following guideline: If the pulse of an Element is at its natural depth and the pulse of the Element which occupies the other half of the same Great Meridian is out of its natural depth, then there is a very strong likelihood that the latter is the constitutionally imbalanced branch of the Meridian.[14] My disagreement with Adams is more terminological than anything else. It concerns the Chi pulse on the right side. I consider this a Fire Element pulse, reflecting the Pericardium and Triple Heater for purposes of constitutional diagnosis, but its natural depth is at the same deep level as the Water Element pulse. Adams treats both Chi pulses as Kidney pulses, so he expects the level to be deep, but if it is more superficial on the right side, he treats the Water Element while I treat the Fire Element (Pericardium or Triple Heater). While the depth evaluation aspect of pulse examination contributes useful energetic information, it is not necessarily reflective of the constitutional versus the conditional status in any given case. After carrying out all these exams, there may still be occasions where it is unclear which branch of Taiyang or Shaoyin is the constitutional focus. The two possible Elements in each case are Fire and Water. Although I am jumping the gun by describing my way of resolving this issue here, it is important enough to merit early mention: I place a good deal of weight on the Subdoshas in the Vikruti pulse. In Part Two I will describe how I correlate the Elements with the Subdoshas, and one can see that Fire and Water Subdoshas are quite different in their manifestation. Although the Subdoshas are at the Vikruti level, it is frequently the case that the Element of the CF appears in the Subdosha pulses on at least one side of the body. Thus Fire and Water CFs can be more easily distinguished by this observation.

---

13   *Nanjing*, Chapter 5.

14   A common finding, in my experience, is that the constitutional Element, as revealed by the SEL pulse, will be out of its proper depth, and the Element corresponding to the depth of the pulse at the constitutional Element will be involved in the conditional imbalance. Moreover, this conditional Element's pulse will usually have its own pulse depth displaced to that of the constitutional Element. For example, if the constitution is found to be Earth, but the right Guan pulse is biggest at the superficial depth (Metal), then one will often find that the right Cun pulse will be biggest at the middle depth (Earth). These deflections might appear either at the Yang or Yin locations of the pulses.

CHAPTER 7

DETERMINING THE CAUSATIVE FACTOR (CF)

Before returning to the expanded forms of the Sasang tradition in constitutional diagnosis, let me summarize what can be determined about the constitution from the methods and theories already presented.

The SEL pulse determination will usually indicate the CF, if it is viewed in the context of the depth of the pulse at the putative CF location. First one determines the Great Meridian or Warp indicated by the pulse, then one selects the Hand or Foot branch of this Meridian using the pulse depth method.[1] The CF will be the Element associated with this branch of the Great Meridian. For example, if the Chi pulse (on either hand, but ideally one should be able to detect it on both sides) is radially deflected in someone, the CF will be in either the Fire or the Wood Element (Shaoyang). To confirm this, check the pulse depth at both the left Guan (GB) and right Chi (TH). These are the two branches of the Shaoyang Meridian. In this case, if the right Chi pulse is at the deepest level (its normal state), while the left Guan pulse is away from the Wood Element depth (which is slightly more superficial than the Water Element depth), then the CF is in the Wood Element and Gall Bladder (GB) Official. One can double check this determination with the Ayurvedic Prakriti pulse which will permit at most two possible Elements for the CF. In this hypothetical case, one would expect either a Kapha pulse (GB Excess) or a Pitta/Vata pulse (GB Deficiency). If there is a discrepancy between these

---

1   The displacement of the depth of the widest part of the pulse might occur in either the Yang or Yin locations of Cun, Guan, and Chi, so both must be checked.

findings, then both SEL and Ayurvedic pulses must be reexamined. In such a case, I rely heavily on the SCM pulse for clarification. Since these are new techniques for many readers of this text, it is important to remember that what I am describing is the result of decades of checking pulses, and at the beginning it is easy to make mistakes, but the mistakes become less frequent with practice. The benefit of having several different methods of cross checking the pulse is that mistakes are caught much more quickly. As I have just shown, there is another piece of information that the Ayurvedic pulse adds to the SEL pulse, and that is the recognition of whether the Organ/Official/Meridian of the CF inherently tends towards Excess or Deficiency. The SEL pulse alone does not tell you this. For example, if you find a radially deflected pulse in the Guan position, and the right Cun is biggest at the deep level, what can you say? The correct answer is that it is a case of a Metal CF with the imbalance in the Large Intestine. There are only two Ayurvedic pulses compatible with this finding: either the Prakriti pulse is Pitta or it is Kapha/Vata. The Pitta version reflects a tendency to Large Intestine Excess while the Kapha/Vata version reflects a tendency towards Large Intestine Deficiency. Table 2.1 in Chapter 2 gives a complete listing of the Ayurvedic pulses associated with both an Excess and a Deficiency of each of the 12 Organs/Officials/Meridians, and the reader is encouraged to work through the reasoning behind each of these findings.

I have selected a case of either Large Intestine Excess or Large Intestine Deficiency as an illustration of what the various pulse procedures discussed so far can reveal, because it happens to be that each of those possible constitutions is one of the eight that were originally proposed by Kuon in his seminal paper on Korean Constitutional Acupuncture, which is the subject of the next chapter. Although his methodology is a powerful one, it seems clear to me, however, that based on the material presented so far, there must be more than eight basic constitutional types. What I've determined is that each of Kuon's pulse types really represents the possibility of three different constitutions, but because they are closely related by their Sasang characteristics and their pulse images, treatment directed at one subtype is often fairly effective for problems of another of the subtypes; however, it is not the optimum treatment. This will be illustrated in the case presentations in Chapter 19. Most recently, I have discovered another reason why these three subtypes might show benefit from treatment directed at partner subtypes: they all share the same set of Excess and Deficient Elements. I will introduce this in Chapter 8 and explain it more fully in Chapter 10.

EIGHT CONSTITUTIONS MEDICINE (ECM OR KCA)

When Lee Je-Ma wrote *Longevity and Life Preservation* in 1894, he predicted that someone would eventually discover a method of acupuncture treatment consonant with the herbal strategies he proposed for Sasang medicine. Lee also predicted that 100 years following his death, Sasang medicine would become a worldwide method of healthcare. Fortuitously, in 1965 Kuon Dowon first described a method of acupuncture applying Sasang principles (Korean Constitutional Acupuncture or KCA), which was introduced at an international acupuncture congress.[1] His method was the first form of constitutional acupuncture to which I was exposed and, in the years since, Kuon's work has inspired many other followers, both of his particular methodology, but also of many individual variants. In his work Kuon made a number of significant contributions, but there are two that stand out as the most remarkable. The first was his discovery of a method of pulse examination that revealed eight, and only eight, patterns, which were permanent characteristics of every individual, not varying over the life of the individual despite changes in environment, behavior, age, or health status. The second was his discovery that the Four Needle Technique, a Five Element based acupuncture method developed by

---

1   Kuon Dowon, "A Study of Constitution-Acupuncture." *Journal of the International Congress of Acupuncture and Moxibustion*, 10, 1965, pp.149–167.

the medieval Korean monk Sa Am, could successfully address many health problems of individuals classified by these eight pulse types, without the need for further diagnostic information.[2]

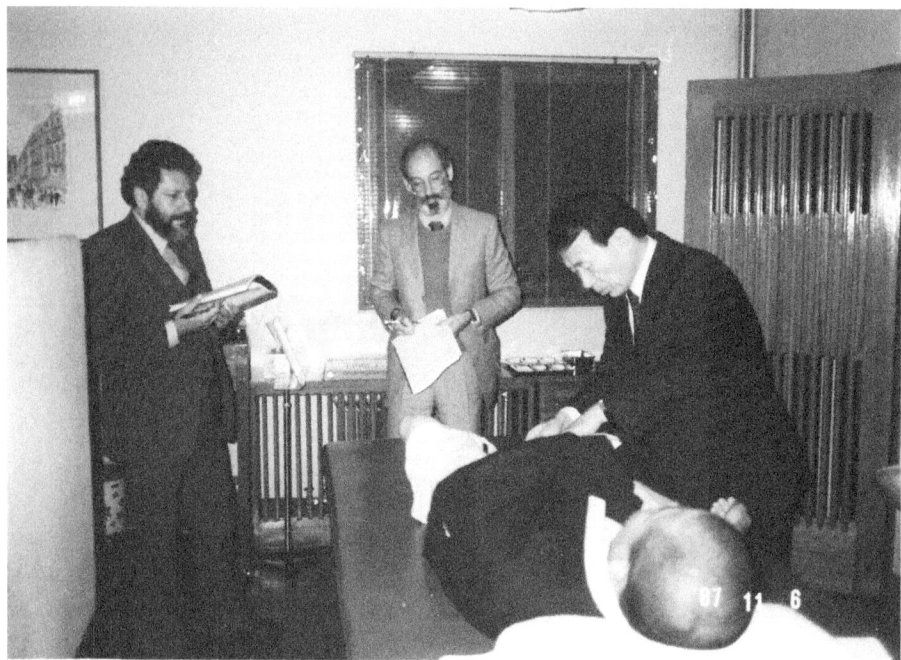

Figure 8.1 Kuon Dowon treating a Buddhist monk in Seoul[3]

These eight pulse patterns form the next component of the diagnostic methodology that I employ, and while there are differences between Kuon's interpretation of the meaning of these pulses and my own, his discovery that there are eight and only eight of these constitutional pulse patterns is consistent with my own observations. Before describing Kuon's methodology, I should point out that although he formulated his approach based on Sasang medical principles, he combined them with aspects of Chinese and Western medicine that are rejected by orthodox Sasang practitioners, and thus most of

---

2   Sa Am is the pen name of an anonymous Buddhist monk, who lived in the Yi dynasty, c. 1600 CE, and was a disciple of Sa Myong Dai Sa (1544–1610), a famous patriot and high priest. Sa Am is considered to be the "grandfather of Korean acupuncture," and was perhaps the first practitioner to extensively describe the concrete details of Point selection in applying Five Element treatment, using both the Creative and Control Cycles of the Elements in each instance. Kuon was not alone, nor necessarily the first modern acupuncturist to revive Sa Am's methodology. Yanagiya Sorei (1906–1959), the inspiration behind the Japanese school of Meridian Therapy, used the Four Needle Technique as his basic root treatment method. In his original paper, Kuon cited the work of Honma Shohaku, one of Yanagiya's disciples, who happened to read Korean. Thus it is reasonable to speculate that Kuon was influenced by the Meridian Therapy school in developing his approach to constitutional acupuncture.

3   The author and Stuart Kutchins are taking notes on Kuon's unpublished methods.

Lee's followers do not accept the validity of Kuon's pulse diagnostic method. After presenting Kuon's theory and methodology, I will address the work of practitioners who abide by a more strict adherence to Sasang principles, because it has led me to another crucial step in the development of my own approach to constitutional theory and diagnostic methodology.

Since there are reliable texts in English concerning Ayurveda, FEA, and KHA, I tried not to go into too much detail in my remarks about them, confining myself to what is directly applicable to the constitutional pulse diagnostic methodology I am proposing. Readers interested in knowing more about those disciplines may consult the relevant texts. Such is not the case with Kuon's methods, variously referred to as Korean Constitutional Acupuncture (KCA) or Eight Constitutions Medicine (ECM), which lack a text not only in English, but in Korean as well. For this reason I feel the need to present a broader description of his work, although it will still be far from a complete exposition. His concept of constitutional dynamics is so radically different from the conventional viewpoint that it becomes difficult to describe, which may be another reason why he has yet to publish a textbook himself. Also, his choice of terminology is arcane and highly idiosyncratic, which makes even his journal articles difficult to understand, but the material itself strikes me as the work of a genius.

Perhaps the best way to present his work is to proceed chronologically, starting with the material in his 1965 journal article.[4] The first salient point in this article is that Kuon's ideas are based on a synthesis of Sasang medicine, the Korean Five Element tradition in acupuncture, Chinese medicine, and Western medicine.[5] Kuon proposed that each of Lee's constitutional types is further divisible into two "temperaments," one reflecting the Zang Organs and Meridians, with the other reflecting the Fu Organs and Meridians. Thus there are eight constitutional types, which are identified by discrete pulse patterns, following a new protocol for pulse taking that he discovered (see Figure 8.2). I've also included an illustration from one of Kuon's disciples, M. B. Lee (see Figure 8.3), to try to transmit as much information as possible about this unique approach to pulse examination.

---

4   Kuon Dowon, op. cit.

5   He cites Lee Je-Ma and Sa Am as Korean influences; Chapter 16 of the Jin dynasty Chinese text *Jiayijing* (as recommending differential acupuncture treatment by constitution); mentions the Japanese author Honma Shohaku; and from Western medicine the splanchnic interrelational theory, which he associates with the endocrine system, and the work of Dr. Hans Selye.

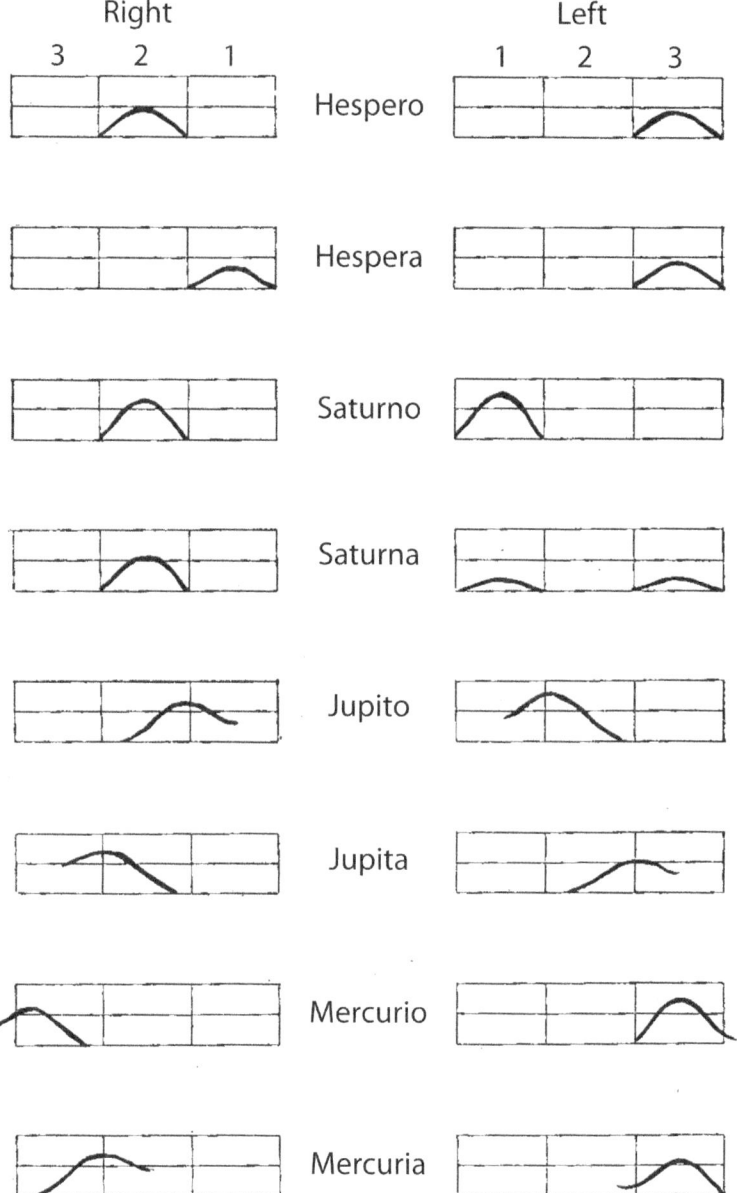

Figure 8.2 Kuon's pulse images[6]

6   Image: Neal White and Elisabeth Waller-White. Based on Kuon Dowon, "Studies on Constitution-Acupuncture Therapy." *Korean Central Journal of Medicine*, 25 (3), 1973, pp.327–342. 1 is the index finger, 2 is the middle finger, and 3 is the ring finger of the examiner.

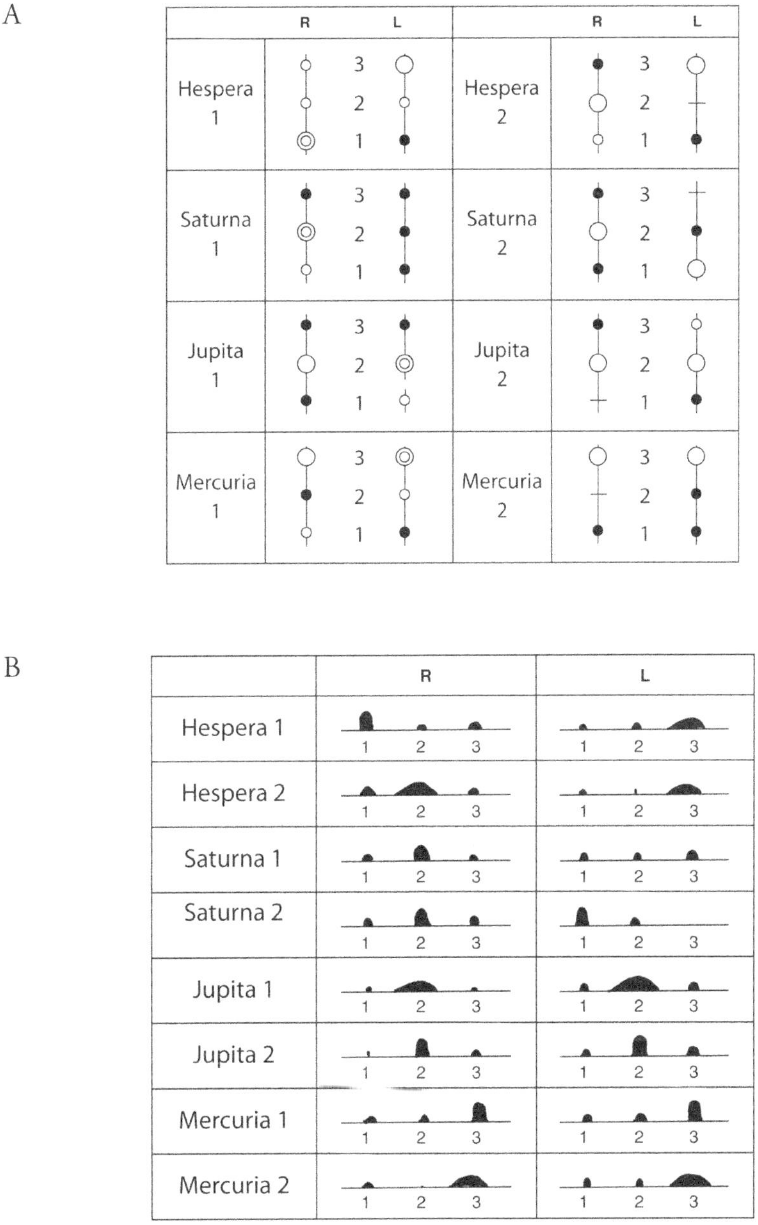

A

	R		L		R		L
Hespera 1		3	○	Hespera 2	●	3	○
		2			○	2	┼
	◎	1	●		○	1	●
Saturna 1	●	3	●	Saturna 2	●	3	┼
	◎	2	●		○	2	●
	○	1	●		●	1	○
Jupita 1	●	3	●	Jupita 2	●	3	○
	○	2	◎		○	2	○
	●	1	○		┼	1	●
Mercuria 1	○	3	◎	Mercuria 2	○	3	○
	●	2	○		┼	2	●
	○	1	●		●	1	●

B

Figure 8.3 The eight KCA pulse patterns[7]

7   Image: Neal White and Elisabeth Waller-White. Based on Lee, M. B., *On Constitution-Acupuncture*. Seoul: New Medical, 1973. Lee's type 1 corresponds to Kuon's Fu constitutions; thus Hespero 1 for Lee is the same as Hespera for Kuon. The pulse positions 1, 2, and 3 represent index, middle, and ring fingers respectively. These two ways of showing the pulse images makes the information somewhat clearer. The differences in Lee's representation from Kuon's is most notable in the Greater Yin and Lesser Yin types. Kuon's Jupita pulses are felt on the proximal part of the middle finger, while his Jupito pulses are felt on the distal part of the middle finger. Kuon's Mercuria pulses are felt on the distal part of the ring finger, and his Mercurio pulses are felt on the proximal part of the ring finger.

Kuon described these eight constitutions as being characterized by the following cardinal imbalances:

Strong Large Intestine	Hespera	(Greater Yang–1)
Weak Liver	Hespero	(Greater Yang–2)
Strong Stomach	Saturna	(Lesser Yang–1)
Weak Kidney	Saturno	(Lesser Yang–2)
Weak Large Intestine	Jupita	(Greater Yin–1)
Strong Liver	Jupito	(Greater Yin–2)
Weak Stomach	Mercuria	(Lesser Yin–1)
Strong Kidney	Mercurio	(Lesser Yin–2)

There are several further points that Kuon emphasized. These constitutional imbalances exist even in the healthy individual. What occurs in the development of an illness is that the normally strong Organ becomes not just strong, but Excessive, or the normally weak Organ becomes not just weak, but Deficient. Thus the goal of treatment is to return the constitutional Organ to its premorbid state, which will still be either stronger or weaker than the other Organs, depending on the constitution. For each of these eight types, Kuon also determined the relative strengths of the non-constitutional Organs, which explained the choice of treatment points for each constitution. For example, the energetic state of the Lesser Yang Saturno constitution is illustrated in Figure 8.4.

Kuon initially used only Sa Am's Four Needle technique for Tonification or Sedation (Fundamental Formula) as his treatment, but later appended an Auxiliary Formula to direct the effect of treatment towards a specific pathomechanism.[8] These Auxiliary Formulae will be described below. While Kuon used the pulse as his ultimate criterion for determining the constitution, he did recognize that morphological and psychophysiological characteristics could be helpful as well. One of the most important of these was the observation that individuals with Zang constitutions tended to develop symptoms mainly on their left sides, and they were most effectively treated on their "healthy" right

---

8   See Kuon Dowon, 1973 and Lee, 1973, in the References.

sides. Conversely, individuals of Fu constitutions tended to develop symptoms mainly on their right sides, and were most effectively treated on their "healthy" left sides. Since Zang/Fu and left/right are examples of Yin/Yang dualities, such a finding is not surprising.[9] His thorough integration of Five Element and Yin/Yang analysis is undoubtedly part of what makes Kuon's work so appealing to me, in my search for a unified understanding of Oriental medicine.

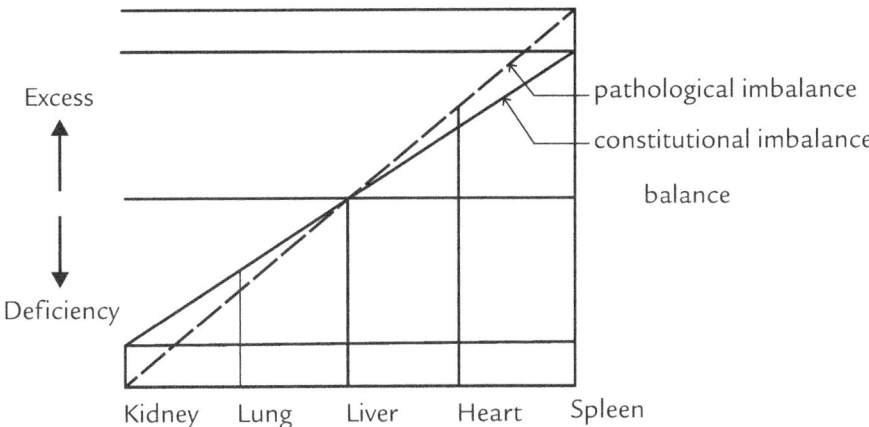

Figure 8.4 Organ states in the Saturno constitution[10]

---

9   Opposite side needling is found in many acupuncture traditions, and is mentioned in *Suwen* 4 (and 20): "a capable acupuncturist…will know how to needle the right side for treatment of disease on the left side, and how to needle the left side for disease on the right side." The only attempt at formulating a physiological rationale for this, of which I am aware, was proposed by Yoo Tae Woo, and I have adapted it as follows: Most physical symptoms are connected to the opposite side of the brain by the crossing (decussation) of sensory and motor nerve tracts from left to right and vice versa. The brain function itself is regulated by its blood flow distribution, which is governed by the balance between the carotid and vertebral arteries (supplying the anterior and posterior parts of the brain respectively). Yoo chose the radial artery as a surrogate for the vertebral artery, because they share a common origin, and the vertebral artery is not itself accessible for palpation. When we compare radial and carotid arteries, we are evaluating the health of the brain's functions on that side of the body, which is opposite to the side of the body that it senses and controls. Yoo also determined that needling one side of the body influenced the radial/carotid ratio on the same (needled) side (and therefore the brain on the same side), which would impact symptoms on the opposite side of the body. My own addition to this line of speculation is that the influence on radial/carotid flow is ipsilateral to the side needled because the acupunctural effect is not a result of conventionally described neurological functions, but is carried by a different mechanism (perhaps direct currents or potential differences), which do not decussate, or cross sides, as they are transmitted to the vascular network and ultimately to the brain. In summary then, left side treatment affects the left side radial/carotid balance, which in turn affects the right side of the body.

10   Eckman, P., "Korean Acupuncture." *Trad. Ac. Soc. J.* (UK), 7, 1990, pp.1–6. Although Figure 8.4 shows the Liver as being balanced, which was Kuon's original hypothesis, he later developed treatment protocols that included Tonification of the Liver for certain maladies of Saturno individuals. This revision agrees with my own experience, that each of the Elements in any constitution will tend either towards Excess or Deficiency, albeit to different degrees. The description of these inherent Elemental tendencies can be found in Chapter 10.

Before going into more detail about Kuon's methodology, I should describe how his constitutional pulse is palpated. The position of the fingers on the radial artery is similar to that used in the other constitutional pulse exams. The index, middle, and ring fingers are adjoined, and positioned ulnar to the flexor pollicis tendon. Kuon's method of pulse taking involves pressing down on the radial artery with all three fingertips, while pulling the flexor tendon over the radial artery, and then compressing the artery with the *pads* of the fingers until the pulse is completely obliterated.[11] The constitutional pulse is the first pattern felt as the pressure is evenly released on all three fingers. This must be carried out on both left and right radial arteries in order to arrive at the correct constitutional pattern. I have found that the results are more reliable if the pads of the fingers close to their tips press straight down on the flexor tendon, while the pulse is felt with the part of the finger that is just a bit more proximal. Skill in determining this pulse is not easy to acquire, so repeated practice is a necessity, but it becomes easier to feel if one already has some information about the Sasang diagnosis and/or the Ayurvedic diagnosis, as each determination limits the remaining possibilities.

Because Sa Am's Four Needle technique for Tonification or Sedation was the treatment method originally advocated by Kuon for the Fundamental Formulae, the specific rules for Point selection in this protocol are reviewed as follows (making use of the Five Element Creation (Sheng) and Control (Ke) cycles): To Tonify a Deficient Meridian, its Mother Meridian is Tonified at its own Element Point, and this same Element Point is Tonified on the Deficient Meridian. In addition, the Controlling Meridian's own Element Point is Sedated, as is this Element Point on the Deficient Meridian. Tonification and Sedation are accomplished by puncturing either with or against the direction of the Meridian flow respectively, at an angle of 45 degrees. An analogous protocol is used to Sedate Excess Meridians: The own Element Point on the Son Meridian is Sedated, as is the same Element Point on the Excess Meridian, and in addition the own Element Point on the Controlling Meridian is Tonified, as is this Element Point on the Excess Meridian. These simple rules do not necessarily hold for the Auxiliary Formulae, whose Point selection depends on the relative strengths and weaknesses of the other (non-constitutional) Organs and Elements. The rationale for Kuon's choice of Points in these Formulae can be appreciated by studying these strengths and weaknesses, but the structure of each Formula still comprises four needles and employs both Mother-Son

---

11   The crucial difference between the SCM pulse and the KCA pulse is that the former is felt with the tips of the fingers pressing straight down, while the latter is felt with the pads of the fingers, pulling radially at the same time as they are pushing down towards the bone. I try to feel this pulse with the segment of my distal phalanx that is just distal to the DIP (distal inter-phalangeal) joint, which is actually proximal to the finger pad.

and Controller-Controlled dynamics.[12] The classical Four Needle technique was chosen as the Fundamental formula for each constitution by Kuon in his initial paper; however, he later revised the choice of Points for the Fundamental Formula in some of the constitutional types, presumably based on clinical responses.

Kuon's only other publication giving specific details about constitutional acupuncture was in 1973.[13] In this paper he introduced the concept of Auxiliary treatments of the Meridians in fixed relationships to the constitutional Meridian, which could specifically treat problems that Kuon called issues of Zang inflammation (e.g. hepatitis, carditis, pancreatitis, pneumonitis, nephritis, arthritis, and osteomyelitis), Fu inflammation (e.g. cholecystitis, ileitis, gastritis, colitis, cystitis, skin diseases, vasculitis, gynecological problems, ENT diseases, and epilepsy), devitalization (e.g. senile atrophic changes, hypotonia, ptosis, and neuralgia), infection (initially limited to bacterial diseases, but possibly also effective for viral and other pathogens), paralysis (e.g. stroke, Bell's palsy, and polio), and neuropsychology (e.g. all neurological and psychiatric diseases except epilepsy, and all abnormalities of autonomic nerve function, such as certain cases of asthma).[14] All of these Auxiliary Formulae were to be preceded by the Fundamental Formula for the constitution of the individual (Table 8.1).[15] This model is one in which the constitutional Meridian/Organ is at the center of a constellation of related functions whereby, for instance, the Stomach could be the Organ that controls infections in one constitution, revitalizes asthenic conditions in another constitution, and is itself the origin of all imbalances in yet a third constitution.

Figure 8.5 illustrates the constellational relationships in Kuon's original choice of Auxiliary Formulae. The circle on the left represents the cycle of the Five Elements for a patient with a Zang (Yin Organ) constitution, while that on the right represents the cycle for a patient with a Fu (Yang Organ) constitution. The Element treated is arbitrarily situated at the bottom, and all the Organs to be treated by the Auxiliary Formulae are automatically determined by their Five Element relationships. The Yin Organs are given female gender designations (Sister, Grandmother, Granddaughter), while the Yang Organs are considered male (Brother, Grandfather, Grandson). The only Auxiliary

---

12 This rule holds for all Auxiliary Formulae except the Psyche Formulae. Kuon's rationale for choosing Points in the Psyche Formulae remains obscure, and may be purely empirical.

13 Kuon Dowon, 1973.

14 Kuon's original terminology for the Auxiliary Formulae have been editorially altered, as have many of his other choices of nomenclature, for purposes of clarity.

15 Kuon's treatment style involves repetitive in and out shallow needling of all the Points in a fixed sequence, a specific number of times. The whole treatment rarely takes more than a couple of minutes, but he initially treats as often as daily. Other practitioners have found it equally effective to simply retain all the needles for 20 minutes.

Formulae not included in the diagram are the Psyche Formulae; they represent the integration of the Fire Element into what was originally a Four Element, or Sasang, model. Kuon's constellational view of the relativity of the roles of the different Organs/Meridians in each constitution, which he characterized as a field theory, is conceptually an enormous departure from the thinking in any of the other traditions of Oriental medicine of which I am aware, and strikes me as an insight that may eventually lead to a paradigm shift in Oriental medicine itself. I do believe that, in a subtle way, this "constellational" approach was presaged in the *Nanjing*, Chapter 50, where heart disease is used as an illustration of how similar pathology can arise from disturbances in any of the Five Elements. Curiously, Kuon cited the *Nanjing* in his 1973 paper, but referenced only Chapters 69 and 75, which detail fundamental aspects of Five Element treatment theory.

Zang Constitution: Treat		*Formula*		*Treat: Fu Constitution*	
(Se)	Self	– Fundamental	(Fun)	– Self	(Se)
(GM)	Grandmother	– Zang Inflammation	(Z)	– Grandfather	(GF)
(GD)	Grand-daughter	– Fu Inflammation	(F)	– Grandson	(GS)
(GF)	Grandfather	– Vitalisation	(V)	– Grandmother	(GM)
(GS)	Grandson	– Antibiotic	(B)	– Grand-daughter	(GD)
(Br)	Brother	– Anti-paralytic	(P)	– Sister	(Si)

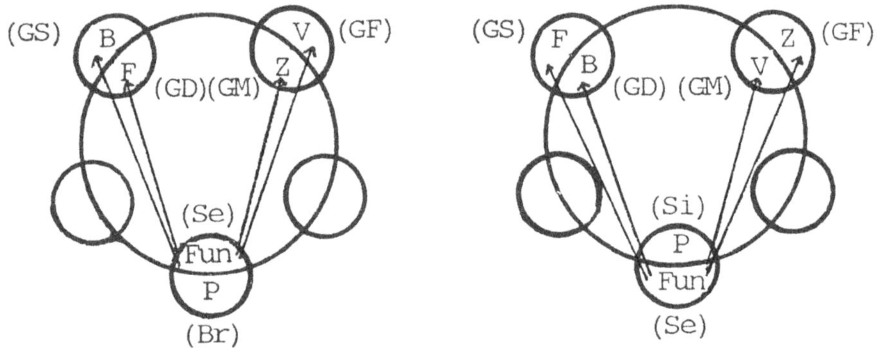

Figure 8.5 Constellations for Zang and Fu constitutions[16]

The observant reader, in studying Table 8.1, will quickly realize that, although the basic form of the Four Needle technique is maintained in all Formulae (except the Psyche Formulae), Kuon has taken some liberties with the dogma for Tonification and Sedation. Sometimes he uses the Son Point rather than the Mother Point for Tonification, and sometimes he uses the Mother Point rather than the Son Point for Sedation. Likewise, his use of the Grandmother and Grandson Points do not always follow Sa Am's rules for Tonification and

---

16   Eckman, 1990.

Sedation. Actually, Sa Am himself posited some of these variant prescriptions as methods for Cooling or Heating, rather than Tonifying or Sedating, so what Kuon has been experimenting with is entirely within traditional approaches to the Five Elements. Although Kuon has not published any further instructional material in English, he has taught some of his newer material to Korean practitioners in a public forum, and in Table 8.2, I have shown some of the changes in Nomenclature and Formulae, as I understand them, which illustrate the way his thinking has been evolving.[17] In my experience, there are some patients who respond better to the original Formulae, and others who respond better to the newer Formulae. I believe this reflects subtypes within the constitutions, but that is a subject for later exploration.

---

17 Several Korean commentators also have noted that Kuon's Fundamental Formulae for individuals with a Fu constitution are now what I've labeled as the Paralysis Formulae in Table 8.2, confirmed by Kuon Wujon's website: www.ecmed.org. In the next chapter I will present a table that shows these former Paralysis Formulae as the new Fundamental Formulae.

Table 8.1 Kuon's original Constitutional Formulae (1973)[a]

	Fundamental	Zang	Fu	Vitality	Infection	Paralysis	Psyche
LI+	UB 66, LI 2-	UB 66, SI 2-	LI 1, GB 44-	KI 10, HE 3-	LU 8, LV 4-	KI 10, LU 5-	SI 1-
	SI 5, LI 5+	GB 41, SI 3+	SI 5, GB 38+	LV 1, HE 9+	HE 8, LV 2+	HE 8, LU 10+	SI 3+
LV-	LU 8, LV 4-	SP 3, LU 9-	LU 8, SP 5-	ST 36, LI 11-	LI 1, ST 45-	LI 1, GB 44-	PE 7-
	KI 10, LV 8+	LV 1, LU 11+	KI 10, SP 9+	GB 41, LI 3+	UB 66, ST 44+	UB 66, GB 43+	PE 3+
ST+	LI 1, ST 45-	LI 1, GB 44-	ST 36, UB 40-	LU 8, LV 4-	SP 3, KI 3-	LU 8, SP 5-	TH 1-
	GB 41, ST 43+	UB 66, GB 43+	GB 41, UB 65+	KI 10, LV 8+	LV 1, KI 1+	LV 3, SP 3+	TH 3+
KI-	SP 3, KI 3-	HE 8, SP 2-	SP 3, HE 7-	SI 5, ST 41-	ST 36, SI 8-	ST 36, UB 40-	HE 7-
	LU 8, KI 7+	KI 10, SP 9+	LU 8, HE 4+	UB 66, ST 44+	LI 1, SI 1+	LI 1, UB 67+	HE 3+
LI-	ST 36, LI 11+	LI 1, SI 1+	ST 36, GB 34+	LU 8, HE 4+	SP 3, LV 3+	SP 3, LU 9+	SI 1+
	SI 5, LI 5-	GB 41, SI 3-	SI 5, GB 38-	LV 1, HE 9-	HE 8, LV 2-	HE 8, LU 10-	SI 3-
LV+	LU 8, LV 4+	SP 3, LU 9+	LU 8, SP 5+	ST 36, LI 11+	LI 1, ST 45+	LI 1, GB 44+	PE 7+
	HE 8, LV 2-	LV 1, LU 11-	LV 1, SP 1-	SI 5, LI 5-	GB 41, ST 43-	SI 5, GB 38-	PE 3-
ST-	SI 5, ST 41+	ST 36, GB 34+	SI 5, UB 60+	SP 3, LV 3+	HE 8, KI 2+	HE 8, SP 2+	TH 1+
	GB 41, ST 43-	UB 66, GB 43-	GB 41, UB 65-	KI 10, LV 8-	LV 1, KI 1-	LV 3, SP 3-	TH 3-
KI+	SP 3, KI 3+	HE 8, SP 2+	SP 3, HE 7+	SI 5, ST 41+	ST 36, SI 8+	ST 36, UB 40+	HE 7+
	LV 1, KI 1-	LV 1, SP 1-	KI 10, HE 3-	GB 41, ST 43-	UB 66, SI 2-	GB 41, UB 65-	HE 3-

a I have taken the liberty of translating Kuon's nomenclature for the Points into their corresponding designations by Organ system and Point number familiar to the broader acupuncture profession. It should be noted that Kuon uses his own nomenclature because he does not accept all aspects of traditional teachings, and indeed has developed his system based on an entirely novel perspective described in detail in *Pyrologos: A New Theory of Life and the Universe*. IMKS Occasional Paper No. 1, Yonsei University Press, 2002, first enunciated in 1983.

Table 8.2 Kuon's revised Constitutional Formulae

	Fundamental	Zang	Fu	Vitality	Infection	Paralysis	Psyche
Colonotonia (LI+)	UB 66, LI 2-	KI 10, HE 3-	LU 8, LV 4-	UB 66, SI 2-	LI 1, GB 44-	KI 10, LU 5-	SI 1-
	GB 41, LI 3+	LV 1, HE 9+	HE 8, LV 2+	GB 41, SI 3+	SI 5, GB 38+	LV 1, LU 11+	SI 3+
Pulmotonia (LV-)	LU 8, LV 4-	SP 3, LU 9-	LU 8, SP 5-	ST 36, LI 11-	LI 1, ST 45-	LI 1, GB 44-	PE 7-
	KI 10, LV 8+	LV 1, LU 11+	KI 10, SP 9+	GB 41, LI 3+	UB 66, ST 44+	UB 66, GB 43+	PE 3+
Gastrotonia (ST+)	LI 1, ST 45-	LU 8, LV 4-	SP 3, KI 3-	LI 1, GB 44-	ST 36, UB 40-	LU 8, SP 5-	TH 1-
	UB 66, ST 44+	KI 10, LV 8+	LV 1, KI 1+	UB 66, GB 43+	GB 41, UB 65+	KI 10, SP 9+	TH 3+
Pancreatonia (KI-)	SP 3, KI 3-	HE 8, SP 2-	SP 3, HE 7-	SI 5, ST 41-	ST 36, SI 8-	ST 36, UB 40-	HE 7-
	LU 8, KI 7+	KI 10, SP 9+	LU 8, HE 4+	UB 66, ST 44+	LI 1, SI 1+	LI 1, UB 67+	HE 3+
Cholecystonia (LI-)	UB 66, LI 2+	KI 10, HE 3+	LU 8, LV 4+	UB 66, SI 2+	LI 1, GB 44+	KI 10, LU 5+	SI 1+
	GB 41, LI 3-	LV 1, HE 9-	HE 8, LV 2-	GB 41, SI 3-	SI 5, GB 38-	LV 1, LU 11-	SI 3-
Hepatonia (LV+)	LU 8, LV 4+	SP 3, LU 9+	LU 8, SP 5+	ST 36, LI 11+	LI 1, ST 45+	LI 1, GB 44+	PE 7+
	KI 10, LV 8-	LV 1, LU 11-	KI 10, SP 9-	GB 41, LI 3-	UB 66, ST 44-	UB 66, GB 43-	PE 3-
Vesicotonia (ST-)	LI 1, ST 45+	LU 8, LV 4+	SP 3, KI 3+	LI 1, GB 44+	ST 36, UB 54+	LU 8, SP 5+	TH 1+
	UB 66, ST 44-	KI 10, LV 8-	LV 1, KI 1-	UB 66, GB 43-	GB 41, UB 65-	KI 10, SP 9-	TH 3-
Renotonia (KI+)	SP 3, KI 3+	HE 8, SP 2+	SP 3, HE 7+	SI 5, ST 41+	ST 36, SI 8+	ST 36, UB 40+	HE 7+
	LU 8, KI 7-	LV 1, SP 1-	KI 10, HE 3-	GB 41, ST 43-	LI 1, SI 1-	LI 1, UB 67-	HE 3-

There have been many further developments in Kuon's approach that I am not at liberty to discuss yet, so it would not be fair to characterize Table 8.2 as representing his current methodology, but rather as an intermediate stage of his treatment style. I have chosen to present the material in Table 8.2 so that the reader will at least be able to follow the logic of the treatments that appear in some of my case histories in Chapter 19.

In 1973 one of Kuon's disciples, Myung-Bok Lee M.D., who was a professor of anatomy at the College of Medicine of Seoul National University, published a paper (privately) in which he listed the harmful and beneficial foods for each of the eight constitutional types, material which he had learned from Kuon. I interviewed him on a visit to Korea, and discovered that while he did not practice acupuncture (although he detailed the Fundamental and Auxiliary Formulae in his 1973 paper), he used these food recommendations, based on Kuon's constitutional pulse diagnostic method, as the sole basis for a successful practice. Kuon subsequently published a collaborative paper in which he used Western medical laboratory results to confirm the dietary aspect of Eight Constitutions Medicine.[18] Although these dietary instructions were never published by Kuon (in English), the following material from Lee's paper is included to allow practitioners interested in KCA to incorporate this aspect of therapy and to confirm the accuracy of KCA teachings:[19]

Large Intestine Excess (Hespera)

Harmful foods: wheat, millet, beans, beef, pork, other meats, coffee, butter, sugar, pear, watermelon, walnut, pine nut, chestnut, ginko nut, platycodon, lotus root, radish, garlic, red pepper, alcohol.

Beneficial foods: buckwheat, rice, shellfish, fish, cabbage, lettuce, potato, seaweed, grape, orange, mustard.

Liver Deficiency (Hespero)

Harmful foods: wheat, millet, beans, beef, chicken, milk, coffee, butter, sugar, pear, watermelon, walnut, pine nut, chestnut, ginko nut, sesame seed, sesame oil, platycodon, lotus root, radish, garlic, red pepper, alcohol.

Beneficial foods: rice, non-glutinous millet, buckwheat, red bean, shellfish, fish, cabbage, lettuce, grape, banana, cherry, Chinese quince.

---

18 Kim, S. H. *et al.*, "A Comparison of Nutritional Status Among Eight Constitutional Groups in Relation to Food Preference on the View Point of Constitutional Medicine." *Korean Nutrition Society Journal*, 18, 1985, pp.155–166. Kuon Dowon's son, Kuon Wujon, has more recently provided an expanded version of his father's dietary guidelines and lots of other information about ECM at www. ecmed.org.

19 Essentially similar diets can be found on Puramo's website, www.puramo.com, as this information is now pretty standard among Sasang practitioners in Korea.

Stomach Excess (Saturna)

Harmful foods: glutinous rice, glutinous millet, chicken, venison, sheep's milk, potato, sweet potato, sesame seed, sesame oil, honey, apple, orange, alcohol.

Beneficial foods: rice, red bean, green bean, barley, cabbage, cucumber, pork, egg, oyster, squid, shrimp, lobster, crab, herring, melon, strawberry, persimmon, ice.

Kidney Deficiency (Saturno)

Harmful foods: glutinous rice, glutinous millet, chicken, venison, sheep's milk, potato, sesame seed, sesame oil, mustard, honey, apple, orange, alcohol.

Beneficial foods: rice, red bean, green bean, barley, cabbage, cucumber, pork, beef, egg, oyster, squid, shrimp, lobster, herring, melon, strawberry, persimmon, pear.

Large Intestine Deficiency (Jupita)

Harmful foods: alcohol, buckwheat, shellfish, grape, cherry.

Beneficial foods: rice, beans, wheat, millet, tofu, beef, milk, egg, radish, platycodon, lotus root, pear, watermelon, walnut, sugar, miso, garlic.

Liver Excess (Jupito)

Harmful foods: alcohol, buckwheat, shellfish, grape, cherry.

Beneficial foods: rice, beans, wheat, millet, tofu, beef, milk, egg, radish, platycodon, lotus root, chestnut, pine nut, ginko nut, watermelon, sugar, miso, garlic.

Stomach Deficiency (Mercuria)

Harmful foods: barley, red bean, pork, melon, cucumber, oyster, shrimp, crab, squid, beer, ice.

Beneficial foods: glutinous rice, glutinous millet, sheep's milk, potato, carrot, radish, venison, beef, sesame oil, ginger, garlic, black pepper, mustard, tomato, peach, orange, honey.

Kidney Excess (Mercurio)

Harmful foods: barley, red bean, green bean, wheat, pork, egg, melon, cucumber, banana, strawberry, oyster, lobster, shrimp, crab, squid, beer, ice.

Beneficial foods: glutinous rice, glutinous millet, potato, carrot, radish, spinach, chicken, venison, sesame oil, ginger, black pepper, mustard, peach, apple, honey.

In spite of the fact that Kuon's treatment style has evolved over the years, and his nomenclature has changed, his basic methodology has remained true to his original vision. When I've visited him in clinic, I've seen the use of complex combinations of Auxiliary treatments, but they always center around the constitutional typology. He has seen countless thousands of patients, and his methodology has evolved to reflect the choice of Points and Auxiliary Formulae that give the best results. I cannot say much more about Kuon's methods, other than to mention that he presently specializes in using constitutional acupuncture to treat cancer, and has had some remarkable successes with supposedly incurable cases. He also participates in Western medical research aimed at elucidating the biochemical changes that occur in these cancer patients who receive constitutional acupuncture treatment.[20]

Having lauded Kuon's methodology, I should also point out that, as his approach is in a continual state of evolution, one can imagine that his treatments are not always successful, an observation that I could make equally well regarding any of the masterful teachers under whom I have studied. I do not believe that anyone has yet discovered an infallible system of diagnosis or treatment, certainly myself included. This should be kept in mind when I propose an alternate interpretation of the meaning of Kuon's eight pulse types, but first the intervening steps that led me in that direction should be described.

---

20 In 2003, Kuon collaborated on a paper titled "Therapeutic Monitoring on Urinary Nucleoside and Polyamine Levels of Cancer Patients by Capillary Electrophoresis and Gas Chromatography under Acupuncture Treatment," published in the *Proceedings of the Convention of the Pharmaceutical Society of Korea*. In this study, Kuon diagnosed and treated the patients by ECM acupuncture. The results showed that the abnormal urinary levels of 14 nucleosides and 9 polyamines were markedly decreased after two treatments, and had returned to the normal range. In a personal communication to me about this study in 2006, Kuon explained that this was the first type of intervention that had returned the nucleoside markers to normal in cancer treatment. Even surgical removal of cancers or chemotherapy, which returned other markers such as alpha-fetoprotein to normal, did not influence the abnormal nucleoside levels. Kuon's interpretation of these results was that constitutional acupuncture not only caused the cancers to regress, but also suggested that it would also reduce the recurrence rate, because it was acting at the causal level. For further information on the use of ECM in treating cancer, contact the Dawnting Cancer Research Institute, 236–378, Shindang-dong, Chung-ku, 100–823, Seoul, Korea. A complete listing of Kuon's English language publications can be found in the bibliography, including a brief theoretical overview that he published in 2011 at the age of 90!

CHAPTER 9

EXPANDING SCM (THE 16 CONSTITUTIONS HYPOTHESIS)

In 2004, I began corresponding with a highly respected practitioner of SCM, Puramo Chong,[1] and discovered that his personal model of constitutional typology, while following Lee Je-Ma's theory, discerned 16 different constitutions, four in each Sang. Chong, a Korean Oriental Medical Doctor (OMD), had originally learned about constitutional acupuncture from Lee Dong Woong,[2] a former banker who had been inspired by the work of Lee Je-Ma and Kuon Dowon. The 16 type model was Lee Dong Woong's idea, but Chong developed a rationale for it based on the differences in body shape, physiology, and temperament in members of the same Sang, attributing them to differences in the physical size of the associated organs. Initially, the four Sang were divided into eight, based on their Hot or Cold tendencies. This produced very similar results to Kuon's typology,[3] but only dealt with imbalances of the Zang Organs. Thus instead of naming the two forms of Greater Yang as Liver Deficiency and Large Intestine Excess, Lee classified them as Liver Deficiency

---

1   That's his "style name." He is Dr. Woncho Chong.

2   Lee Dong Woong wrote two books that have not been translated into English yet. They are: *Physical Constitution by Yin-Yang Theory*. Seoul, 1999, and *Acupuncture by Constitution Medicine*. Seoul, 2002 (personal communication from acupuncturist David Lee, 2013).

3   Not surprising, as Lee took his inspiration from Kuon's published work.

and Lung Excess.[4] This may appear to be a trivial distinction, but it actually is not, because the Large Intestine is part of the Kidney system in SCM, and therefore does not readily fit a Greater Yang classification. In this model, Lung Excess is a Hot type of Greater Yang, while Liver Deficiency is a Cold type of Greater Yang.[5] The model which Lee and Chong used further divided these into four subtypes: Hot, Warm, Cool, and Cold. This type of analysis is much easier to correlate with Sasang herbal medicine, which deals with illnesses of each Sang on the basis of such thermal distinctions. The 16 types are shown in Table 9.1.

Morphologically, the types were distinguished by associating the Hot types with a tendency towards obesity and the Cold types with a tendency towards skinniness, with the other types in between. Since the same Organ imbalances showed up in different Sang (Liver Excess is in both Greater Yin and Lesser Yin, for example), Chong used different modifications of the Four Needle technique to treat them. His website gives a comprehensive rationale for these treatments, and an as yet unpublished manuscript of his delineates the specific acupuncture Point prescriptions he uses.[6]

While I am very impressed with this theoretical approach (and I must say that Puramo's results were equally impressive when I visited his clinic in 2005),[7] there are a number of reasons why I am not completely satisfied with such a model. These include the obvious one of several different constitutions having the same fundamental imbalance, and the asymmetry of constitutions such that the Lung and Kidney have half as many types as the Liver, Spleen, and Heart. In fact, the presence of Heart imbalanced constitutions seems to me to be in direct conflict with Sasang principles. Also, it is difficult for me to believe

---

4   Interestingly, in reports of Kuon's most recent thinking, the Fu constitutions have been reclassified (based on the Fundamental treatment formulae) as their coupled Zang Organ constitutions. Thus, what was originally Large Intestine Excess is now treated as Lung Excess by Kuon, although he still calls it Large Intestine Excess (Colonotonia). Thus Kuon and Lee have apparently arrived at the same conclusion in this regard. Kuon's nomenclature is often confusing. In Table 9.1, I have listed Kuon's most recent ideas merely to show their relationship to SCM typology.

5   In Chong's approach to SCM, the Upper Jiao and Upper Middle Jiao Organs (Lung and Spleen respectively) are hot, and the Lower Middle Jiao and Lower Jiao Organs (Liver and Kidney respectively) are cold. This follows traditional Yin/Yang attributes but is also consistent with Kuon's original finding that Liver and Kidney constitutions benefited by right side treatment, while Stomach and Large Intestine constitutions (which Chong classifies as Spleen and Lung) benefit by left side treatment. Thus Chong treats Hot types on the left side and Cold types on the right side, while Kuon treats Fu types on the left side and Zang types on the right side.

6   P. Chong, personal communication.

7   Chong did explain that there were definitely some cases he encountered where his approach to treatment did not work, even with typically responsive problems like sciatica, shoulder pain, and low back sprain. He attributed this to psychological problems in the patient's life for the most part. This finding is not meant to disparage Chong's clinical skills. Every practitioner I have ever studied under has had similar treatment failures. Personally, however, I do not think the explanation is psychological, but rather reflects the lack of perfection in all "systems" so far developed; thus they are unable to capture the potentially unlimited variability in living organisms.

that there are no constitutions based on the Pericardium (since Ministerial Fire is frequently found to be the CF in FEA), let alone the absence of any Fu constitutions, the presence of which accounted for many of Kuon's successful treatments. Thus I am left with the feeling that the 16 type constitutional model is incomplete, and still needs modification.

Table 9.1 Classification and treatment of the 16 constitutional types

Sasang type	Puramo root[a] treatment	Kuon type	Root treatment
Hot Greater Yang	Lung Excess	Colonotonia	Lung Excess
Warm Greater Yang	Heart Deficiency		
Cool Greater Yang	Spleen Excess		
Cold Greater Yang	Liver Deficiency	Pulmotonia	Liver Deficiency
Hot Greater Yin	Lung Deficiency	Cholecystonia	Lung Deficiency
Warm Greater Yin	Heart Excess		
Cool Greater Yin	Spleen Deficiency		
Cold Greater Yin	Liver Excess	Hepatonia	Liver Excess
Hot Lesser Yang	Spleen Excess	Gastrotonia	Spleen Excess
Warm Lesser Yang	Liver Deficiency		
Cool Lesser Yang	Heart Excess		
Cold Lesser Yang	Kidney Deficiency	Pancreatonia	Kidney Deficiency
Hot Lesser Yin	Spleen Deficiency	Vesicotonia	Spleen Deficiency
Warm Lesser Yin	Liver Excess[b]		
Cool Lesser Yin	Heart Deficiency		
Cold Lesser Yin	Kidney Excess	Renotonia	Kidney Excess

a   I am using the terms Root and Fundamental Formulae synonymously.

b   This Hot, Warm, Cool, and Cold model does not appear to be entirely consistent, because the Heart is not so classifiable in SCM, but also the Warm and Cool types do not always follow their theoretical order, e.g. Warm Lesser Yin is attributed to Liver Excess, which should be a Cool or Cold type of constitution.

CHAPTER 10

A COMPLETE MODEL
THE 24 CONSTITUTIONS

Although I had trouble with some of the theoretical aspects of Chong's approach, I was impressed enough with his clinical results to try and reformulate his work in a way to bring it into greater congruence with Kuon's constellational approach. The first thing I did was to restore the Fu constitutions, recognizing that Kuon's experience validated their existence. As a result, now there were the additional Fu constitutions that are implicit in Chong's analysis, leading to the following list:

Hespera Greater Yang: Large Intestine Excess and Small Intestine Deficiency

Hespero Greater Yang: Liver Deficiency and Spleen Excess

Jupita Greater Yin: Large Intestine Deficiency and Small Intestine Excess

Jupito Greater Yin: Liver Excess and Spleen Deficiency

Saturna Lesser Yang: Stomach Excess and Gall Bladder Deficiency

Saturno Lesser Yang: Kidney Deficiency and Heart Excess

Mercuria Lesser Yin: Stomach Deficiency and Gall Bladder Excess

Mercurio Lesser Yin: Kidney Excess and Heart Deficiency

Looking over this list, it is notable that there are eight Organs/Officials represented, each having an Excess and a Deficient constitution associated. As there are 12 Organs/Officials described in the classics, there are four missing from this list. If each of these four also had an Excess and a Deficient constitutional type, then there would be eight more constitutions and, to distribute them evenly, each of the above pairs should have one more member. If this were so, it would be consistent with Kuon's experience that there are only eight constitutional pulse types, assuming that all three members of each set produced the same constitutional pulse.

Starting from this premise, I considered what the similar characteristics of the Four Sang were, in terms of their Ayurvedic analogs. All the Greater Yang constitutions can be seen to lack Vata in their make-up, and all the Greater Yin constitutions include Vata in their make-up. If this finding reflects an expression of Greater Yang energetics, then the only possibilities for the missing Hespera constitution would be Bladder Excess or Triple Heater Deficiency (both being Pitta/Kapha types). I used two theoretical considerations to choose between them as follows: Both of the Hespera constitutions already identified belong to arm Meridians, but the Saturno and Mercurio constitutions were divided between arm and leg Meridians, so to keep a consistent pattern it would be preferable to pick Bladder Excess in this case. Also, in Kuon's treatment formulae for Greater Yang constitutions, Ministerial Fire is always Sedated, so again it would be preferable to pick Bladder Excess. Notwithstanding these theoretical considerations, I also tried seeing which constitutional treatment gave better results in the clinical setting when someone with a Hespera pulse did not respond to treatments for Large Intestine Excess or Small Intestine Deficiency, and it turned out that Bladder Excess treatments worked better. In a similar fashion Pericardium Excess was identified as the missing Hespero constitution. The missing Greater Yin constitutions are simply their mirror images: Bladder Deficiency for Jupita and Pericardium Deficiency for Jupito.

Using a similar method I analyzed the Lesser Yin constitutions and discovered that they all lacked Pitta in their Ayurvedic make-up, while the Lesser Yang constitutions all included Pitta in their make-up. Applying the same rule of symmetry, the only possibility for Mercuria was Triple Heater Excess, and this again agreed with Kuon's finding that Mercuria types needed Sedation of Ministerial Fire when it required treatment. The missing Mercurio constitution could only be Lung Excess, and finally the missing Saturna constitution must be Triple Heater Deficiency and the missing Saturno constitution must be Lung Deficiency.

These conclusions lead to a constitutional theory with the following characteristics: All the Organs/Officials are represented in both Excess and Deficient possibilities and the existence of the four "Sasang" classifications is maintained, as is the limitation of KCA constitutional pulse types to the eight possibilities empirically discovered. Each of the Sasang groupings shares similar Ayurvedic energetics, and each of the eight pulse types include Meridians on both the upper and lower extremities.

Having arrived at this arrangement of 24 constitutions, divided into eight groups of three similar subtypes, I wondered if there was any simpler way of visualizing these eight groups, especially from a therapeutic perspective. I am indebted to David Lee, another Korean Sasang practitioner, for suggesting an approach that has proven quite useful in my current practice: He surmised that each constitutional type could be classified by which of its Elements were Excessive in tendency, and which were Deficient in tendency. While I have come to different conclusions from David in this regard, his insight was an important stepping stone for me. In applying this concept, I was forced to acknowledge that the Fire Element can't be treated as a single Element, since in some constitutions Imperial Fire (Heart and Small Intestine) tends towards Excess at the same time that Ministerial Fire (Pericardium and Triple Heater) tends towards Deficiency, and vice-versa. Thus for this kind of analysis, one must envision six Elements, rather than five. What I discovered was that each of the eight constitutional subtypes shares the same three Excess and three Deficient Elements, thus creating a rationale for their existence as discrete groups. Recognizing this situation immediately leads to practical choices for acupuncture treatment via allowable variants of the Four Needle technique. The Elemental makeup of these eight distinct types is as follows:

1. Lesser Yang Zang Constitutions (HT+, KI-, LU-) have the Elements of Earth, Imperial Fire, Ministerial Fire in Excess and the Elements of Metal, Water, Wood in Deficiency.

2. Lesser Yang Fu Constitutions (ST+, GB-, TH-) have the Elements of Imperial Fire, Earth, Metal in Excess and the Elements of Water, Wood, Ministerial Fire in Deficiency.

3. Greater Yin Zang Constitutions (LV+, SP-, PE-) have the Elements of Water, Wood, Imperial Fire in Excess and the Elements of Earth, Metal, Ministerial Fire in Deficiency.

4. Greater Yin Fu Constitutions (LI-, SI+, UB-) have the Elements of Wood, Imperial Fire, Ministerial Fire in Excess and the Elements of Earth, Metal, Water in Deficiency.

5. Lesser Yin Zang Constitutions (KI+, HE-, LU+) have the Elements of Metal, Water, Wood in Excess and the Elements of Earth, Imperial Fire, Ministerial Fire in Deficiency.

6. Lesser Yin Fu Constitutions (ST-, GB+, TH+) have the Elements of Water, Wood, Ministerial Fire in Excess and the Elements of Imperial Fire, Earth, Metal in Deficiency.

7. Greater Yang Zang Constitutions (LV-, SP+, PE+) have the Elements of Earth, Metal, Ministerial Fire in Excess and the Elements of Water, Wood, Imperial Fire in Deficiency.

8. Greater Yang Fu Constitutions (LI+, SI-, UB+) have the Elements of Earth, Metal, Water in Excess and the Elements of Wood, Imperial Fire, Ministerial Fire in Deficiency.

Undoubtedly, the various constitutions within each of the above groups will have different orderings within the Excess and Deficient Elements that they share, but that is a subject for future research. This allocation of Elemental assignments, arrived at by clinical observation, is certainly controversial, as it differs from those proposed by Kuon and others. I have found that by using this schema, however, it is possible to construct the most effective Four Needle type combinations to treat any Meridian that is found to be energetically imbalanced, after carrying out a complete pulse diagnosis, as presented in this text. This Elemental distribution of Excess and Deficient Elements within any constitution is the most recent component of my theoretical interpretation of constitutional makeup. The case histories to be presented illustrate all the techniques and interpretations introduced in this text, excepting only this final "inner Elemental makeup," which was recognized only after the case history chapter was already completed. I have added this material on the inner Elemental makeup of the eight constitutional pulse types for several reasons. Not only is it of major importance for a thorough understanding of constitutional pulse diagnosis and treatment formulation, but it also nicely illustrates the evolving nature of my own research.

Looking back, I might compare my theory of Constitutions with Worsley's concept of the Causative Factor (CF). I posit 24 types, while he taught five. At first glance it might seem that these models are worlds apart, but the differences are more apparent than real. The CF is taught as an Elemental issue, while I see the Constitutions as reflecting more specifically the Organs/Officials/Meridians. In the time I spent studying with Worsley, I remember a number of occasions when he described pulse taking as "communicating with the Officials." In particular I remember one patient whose case was either a perfect example of the dictum "the exception that proves the rule," or an instance where Worsley's clinical skills led him to a diagnosis that makes sense in my typology, but not in his own! The patient was a gentleman with color, sound, odor, and emotion all in the same Element, but Worsley claimed it wasn't his CF![1] When we enquired how he could possibly have arrived at such a conclusion, he simply stated, "I asked the Officials." Knowing how adamant he was about not being fooled by symptomatology, the only interpretation I can put on this statement is that it either reflected a psychic level of diagnosis, or he had felt something in the pulse that pointed to a particular Official. Since he had described pulse taking as communicating with the Officials, I prefer to believe that the latter explanation is the correct one, and that in actuality, his notion of the CF was a reflection of a more basic assessment of the Officials. In this light, we may have been in total agreement. Knowing which of the 24 Constitutions is present automatically tells one the CF. Thus rather than replacing the notion of the CF, the "Constitution" expands it and opens up more possibilities for treatment strategies.

There is a certain mathematical symmetry to the Constitutional model that I find compelling.[2] Each Element is represented once, and only once, in each one of the four (Sa) Sang. Conversely, knowing which Sang someone belongs to tells you nothing about their CF. Each one of Kuon's eight pulse types represents three possible Constitutions. Each one of the six Ayurvedic pulse types is specific for no more than two Elements. By themselves, the diagnoses based on two, four, five, six, or eight part systems are partial, whereas the 24 type Constitutional diagnosis is comprehensive, and includes all the others. The list below describes these Constitutions, with all their relationships.

1. *Lung Excess.* This belongs to the Lesser Yin Sang and the Metal Element. The Prakriti pulse is Kapha/Vata and is of Kuon's Mercurio type. The Guan pulse shows ulnar deviation. The combination of a Kapha/Vata Prakriti pulse *and* either a Lesser Yin pulse or a Mercurio pulse is diagnostic. Metal, Water, Wood are in Excess and Earth, Imperial Fire, Ministerial Fire are in Deficiency. (I might point out that while Metal is in Excess, its mother, Earth, is in Deficiency. This finding differs from the Mother-Son law employed by Sa Am in the Four Needle technique, but instead obeys the Sasang dictum that Lesser Yin types are characterized by Deficient Earth and Excess Water Elements. A similar analysis can be made for the ensuing 23 constitutions.)

2. *Lung Deficiency.* This belongs to the Lesser Yang Sang and the Metal Element. The Prakriti pulse is Pitta and is of Kuon's Saturno type. The Guan pulse shows ulnar deviation. The combination of a Pitta Prakriti

---

1   After this many years, I can't recall if the signs were all in Fire, but the CF was in Earth, or the other way around.

2   See Walton's first remark in the dedication. For the purpose of mathematical analysis, the two aspects of the Fire Element, Imperial Fire (Jun Huo—Heart and Small Intestine) and Ministerial Fire (Xiang Huo—Pericardium and Triple Heater), are treated as separate Elements.

pulse *and* either a Lesser Yang pulse or a Saturno pulse is diagnostic. Earth, Imperial Fire, Ministerial Fire are in Excess and Metal, Water, Wood are in Deficiency.

3. *Large Intestine Excess.* This belongs to the Greater Yang Sang and the Metal Element. The Prakriti pulse is Pitta and is of Kuon's Hespera type. The Guan pulse shows radial deviation. Internally generated symptoms tend to be predominantly right sided.[3] The combination of a Pitta Prakriti pulse *and* either a Greater Yang pulse or a Hespera pulse is diagnostic. Earth, Metal, Water are in Excess and Wood, Imperial Fire, Ministerial Fire are in Deficiency.

4. *Large Intestine Deficiency.* This belongs to the Greater Yin Sang and the Metal Element. The Prakriti pulse is Kapha/Vata and is of Kuon's Jupita type. The Guan pulse shows radial deviation. Internally generated symptoms tend to be predominantly right sided. The combination of a Kapha/Vata Prakriti Pulse *and* either a Greater Yin pulse or a Jupita pulse is diagnostic. Wood, Imperial Fire, Ministerial Fire are in Excess and Earth, Metal, Water are in Deficiency.

5. *Stomach Excess.* This belongs to the Lesser Yang Sang and the Earth Element. The Prakriti pulse is Pitta/Vata and is of Kuon's Saturna type. The Guan pulse shows radial deviation. Internally generated symptoms tend to be predominantly right sided. The combination of a Pitta/Vata Prakriti pulse, a radially deviated Guan pulse, *and* either a Saturna pulse or a Lesser Yang pulse is diagnostic. Imperial Fire, Earth, Metal are in Excess and Water, Wood, Ministerial Fire are in Deficiency.

6. *Stomach Deficiency.* This belongs to the Lesser Yin Sang and the Earth Element. The Prakriti pulse is Kapha and is of Kuon's Mercuria type. The Guan pulse shows radial deviation. Internally generated symptoms tend to be predominantly right sided. The combination of a Kapha Prakriti pulse, a radially deviated Guan pulse, *and* either a Mercuria pulse or a Lesser Yin pulse is diagnostic. Water, Wood, Ministerial Fire are in Excess and Imperial Fire, Earth, Metal are in Deficiency.

7. *Spleen Excess.* This belongs to the Greater Yang Sang and the Earth Element. The Prakriti pulse is Kapha and is of Kuon's Hespero type. The Guan pulse shows ulnar deviation. The combination of a Kapha Prakriti pulse, an ulnarly deviated Guan pulse, *and* either a Greater Yang pulse or a Hespero pulse is diagnostic. Earth, Metal, Ministerial Fire are in Excess and Water, Wood, Imperial Fire are in Deficiency.

---

3   By internally generated symptoms I mean to exclude all symptoms related to trauma or surgery, and their sequellae, no matter how long afterwards they make their appearance.

8. *Spleen Deficiency.* This belongs to the Greater Yin Sang and the Earth Element. The constitutional pulse is Pitta/Vata and is of Kuon's Jupito type. The Guan pulse shows ulnar deviation. The combination of a Pitta/Vata Prakriti pulse, an ulnarly deviated Guan pulse, *and* either a Greater Yin pulse or a Jupito pulse is diagnostic. Water, Wood, Imperial Fire are in Excess and Earth, Metal, Ministerial Fire are in Deficiency.

9. *Heart Excess.* This belongs to the Lesser Yang Sang and the Fire Element. The Prakriti pulse is Pitta/Kapha and is of Kuon's Saturno type. The Chi pulse shows ulnar deviation. The combination of a Pitta/Kapha Prakriti pulse *and* either a Lesser Yang pulse or a Saturno pulse is suggestive, but must be confirmed by a pulse at the Cun position on the left wrist that is not biggest at the Fire depth. Earth, Imperial Fire, Ministerial Fire are in Excess and Metal, Water, Wood are in Deficiency.

10. *Heart Deficiency.* This belongs to the Lesser Yin Sang and the Fire Element. The Prakriti pulse is Vata and is of Kuon's Mercurio type. The Chi pulse shows ulnar deviation. The combination of a Vata Prakriti pulse *and* either a Lesser Yin pulse or a Mercurio pulse is suggestive, but must be confirmed by a pulse at the Cun position on the left wrist that is not biggest at the Fire depth. Metal, Water, Wood are in Excess and Earth, Imperial Fire, Ministerial Fire are in Deficiency.

11. *Small Intestine Excess.* This belongs to the Greater Yin Sang and the Fire Element. The Prakriti pulse is Vata and is of Kuon's Jupita type. The Cun pulse shows radial deviation. The combination of a Vata Prakriti pulse *and* either a Greater Yin pulse or a Jupita pulse is suggestive, but must be confirmed by a pulse at the Cun position on the left wrist that is not biggest at the Fire depth. Wood, Imperial Fire, Ministerial Fire are in Excess and Earth, Metal, Water are in Deficiency.

12. *Small Intestine Deficiency.* This belongs to the Greater Yang Sang and the Fire Element. The Prakriti pulse is Pitta/Kapha and is of Kuon's Hespera type. The Cun pulse shows radial deviation. The combination of a Pitta/Kapha Prakriti pulse *and* either a Greater Yang pulse or a Hespera pulse is suggestive, but must be confirmed by a pulse at the Cun position on the left wrist that is not biggest at the Fire depth. Earth, Metal, Water are in Excess and Wood, Imperial Fire, Ministerial Fire are in Deficiency.

13. *Bladder Excess.* This belongs to the Greater Yang Sang and the Water Element. The Prakriti pulse is Pitta/Kapha and is of Kuon's Hespera type. The Cun pulse shows radial deviation. The combination of a Pitta/Kapha Prakriti pulse *and* either a Greater Yang pulse or a Hespera pulse is suggestive, but must be confirmed by a pulse at the Chi position on

the left wrist that is not biggest at the Water depth. Earth, Metal, Water are in Excess and Wood, Imperial Fire, Ministerial Fire are in Deficiency.

14. *Bladder Deficiency.* This belongs to the Greater Yin Sang and the Water Element. The Prakriti pulse is Vata and is of Kuon's Jupita type. The Cun pulse shows radial deviation. The combination of a Vata Prakriti pulse *and* either a Greater Yin pulse or a Jupita pulse is suggestive, but must be confirmed by a pulse at the Chi position on the left wrist that is not biggest at the Water depth. Wood, Imperial Fire, Ministerial Fire are in Excess and Earth, Metal, Water are in Deficiency.

15. *Kidney Excess.* This belongs to the Lesser Yin Sang and the Water Element. The Prakriti pulse is Vata and is of Kuon's Mercurio type. The Chi pulse shows ulnar deviation. Internally generated symptoms tend to be predominantly left sided. The combination of a Vata Prakriti pulse *and* either a Lesser Yin pulse or a Mercurio pulse is suggestive, but must be confirmed by a pulse at the Chi position on the left wrist that is not biggest at the Water depth. Metal, Water, Wood are in Excess and Earth, Imperial Fire, Ministerial Fire are in Deficiency.

16. *Kidney Deficiency.* This belongs to the Lesser Yang Sang and the Water Element. The Prakriti pulse is Pitta/Kapha and is of Kuon's Saturno type. The Chi pulse shows ulnar deviation. Internally generated symptoms tend to be predominantly left sided. The combination of a Pitta/Kapha Prakriti pulse *and* either a Lesser Yang pulse or a Saturno pulse is suggestive, but must be confirmed by a pulse at the Chi position on the left wrist that is not biggest at the Water depth. Earth, Imperial Fire, Ministerial Fire are in Excess and Metal, Water, Wood are in Deficiency.

17. *Pericardium Excess.* This belongs to the Greater Yang Sang and the Fire Element. The Prakriti pulse is Pitta/Kapha and is of Kuon's Hespero type. The Cun pulse shows ulnar deviation. The combination of a Pitta/Kapha Prakriti pulse *and* a Hespero pulse is diagnostic. Earth, Metal, Ministerial Fire are in Excess and Water, Wood, Imperial Fire are in Deficiency.

18. *Pericardium Deficiency.* This belongs to the Greater Yin Sang and the Fire Element. The Prakriti pulse is Vata and is of Kuon's Jupito type. The Cun pulse shows ulnar deviation. The combination of a Vata Prakriti pulse *and* a Jupito pulse is diagnostic. Water, Wood, Imperial Fire are in Excess and Earth, Metal, Ministerial Fire are in Deficiency.

19. *Triple Heater Excess.* This belongs to the Lesser Yin Sang and the Fire Element. The Prakriti pulse is Vata and is of Kuon's Mercuria type. The Chi pulse shows radial deviation. The combination of a Vata Prakriti pulse *and* a Mercuria pulse is diagnostic. Water, Wood, Ministerial Fire are in Excess and Imperial Fire, Earth, Metal are in Deficiency.

20. *Triple Heater Deficiency.* This belongs to the Lesser Yang Sang and the Fire Element. The Prakriti pulse is Pitta/Kapha and is of Kuon's Saturna type. The Chi pulse shows radial deviation. The combination of a Pitta/Kapha Prakriti pulse *and* a Saturna pulse is diagnostic. Imperial Fire, Earth, Metal are in Excess and Water, Wood, Ministerial Fire are in Deficiency.

21. *Gall Bladder Excess.* This belongs to the Lesser Yin Sang and the Wood Element. The Prakriti pulse is Kapha and is of Kuon's Mercuria type. The Chi pulse shows radial deviation. The combination of a Kapha Prakriti pulse, a radially deviated Chi pulse, *and* either a Lesser Yin pulse or a Mercuria pulse is diagnostic. Water, Wood, Ministerial Fire are in Excess and Imperial Fire, Earth, Metal are in Deficiency.

22. *Gall Bladder Deficiency.* This belongs to the Lesser Yang Sang and the Wood Element. The Prakriti pulse is Pitta/Vata and is of Kuon's Saturna type. The Chi pulse shows radial deviation. The combination of a Pitta/Vata Prakriti pulse, a radially deviated Chi pulse, *and* either a Lesser Yang pulse or a Saturna pulse is diagnostic. Imperial Fire, Earth, Metal are in Excess and Water, Wood, Ministerial Fire are in Deficiency.

23. *Liver Excess.* This belongs to the Greater Yin Sang and the Wood Element. The Prakriti pulse is Pitta/Vata and is of Kuon's Jupito type. The Cun pulse shows ulnar deviation. Internally generated symptoms tend to be predominantly left sided. The combination of a Pitta/Vata Prakriti pulse, an ulnarly deviated Cun pulse, *and* either a Greater Yin pulse or a Jupito pulse is diagnostic. Water, Wood, Imperial Fire are in Excess and Earth, Metal, Ministerial Fire are in Deficiency.

24. *Liver Deficiency.* This belongs to the Greater Yang Sang and the Wood Element. The Prakriti pulse is Kapha and is of Kuon's Hespero type. The Cun pulse shows ulnar deviation. Internally generated symptoms tend to be predominantly left sided. The combination of a Kapha Prakriti pulse, an ulnarly deviated Cun pulse, *and* either a Greater Yang pulse or a Hespero pulse is diagnostic. Earth, Metal, Ministerial Fire are in Excess and Water, Wood, Imperial Fire are in Deficiency.

PART TWO

CONDITIONAL PULSE DIAGNOSIS

CHAPTER 11

CAROTID/RADIAL PULSES (YIN/YANG, SIX LEVELS, AND EIGHT EXTRAS)

My introduction to carotid/radial artery pulse diagnosis was via personal instruction by Yoo Tae Woo, the originator of KHA. Although KHA is a modern approach to acupuncture, Yoo is a classically trained practitioner, and incorporated many traditional methods in KHA, including some that appear in the earliest writings, but are no longer included in other "traditional" styles such as TCM. The primary method of pulse diagnosis that he uses is the comparison of the carotid and radial pulses on each side of the body, first described in the *Neijing*.[1] Yoo's interpretation of this pulse finding follows that of the *Neijing* exactly, but he also devised a new method for using these pulses, together with the abdominal sensitivity pattern, to diagnose imbalances of the Eight Extraordinary Meridians. Because it is repeatedly presented in the *Neijing*, I will briefly describe the Six Level diagnostic system based on these pulses, but I have not found this methodology to be sufficiently accurate to be clinically

---

1   *Suwen* 9 and 40, and *Lingshu* 9 and 10.

useful in my own experience.[2] Afterwards, I will describe Yoo's Extraordinary Meridian diagnostic methodology, which I find to be relatively more reliable, and I will also introduce and explain the corroborating techniques I use, which I believe increase its accuracy.

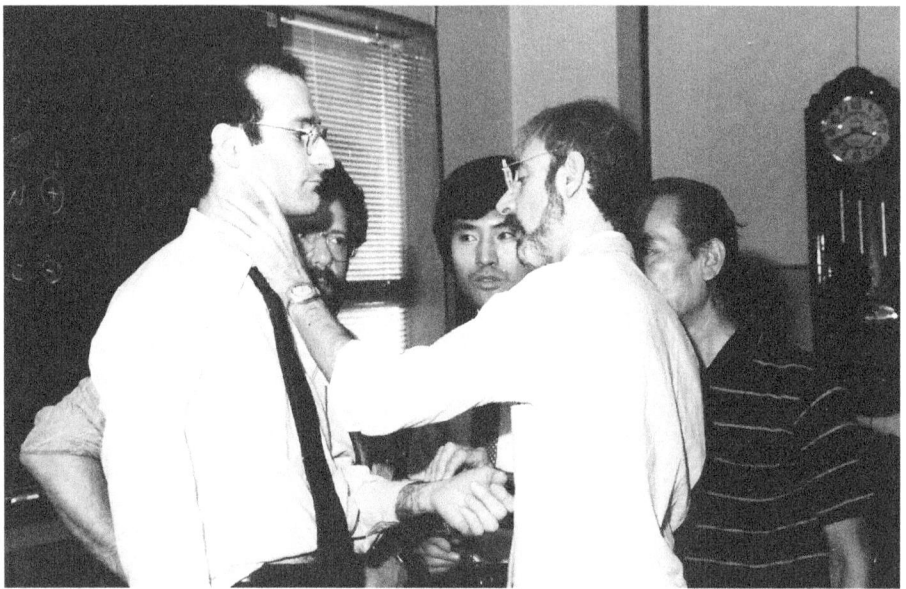

Figure 11.1 The author learning carotid/radial pulse diagnosis from Yoo Tae Woo (center)

Since carotid/radial pulse diagnosis of the Six Levels is given such importance in the *Neijing*, what might possibly explain the difficulty that I and other acupuncturists have found in applying this technique successfully? There is a fair amount of obscurity in the presentation given in *Lingshu* 9. One passage equates the Yang with Xie Qi (Perverse Energy) and the Yin with Zheng Qi (Righteous Energy), and recommends Dispersing the Yang and Tonifying the

---

2   After studying with Yoo, I subsequently studied an alternative carotid/radial pulse diagnostic system practiced by a Japanese school, at a Jingei pulse diagnosis class with Master Ogawa in Tokyo in 1982. The two approaches are quite divergent in their interpretation of the meaning of these pulses, and I should acknowledge that my impression is that Yoo's interpretation, while not completely reliable in my hands, is the more accurate of the two. The difference between these two schools relates specifically to Six Level Meridian diagnosis, as described in the *Neijing*. According to Yoo, a healthy state is reflected in equally large carotid and radial pulses, while the Japanese school teaches that the healthy state is reflected in carotid pulses that are four times as large as the radial pulses. See Van Meter, S., *Jingei Pulse Diagnosis*. Portland, OR: Working Class Acupuncture, 2007, for a published account of this Japanese interpretation. Clearly, these interpretations could not be more antithetical. Both approaches correlate the four times bigger carotid with the Yangming Level, but the Korean interpretation is that this is pathologic, while the Japanese interpretation is that it is physiologically normal. My reading of the *Neijing* clearly supports the Korean view; however, the clinical success claimed by the Japanese school inclines me to be very cautious about applying this diagnostic technique altogether.

Yin. Such an approach could conceivably make sense when the carotid pulse is bigger than the radial pulse, but makes no sense at all if the radial pulse is the larger one. In such a case it is the Yin that should be Dispersed and the Yang Tonified, but why would one ever Tonify Xie Qi? Perhaps scholarly commentaries on this topic by practitioners who have clinical experience with this method will clarify how to use it properly in the future. One possibility that has occurred to me is that this method is designed to identify which of the three major cycles of Qi flow is being adversely affected. A two to one pulse ratio might implicate the Jue Yin/Shao Yang circuit in one of its four component Meridians; similarly, a three to one ratio might implicate the Shao Yin/Tai Yang circuit, and a four to one ratio might implicate the Tai Yin/Yang Ming circuit. My efforts so far have been unable to confirm even this somewhat broader interpretation, and await further study.

A précis of the Six Level diagnosis is as follows:[3] Yoo's main teaching in this regard is that a preponderance of the carotid artery indicates that the imbalance is located in the Yang Meridians,[4] while a preponderance of the radial artery indicates that the imbalance is located in the Yin Meridians. Following the *Neijing*, he assigns specific Meridians as being correlated with different ratios of size between these arteries as follows:[5]

Carotid twice radial—Excess in Shaoyang Meridians or Deficiency in Jueyin

Carotid three times radial—Excess in Taiyang Meridians or Deficiency in Shaoyin

Carotid four times radial—Excess in Yangming Meridians or Deficiency in Taiyin

Radial twice carotid—Excess in Jueyin Meridians or Deficiency in Shaoyang

---

3   This Six Level diagnosis is at the conditional level, in contrast with the SEL diagnostic methodology from the *Maijing* presented in Chapter 6, which is applied to the constitutional diagnosis, in my diagnostic approach. Of course, it is not infrequent that both constitution and condition will point to the same locus of attention in any given situation.

4   Although the imbalance may be diagnosed as being in the Yang Meridians, e.g. Gall Bladder, the treatment Yoo recommends might be either Sedating the Gall Bladder or Tonifying the Liver Meridian. This strategy is explicitly stated in the schema from the *Neijing* to follow, where treatment of both the Yin and Yang coupled Organs of the same Element is recommended for all Six Level rebalancing treatments. I believe what Yoo means by saying bigger carotid pulses imply Yang Meridian imbalances is that the Yang Meridians are in Excess with respect to the Yin Meridians. Almost all of KHA is formulated around the Excess Meridians, as manifested in tender Mo Points, Ah Shi Points, and the diagnostic Points of the "Three Constitutions."

5   Imbalances in one of the two branches of the same Great Meridian can be distinguished by the criteria presented in the *Neijing*: If the bigger pulse is smooth in quality, the imbalance is in the Foot branch. If the bigger pulse has a "bustling" (Zao—Mathews, R. H., *Mathews' Chinese-English Dictionary*. Cambridge, MA: Harvard University Press, 1979, no. 6129) quality, then it is the Arm branch that is imbalanced.

Radial three times carotid—Excess in Shaoyin Meridians or Deficiency in Taiyang

Radial four times carotid—Excess in Taiyin Meridians or Deficiency in Yangming

In KHA, these imbalances are treated as conditions rather than constitutions, and it is not unusual for the ratio to change in the course of treatment, thereby indicating a need to change the focus of further treatment. This approach to Six Level conditional diagnosis remains unreliable in my hands, and so will not appear in the case histories, but I am open to the possibility that my application of the pulse reading techniques, to be described below, is at fault, and I would be glad to hear from readers who have had success with this methodology.

Yoo was the first (to my knowledge) to additionally propose using the carotid/radial (*Jingei* in Japanese) comparison in the diagnosis of imbalances of the Eight Extraordinary Meridians. In his theory, larger carotid pulses indicate an imbalance of a Yang Extraordinary Meridian, while larger radial pulses indicate an imbalance of a Yin Extraordinary Meridian. Yoo's method of determining which of the Yang or Yin Extraordinary Meridians is imbalanced depends on the abdominal discrimination of Yang Excess, Yin Excess, or Kidney Excess presentations according to the following correlations (C = carotid, R = radial):

Yang Excess syndrome, Yang type (C>R) = Yang Qiao Mai

Yang Excess syndrome, Yin type (R>C) = Yin Wei Mai

Yin Excess syndrome, Yang type (C>R) = Dai Mai

Yin Excess syndrome, Yin type (R>C) = Yin Qiao Mai

Kidney Excess syndrome, Yang type (C>R) = Du Mai or Yang Wei Mai

Kidney Excess syndrome, Yin type (R>C) = Ren Mai or Chong Mai

As with all treatment in KHA, Yoo treats Points on the hands alone to address these Extraordinary Meridian imbalances, specifically the Key (Master and Coupled) Points, as they are reflected in the Hand Microsystem. Although this methodology, as taught by Yoo, seems to have exceptions, I suspect that these may be due in general to the inherent imprecision in his method of abdominal diagnosis. It is difficult to always apply an equal degree of pressure at each of the test Points, since individuals differ greatly in how sensitive they are to such palpation, so that light pressure might be needed for one person and quite heavy pressure needed for the next. Also, missing the exact location of the test Points could be another reason for diagnostic error. For these reasons I try to always confirm an Extra Meridian diagnosis by other methods of physical diagnosis. These include making sure that the Dosha corresponding to Yoo's typology is present in the Vikruti pulse and confirming the presence of the *Maijing* pattern of the Extra Meridian radial pulses (which I will describe). One might also employ other methods such as one of the various Japanese approaches taught by Manaka and Matsumoto,[6] and the Chakra correlations taught by Cross,[7] in addition to a judicious application of symptom pictures as presented by Mann[8] and others.

Many teachers have addressed the subject of the diagnosis and treatment of the EEM, but, in addition to Yoo, the most important influences in my own approach have been Jimmy Chang, Jeffrey Yuen, Will Morris, and Felix Mann.[9] I believe that Morris has presented the most useful description (based largely on the *Maijing*) of the pulses of the EEMs and, by adding Yoo's criteria, the diagnosis becomes even clearer. Mann's description of the typical symptomatology of the EEM has been most helpful in cases where there is a choice between Du Mai or Yang Wei Mai for a Yang EEM and Ren Mai or Chong Mai for a Yin EEM. Morris' diagnostic and treatment protocols can be found on his website and listserve, but I will briefly summarize how I use them here. This material is almost identical to what I had previously learned from Chang in a 2006 seminar.

The EEM diagnosis protocol I follow is to first determine if the carotid pulse is larger than the radial pulse (i.e. a Yang EEM) or vice versa (a Yin EEM), and whether this is more pronounced on the left or right side. Then, once knowing whether I am dealing with a Yang or Yin EEM, I can use the following *Maijing* descriptions, which might be expressed on either the Yin or Yang pulses (or both) of Cun, Guan, and Chi, but my clinical experience so far supports the notion that the Yang pulse locations are possibly the more reliable ones to use as the standard. As mentioned in Chapter 6, if the Yang pulses at Cun, Guan, and Chi display a different pattern than is found at the more proximal positions I described for taking the Six Level pulses, then an Extra Meridian problem is a likely finding.[10]

> Du Mai: All three positions (Cun, Guan, and Chi) are felt equally at the superficial or floating (Qi) depth.

> Ren Mai: All three positions are felt equally at the moderate (Blood) depth.

---

6   Manaka, Y., "Extraordinary Meridians." Class notes, San Francisco, 1985, and Matsumoto, K. and Birch, S., *Extraordinary Vessels*. Brookline, MA: Paradigm, 1986.

7   I have also found Cross' associations of specific EEMs with specific Chakras to be of help. These are given in his book, *Acupuncture and the Chakra Energy System*. Berkeley, CA: North Atlantic Books, 2008.

8   Mann, F., *The Meridians of Acupuncture*. London: Heinemann, 1964.

9   Ibid.

10   See Case 33 in Chapter 19.

Chong Mai: All three positions are felt equally at the deep (Jing) level.

Yang Qiao Mai: On first contacting the pulse, only the Cun position can be clearly felt.

Yin Qiao Mai: On first contacting the pulse, only the Chi position can be clearly felt.

Dai Mai: On first contacting the pulse, only the Guan position can be clearly felt.

Yang Wei Mai: The alignment of the pulses shows the distal (Cun) position deviating radially and the proximal position (Chi) deviating ulnarly.

Yin Wei Mai: The alignment of the pulses shows the distal (Cun) position deviating ulnarly and the proximal position (Chi) deviating radially.

Following the logical consequence of equating Vata with Kidney Excess syndrome, Pitta with Yang Excess syndrome, and Kapha with Yin Excess syndrome, it seems evident that when a combination of two Doshas appears on the pulse on one side of the body, then two different Extra Meridians might simultaneously be in need of treatment on the same side of the body. This is only a hypothesis at the present time, but is a departure from Yoo's KHA theory, and my clinical results have not been definitive. I mention it only because I feel it is important to point out areas where "doctrines" might be in need of reinterpretation or modification. For instance, if the Vikruti on the right side is Pitta/Kapha, and the carotid is bigger than the radial on that side, then both the Yang Qiao Mai and the Dai Mai might need treatment on the right side. Of course, it is imperative that other methods of confirmation of the Extra Meridian diagnosis should be employed, and the patient checked after each component of the treatment is in place for signs of clinical improvement. I have used this approach, even adding Manaka style ion-pumping cords (see Figure 11.2) to strengthen the treatment, with some very positive results, as illustrated in the case history chapter.[11]

Morris' and Adams' simple treatment recommendation is to first needle the Opening (Key) Point of the EEM, then to needle the most reactive Ah Shi Point along its pathway, which is an indication of where the Qi is accumulated or stagnant in that Meridian. I have found this to be an effective procedure, but I prefer to Sedate the Opening Point and Tonify the Coupled Point of each chosen EEM with shallow needle insertions, while either applying aluminum and gold plated press pellets on the corresponding KHA Points simultaneously, or attaching Manaka style ion-pumping cords to the needles in order to reinforce their correct polarity. The patient should be checked for a general state

---

11   See Case 27 in Chapter 19.

of relaxation after a few minutes, and the treatment should result in a marked diminution of the initial Vikruti pulse and abdominal sensitivity. Alternatively, KHA needles applied in Tonifying and Sedating directions can be used as the sole treatment, but needling these Points can be more painful than needling body Points because of the presence of more sensory nerve receptors on the fingers than on the rest of the body. A few words of caution: Extraordinary Meridian treatments are very powerful, even when only the two Key Points are treated, and can lead to negative reactions if incorrectly chosen, which is why I recommend using several different diagnostic criteria simultaneously, as well as checking the patient in the first few minutes after treatment is in place, to ascertain that there is a sense of well-being in addition to an improvement in pulses, symptoms, and other signs.

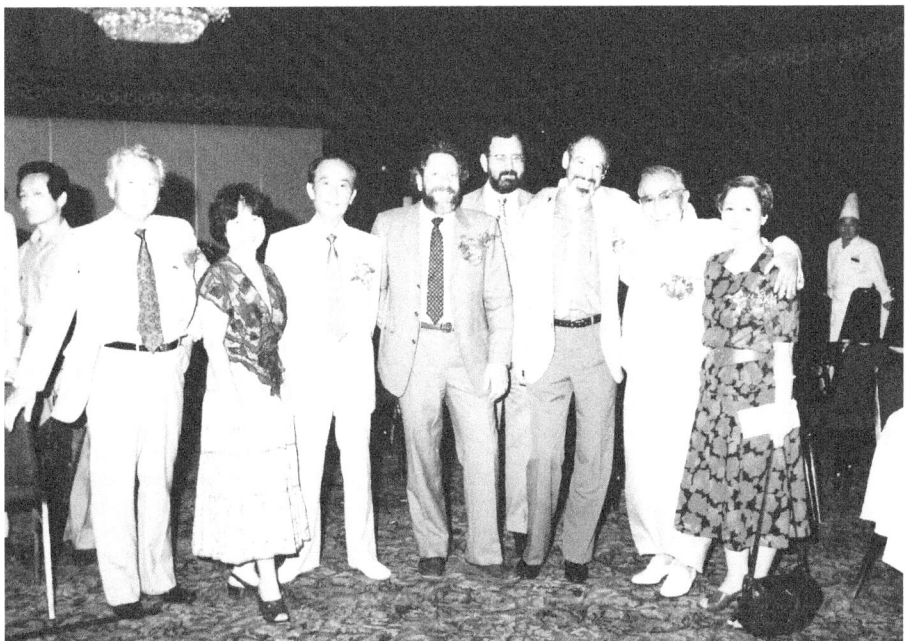

Figure 11.2 The author with Yoshio Manaka (second on the right) in Korea[12]

To reiterate then, I use the carotid/radial size ratio if I suspect there might be an Extraordinary Meridian imbalance present on either side of the body, and I also use these pulses to understand which side of the body is more out of

---

12 Manaka was very influential in the revival of acupuncture in Japan. Although not a member of any of the established traditions, he was respected by all of them. As a Western physician, in addition to being an acupuncturist, he brought a unique point of view to his research and practice. Ion-pumping cords were one of his most well-known innovations, and demonstrate his ability to transcend the limited paradigms of Eastern versus Western medicine. I first met him at a class he taught in San Francisco in 1985 on "The Extraordinary Meridians."

energetic balance. According to Yoo, physical trauma, especially something like a whiplash injury, will frequently lead to an EEM imbalance. Yoo's thinking reflects his idea that the EEMs establish the "grid" or framework around which the Principal Meridians are oriented, and must be correctly balanced in order for these Principal Meridians to properly function. In Chapter 19, I will give some examples of how I incorporate treatment at the EEM level, usually when the imbalances and clinical evolution of the presenting complaints can be clearly traced back to a physical distortion due to trauma or surgery. It is often helpful to start the examination with the carotid/radial comparison, the technique for which I will now describe.

With the patient seated on the side of the exam table, the practitioner compares the size (width) of the neck and wrist arteries separately on each side of the body. The locations of the pulses are at the Points ST 9 (Ren Ying) and LU 9 (Tai Yuan).[13] I usually check the left side first, using my right index finger to feel the pulse at LU 9. Then, using my left thumb, I check the pulse at ST 9, being careful not to keep it compressed more than momentarily. This procedure is then carried out in mirror image symmetry to evaluate the patient's right side pulses. In males, the carotid pulse is felt at the level of the prominence of the Adam's Apple, while in females the ST 9 pulse is felt at the level of the depression between cricoid and thyroid cartilages. In my experience, the most common finding is for patients to have close to even sized pulses on one side, but a definite difference in sizes on the other. I interpret this as indicating that the side with the imbalance is the less healthy side, and that the Extra Meridian system has possibly been activated as a means of compensation; however, the symptoms are more often present on the opposite side. There are numerous references in the classics to treating the opposite side of the body from the symptoms, and Kuon's KCA methodology (see Chapter 8) relies heavily on that approach. I find this to be a useful technique, though not one without exceptions.

Before leaving the discussion of KHA, I'd like to emphasize, once again, that although I've applied Yoo's theories and methodologies as tools in pursuit of information about an individual's constitution, I also use them, as does Yoo himself, to gather information about the individual's present condition. This distinction cannot be repeated too often. As a corollary, in KHA, all treatment is formulated to address the presenting condition. In this way, it is very much like TCM, which treats conditions differentially based on their unique patterns. In my own experience, I have found that even "constitutional systems" get the best results when the treatment chosen is appropriate to the condition. This is true regardless of whether one practices FEA, SCM, KCA, or some other system. As an example, in FEA, it is not enough to know the CF. One must

---

13   LU 9 is at the Yang location of Cun.

also know the strengths and weaknesses of the other Officials if treatments employing transfers are to be used, and the same might be said for the use of any of the "block" clearing protocols, or when making use of the "Spirit of the Point" in choosing an appropriate treatment at any given session. While the focus of Part One of this book was concerned with establishing a more reliable method of constitutional diagnosis, it would be a serious mistake to think that this can be directly translated into the choice of a specific treatment. As was introduced in Chapter 4, for example, SCM is a constitutionally based system of herbal medicine but, once again, in applying it, one needs to know and respond to the presenting condition. I could make virtually the same statement about Ayurveda and KCA, each of which have been presented in some detail, but this preliminary caution seems to me to be essential to the effective practice of Oriental medicine in any of its forms. However, there is a big difference between practicing a therapy that merely addresses the pattern of the presenting condition, and practicing a therapy that does so in the context of knowing the individual's constitution. Very seldom have I encountered a teacher who consciously taught this distinction, and it is often glossed over (in my experience) in FEA and Ayurveda. The one style of acupuncture practice that explicitly integrates constitution and condition into the process by which treatment options are considered is KCA but, unfortunately, its founder Kuon Dowon never explained how he devised any of his formulaic recommendations, leaving the process a total mystery. While I do not expect to ever fully understand the insights that led Kuon to develop such a radically new approach to "traditional" acupuncture, at this point in my own studies, I have come to the conclusion that the very same insights that shed light on the nature of the constitution can also be used to choose treatments which are appropriate to the presenting condition. In Chapters 12 and 13 and in Appendix 2, I will further illustrate how treatment choices are made in light of both the constitution and condition.

CHAPTER 12

INTERPRETING THE VIKRUTI IN AYURVEDA

I've presented a basic outline of the Doshas and Subdoshas which determine the Vikruti. The correspondence of the Doshas and Chinese Five Elements has also been covered. I would like to describe a hypothesis about the relationship of the Subdoshas and their corresponding Chinese Elements which appears to me to provide crucial information in cases where the Prakriti is not perfectly clear. In my experience these correlations appear to be reliable, and I have tentatively incorporated them into my daily pulse taking protocol.

Since there are five Subdoshas for each Dosha (see Figure 3.9), and the fundamental theory in acupuncture at the level of five is the Five Element theory, I tried to discern if there was a meaningful correlation between the two. Let's examine, for instance, the Vata Subdoshas. They are Prana, Udana, Samana, Apana, and Vyana. Prana is the most well known of all the 15 Subdoshas, and is often compared to the Chinese term Qi. It is closely connected with the idea of breath, and so it makes sense to associate it with the Lung Official and the Metal Element. Udana is the upward moving component of Vata, and is commonly imbalanced in conditions of upwardly rebellious energy such as is often found in allergies and headaches, so it makes sense to associate it with the Liver Official and the Wood Element. Samana is the component of Vata in the digestive system, so it makes sense to associate it with the Spleen Official and the Earth Element. Apana is the Vata component that moves downward and is imbalanced in conditions affecting the pelvic cavity or lower abdomen, so it makes sense to associate it with the Kidney Official and the Water Element. Finally, Vyana is the circulatory component of Vata, so it makes sense to associate it with the Heart and Pericardium (Circulation/Sex)

Officials and the Fire Element. In taking the Subdosha pulses, Vyana Vata is diagnosed by finding two Vata Subdoshas that feel equally strong, and which feel as if they are beating together. Interestingly, this idea is reminiscent of the concept in Chinese medicine that Fire is often generated by a transformation of any of the other forms of pathology (Xie Qi) when they become aggravated (similar transformation). This ordering of the Subdoshas is a classical Ayurvedic teaching, and if we look at the corresponding order in terms of the (Chinese) Elements it becomes Metal, Wood, Earth, Water, and Fire. This is none other than the Control Cycle (Xiang Ke) of the Five Elements. Another way of looking at this order is in terms of the body zones associated with the Zang Organs of each Element: Starting from the top, the Lung (Metal) is highest, followed by the Liver (Wood), Spleen (Earth), and then Kidney (Water). The Heart and Circulation (Fire) play a more global role throughout the body. The same analysis can be done for the Pitta and Kapha Subdoshas, but the associations, while suggestive, are not as clear as they are for Vata. It does appear to me, however, that for all three Doshas, the associative order of the Subdoshas is the same: Metal, Wood, Earth, Water, and Fire. The confirmation of this hypothesis is in the finding that the Subdosha presentations match those of the Doshas of both the Vikruti and Prakriti quite frequently, and are another way to clarify the diagnosis, especially in discriminating Taiyang and Shaoyin imbalances that may be either Fire or Water, based on Doshas and SEL pulses alone, but are clearly different based on Subdoshas. For example, if someone has a Vata Vikruti, the Subdoshas may be either a combination of any two (Fire) or Apana alone (Water). Similar reasoning holds for Pitta/Kapha Vikruti differentiations. These considerations will be illustrated in the case histories in Part Three.

One way I apply this information clinically is as follows: If the Constitutional Meridian tends to Excess, I might treat the Element Point on the Constitutional Meridian that corresponds to the most prominent Subdosha in the Vikruti pulse, with the polarity depending on the relationship of this Dosha's Element to that of the constitutional Meridian, Tonifying if it's a Grandparent or Grandchild and Sedating if it's a Parent or Child. It has been my experience that when two different Doshas are showing in the Vikruti, the Subdoshas involved occupy analogous positions. For example, in a Vata/Pitta Vikruti in someone with a Stomach Excess Constitution, it is common to see Udana and Ranjaka (Wood) as the most imbalanced Subdoshas. In such a case, Tonification of ST 43 (Wood Point) on the side of the body where these Subdoshas are felt appears to be the most effective Elemental Point treatment since it increases Kapha (the GB Dosha) to balance the Excess in Vata and Pitta. Tonifying ST 43 also draws Qi from the Liver, thus furthering the decrease in Vata and Pitta. As the

Grandparent Point, Tonifying it should also Sedate the Stomach Meridian.[1] This is not an uncommon scenario in cases of hyperacidity. Contrariwise, in a constitution with a tendency toward Deficiency, one might try to determine which of the Subdoshas is absent from the pulse, compared to the others.[2] For example, in a case of a Stomach Deficient constitution with a Kapha Vikruti, if the first Subdosha is absent (Kledaka) then the best treatment is to Tonify Stomach 45 (Metal Point). This is a common scenario in cases of hypoacidity, which can mimic the symptoms of hyperacidity, although the treatments are quite different. The key, as usual, is in the pulse.

Another way to explain this use of the Doshas of the Vikruti to guide treatment planning was developed by analogy with the transfer techniques used in FEA. For example, taking the previous example where the Vikruti is Pitta/Vata and the constitution is Stomach Excess, even without knowing the Subdoshas, I might Tonify ST 43, the Wood Point, for reasons just mentioned. I believe this transfers Qi from the Yin Wood Organ, the Liver, and when the Liver becomes weaker it diminishes both Pitta and Vata Doshas, thus balancing the Excessive Pitta/Vata situation. ST 43 is a classically indicated Point for hyperacidity, and this type of Doshic thinking provides an interesting rationale for its usefulness. Contrariwise, in a patient with a Stomach Deficient constitution who has a Pitta/Vata Vikruti (not a rare finding!), I might Sedate LV 1, the Wood Point. I believe this reduces the overcontrol of Wood on Earth by the Ke Cycle, and thus reduces the Vata and Pitta Doshas. An alternative treatment would be to Tonify SP 3, the Earth Point. This strategy brings more Qi to the Yin Earth Organ, the Spleen, which will therefore also reduce Pitta and Vata as a result. The Yin and Yang pulses, and the Subdoshas, are the best way to choose which treatment strategy is best.

Having used the case of Stomach Deficiency with a Pitta/Vata Vikruti as an illustration, I should point out that with Stomach Deficiency it is more common to find a Kapha Vikruti. Such a case requires quite a different treatment approach. The Earth Point, ST 36, could be Tonified to increase Pitta and Vata, noting that ST 36 is the most commonly indicated Point to treat Stomach Deficiency conditions. Two other Points on the Stomach Meridian

---

1   The fifth Subdosha in each Dosha represents a special case. It is imbalanced if two or more of the other Subdoshas are showing a simultaneous and equal imbalance. When this is the case, the fifth Subdosha is the one to be treated. Thus, in the case of Stomach Excess with Fire Subdoshas showing in the Vikruti, the Fire Point of the Stomach should be sedated. In Chinese medicine, it is often said that Fire is a result of the evolution of other pathogens that have not been resolved, a strikingly similar notion to the one I am proposing. I realize, however, that this explanation conflates the notions of Fire as an Element, and Fire as a Pathogenic Evil. It is interesting to note that, in Ayurveda, the Doshas (and Subdoshas) are conceptually *both* physiological and pathological descriptions.

2   Actually, my experience is that the deficient Subdosha does not merely feel absent, but usually feels like it is pulling the palpating finger in, rather than pushing it out. The fifth Subdosha, corresponding to the Fire Point, might be Deficient if the other four are equally present. It is possible that the Fire Point is indicated if none of the other positions exhibit this "hollow pulling" phenomenon.

would also be worth considering in such a patient. Tonifying ST 41, the Fire Point, will transfer Qi from the Yang Fire Organs (thus increasing Vata), and Tonifying ST 45, the Metal Point, will transfer Qi from the Yang Metal Organ (thus increasing Pitta). These are of course the classical Tonification and Sedation Points of the Stomach Meridian, and both are used in various Five Element traditions to Tonify the Stomach, because they are in "Mother-Son" relationship to it, and strengthening one will assist the other. It is nice to see that the Ayurvedic perspective again provides a rationale for these clinically effective practices. These "Doshic" methods of Point selection can be confusing, but I will try to give a number of illustrative examples in the case histories.

Having mentioned the use of "transfers" in FEA, I would like to describe the treatment strategy that I often use to balance the Elements and Doshas. In my experience, often one side of the body displays a Vikruti pulse that is reflective of the same Element as the Prakriti. The Vikruti pulse on the opposite side commonly reflects one of the other Elements, with which it is out of coordination or balance. Knowing the constitution, I can presume the polarity of the imbalance in the constitutional and non-constitutional Elements (see Chapter 8 on KCA theory), but it is better to rely on the Yang and Yin pulses at Cun, Guan, and Chi to be sure. The Vikruti pulse on the non-constitutional side will indicate whether it is the Zang or Fu Meridian of the non-constitutional Element that is imbalanced.

As an example, let's say the constitution is found to be Liver Excess (in the 24 types model), and the Vikruti on one side is Kapha (with Avalambaka Subdosha—the Wood Element correlate), and the Wood Yang pulses are Excessive compared to the Wood Yin pulses, which feel relatively normal. This situation indicates an Excess of Gall Bladder Yang. In this case, the effective strategy is to transfer Qi from the Gall Bladder. This will result in transmitting Yang Wood Qi. Where do we want to transfer this Qi, and how do we accomplish that? The answer lies in the Vikruti pulse on the other side of the body. Usually one of the other Elements will show up there. Using the Yin and Yang pulses again together with the Vikruti will give us the information we need. Let's suppose the Vikruti on that side is Pitta/Vata, but the Subdoshas indicate an Earth imbalance (Samana Vata and Sadaka Pitta). This finding implies Deficiency of the Spleen (in the Liver Excess constitution, the Earth Element tends towards Deficiency, and Pitta/Vata determines that it is Spleen rather than Stomach Deficiency). Once again, we check the Yin and Yang pulses, and this time we find the Earth Yin pulses to be Deficient with respect to the Earth Yang pulses. The diagnosis is thus Gall Bladder Yang Excess with Spleen Yin Deficiency. Figure 12.1 illustrates the Qi transfer protocol that can be used to treat this situation.

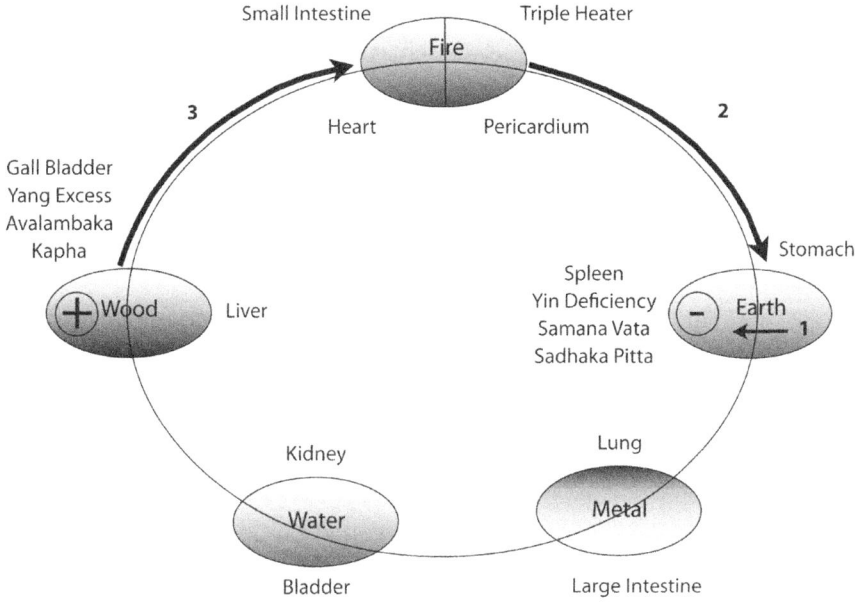

Figure 12.1 Qi transfer from Gall Bladder Yang Excess to Spleen Yin Deficiency[3]

The first needle goes in the Deficient Meridian, at SP 4. Next needles are inserted in ST 41 and SI 3. I usually use a quick Tonifying needle manipulation on SP 4, then remove all the needles in the same order as they were inserted, closing all the holes. This treatment employs two fundamental mechanisms, the Mother/Son relationship embodied in the Sheng (Creation) Cycle, and the Brother/Sister relationship embodied in Coupled Meridians of the same Element via the Luo Mai. In using the Sheng Cycle, the polarity of the Qi being transferred stays the same (Yang to Yang in this case), but in using the Luo Mai, the polarity of the Qi is reversed. So, in this case, Tonifying SP 4 increases Spleen Yin, while simultaneously decreasing Stomach Yang. There are other alternative pathways to accomplish this transfer,[4] but the one that isn't indicated is to Tonify SP 1 (the Wood Point). The reason for not using the Ke (Control) Cycle here is that it transfers Qi of the same polarity from either Yang Organ to Yin Organ or vice versa. In this case, SP 1 would pull Yang Qi from the Gall Bladder, resulting in increased Spleen Yang. As the diagnosis is Spleen Yin Deficiency, such a treatment could worsen the imbalance in the Spleen.

---

3   Image: Neal White and Elisabeth Waller-White.

4   For example, I could have used the combination of SP 2, HE 9, and LV 5, but this would pull Qi from the Gall Bladder to the Liver. Since the Liver here is constitutionally the most vulnerable Organ to Excess, I think it is preferable to avoid protocols that transfer Qi into its Meridian.

This hypothetical case is actually a common finding in my experience, and I have verified that the protocol mentioned is effective. There will be similar examples in the case history chapter, but it is worthwhile to practice devising protocols for any pair of coupled imbalances, in order to reinforce the basic principles of Qi transfers involved. In summary I would like to propose that merely knowing the Elemental status of each Meridian (Excess or Deficient) is not sufficient data to formulate the optimum treatment. Depending on the Doshas and Subdoshas involved, the optimum treatments can be radically different, as was illustrated in the cases of Stomach Deficiency with either Pitta/Vata or Kapha Doshas present. For this reason alone, I encourage practitioners of FEA to learn how to take Ayurvedic pulses.

A word of caution is appropriate here: The Dosha pulses at both the Prakriti and Vikruti levels are not easily mastered. My own experience is that much greater reliability is gained if one identifies the specific Subdoshas involved. I believe, at this time, that the Subdoshas always correlate with the most imbalanced Doshas and Elements of the Vikruti. For example: It may feel, on first palpating, that the Vikruti on one wrist shows a Vata imbalance. However, when checking the Vata Subdoshas, you might discover that only Prana Vata (Metal) is imbalanced. However, Metal imbalances should produce either Pitta or Vata/Kapha Dosha signatures. In such a case, careful study of the Kapha Dosha most often will show a noticeable spike at the Kledaka Kapha location (also Metal). This happens because the Kapha pulses seem naturally softer than those of the other Doshas (they are described as "swanlike," meaning smooth, soft, and graceful, as opposed to the "froglike" pulses of Pitta, which are bounding or jumping, and the "snakelike" pulses of Vata, which tend to be harder and tighter, and thus more easily noticeable, and the softer Kledaka Kapha pulse is easily missed). Alternatively, there may be a second Vata Subdosha in addition to Prana Vata. If either Udana, Samana, or Apana Vata is also present, then this is indeed a Vata Vikruti, but of the Fire Element type (Vyana Subdosha). In my current practice, I find myself relying more and more on the Subdosha presentation to confirm the Vikruti diagnosis, and to lay the groundwork for treatment planning.

CHAPTER 13

REINTERPRETING CLASSICAL CHINESE PULSE DIAGNOSIS (YIN/YANG)

This chapter is essentially a review of material already presented, but as it deals with a core step in both conditional diagnosis and treatment planning, it is worth describing once again. Let me remind the reader that I am primarily discussing pulse volume, rather than pulse quality; however, there are instances where Excess pulses will be smaller than expected, but wiry or tight and hard feeling. Contrarily, it is possible for Deficient pulses to feel large and forceless. These situations are the exception, rather than the rule, but the reader should keep such possibilities in mind, and use all the diagnostic indicators together before drawing a conclusion.

The Yang pulses are taken in the standard position, with the middle finger over the peak of the styloid process, and the index and ring fingers placed adjacently (see Figure 13.1).

Following the Shen/Hammer tradition, the index finger is placed at the base of the thenar eminence. The distance between index and middle fingers should be the same as that between the middle and ring fingers. This protocol will allow for differences in size and shape between individuals, and should result with the ring finger being placed in a definite depression proximal to the styloid process. The pulses felt at these three positions reflect the Yang Qi of the corresponding Zang and Fu Organs associated with each location. I typically use the *Nanjing* five depth analysis here to see if any of the Elements are out of their normal state. To reiterate, the most superficial pulse depth correlates with the Metal Element, then successively deeper pulse depths correspond to the Fire, Earth, Wood, and Water Elements sequentially.[1] Both the tips and the pads of the fingers can be used to evaluate these pulses, and it is often helpful to roll the examining finger around the center of the pulse's location in order to find its widest depth level. For example, if the left Yang Chi pulse is Deficient, but biggest at the Qi depth (Metal Element), it suggests a problem with the Kidney or Bladder Yang. In the same example, if the left Yin Chi pulse is relatively normal, and biggest at the Water Element depth (i.e. normal), then we can diagnose a Deficiency of Water Yang, which is usually most effectively treated via the Bladder Meridian, regardless of whether it is a case of Kidney Yang or Bladder Yang Deficiency. Whatever treatment we decide to use, we should expect that afterwards the left Yang Chi pulse will have returned to the Water Element depth. In this example, it would not be unusual to find the right Yang Cun pulse to be biggest at the Water Element depth. Usually in such cases a simple Tonification of UB 67 will be the best treatment. This maneuver transfers Excess Yang Qi from the Large Intestine to the Bladder via the Sheng Cycle. Pulse volumes can be unreliable in the Yang Cun location, because the radial artery naturally narrows as it approaches the wrist. For this reason, it is even more helpful to notice the depth displacement as an indicator of imbalance here. A good way to check if the Large Intestine is in an Excess state is to test for sensitivity at ST 25 (Mo Point) on both sides. Should there be no sensitivity found there, one must consider the possibility that both the Large Intestine and the Bladder are Deficient in Yang Qi. In that case, I would first Tonify LI 1 (Metal Point) and then Tonify UB 67. Once again, the pulses should be rechecked to make sure that the proper depths have been regained at both places.

In addition to using pulse volumes and pulse depths at each position, it is also helpful to consider the Vikruti pulses on both sides before formulating a diagnosis and treatment plan. In the preceding example, where the left Yang Chi pulse was Deficient and Superficial, one might expect a Vata Vikruti on either the left or right wrist, as Bladder Deficiency and/or Kidney Excess show up as Vata. If there is no Vata Vikruti pulse, but there is a Pitta/Kapha Vikruti pulse, then the indication would be Kidney Yang Deficiency which might be better treated by Tonification of KI 3.[2] In such a case, one might expect

---

1   However, the proper depth of the right Chi position pulse is at the deepest level, even though it is associated with the Fire Element. Perhaps this is one reason some authorities consider the right Chi position as reflecting the Kidney Zang and the Water Element. In my experience, it is more effective to treat Ministerial Fire than to treat the Water Element, in order to return this pulse to the deep level.

2   When Tonification of the Yang of a Yin Organ, or of the Yin of a Yang Organ, is indicated, the Point to choose is the Grandparent Point, using the Control Cycle. Thus, KI 3 transfers Yang Qi from the Stomach to the Kidney. See Thambirajah, R., *Energetics in Acupuncture*. Edinburgh: Churchill Livingstone, 2010, for a fuller presentation of this doctrine.

to find that the right Yang Guan pulse shows an Excess, reflecting Stomach Yang Excess. The Kidney Yang Deficiency occurs because the Control Cycle operating from Stomach to Kidney is not operating properly, and Tonifying KI 3 is a simple way to restart this mechanism and restore balance to the pulses.

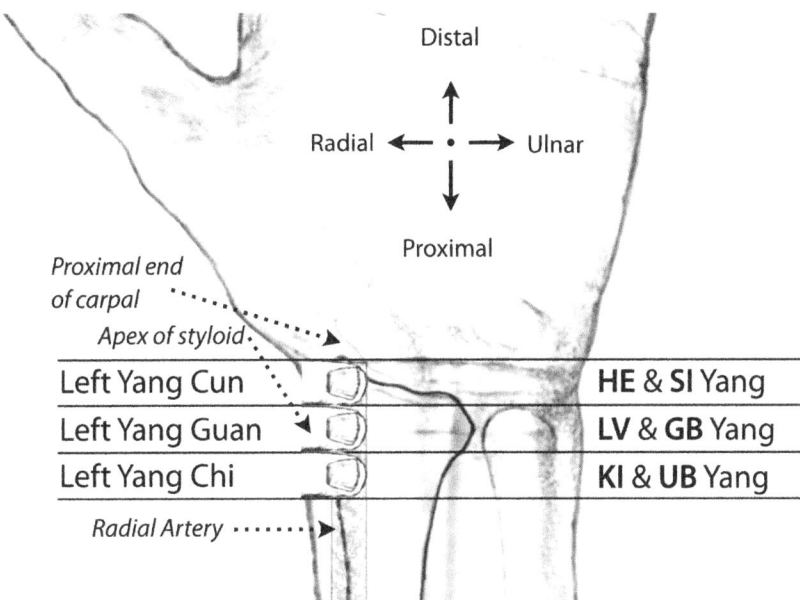

Figure 13.1 Palpating the Yang pulses[3]

The Yin Cun, Guan, and Chi pulses are examined in an analogous fashion. The only difference is that they are located about one half Cun proximally from the Yang pulses (see Figure 13.2).

The criterion is to have the apex of the styloid process exactly between the index and middle fingers of the practitioner's hand. Once again, the pulse depth method gives important information, but it is about the Yin of the Organs/ Meridians, rather than their Yang. An example, frequently found in people of Kidney Deficiency constitution, would be that if the left Yin Chi pulse is Deficient, but widest at the middle depth (Earth), and the right Yin Guan pulse is widest at the deepest level (Water), then we can tentatively diagnose Kidney Yin Deficiency and Spleen Yin Excess. In such a case, typically the right Yin Guan pulse will also be big and feel Excess in quality. The treatment I would use is to first needle KI 7 in Tonification, followed by LU 9 with neutral technique. KI 7 is rapidly Tonified, and then the needles are removed in the same order as they were inserted, with all the holes being closed. This treatment pulls Yin Qi from the Lung Meridian into the Kidney Meridian,

---

3   Image: Neal White and Elisabeth Waller-White.

while simultaneously pulling Yin Qi from the Excessive Spleen Meridian into the Lung Meridian, making sure the Lung is not being deprived of Yin Qi. Theoretically, it would be incorrect to use the Control Cycle here by simply Tonifying KI 3, as explained earlier. My experience matches Thambirajah's teaching that the Control Cycle operates from Yin Meridian to Yang Meridian and vice versa, thus Tonifying KI 3 would Tonify Kidney Yang. Since the diagnosis here is Kidney Yin Deficiency, such a treatment could aggravate the imbalance, rather than correcting it. As always, checking the pulses and the other signs and symptoms after treatment is the best way to know if the treatment was correct or not.

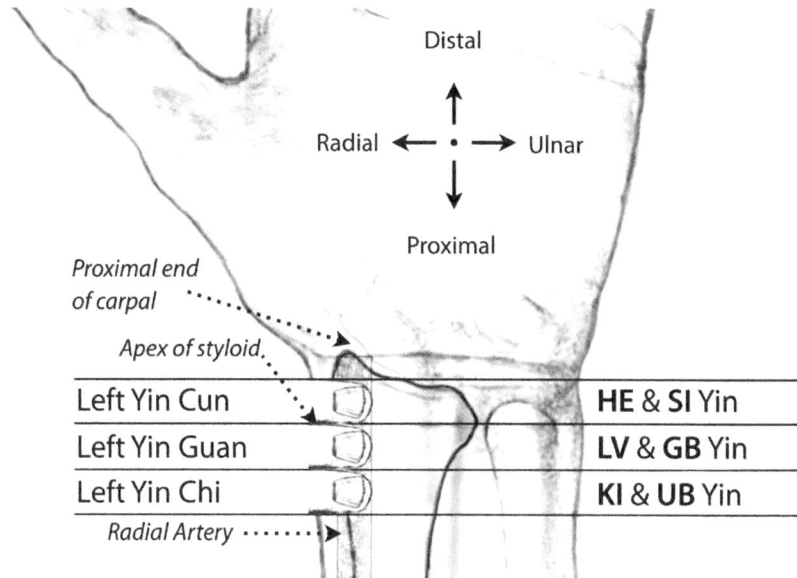

Figure 13.2 Palpating the Yin pulses[4]

The Creative and Control Cycles can also be used with Sedation needling techniques. An example might be someone with a Vata Vikruti of the Water type (Apana Subdosha) on one wrist, and a Kapha Vikruti of the Earth type (Bodaka Subdosha) on the other wrist. I've seen this situation in people with Excess in the left Yang Chi pulse (Kidney Yang Excess, or Kidney Fire), and Deficiency in the right Yang Guan pulse (Stomach Yang Deficiency). I interpret this as a case of the Kidney drawing too much Yang Qi from the Stomach across the Control Cycle, depleting it. The treatment indicated here is simply to Sedate KI 3 (the Grandmother Point), which inhibits the overactivity of the Control Cycle. A similar principle applies to Creative Cycle imbalances, where

---

4   Image: Neal White and Elisabeth Waller-White.

the Son is in Excess and the Mother is Deficient. In such a situation, Sedating the Tonification Point of the Son is the appropriate treatment, although it is also effective to draw the Excess Qi all the way around the Creative Cycle to bring it to the Deficient Mother. The important factor in successfully using these different treatment strategies is to correctly identify both the Vikruti on each wrist, as well as the Excesses and Deficiencies at both the Yin and Yang positions of Cun, Guan, and Chi in the radial pulse.

One common finding I've noticed is that the Yang pulse at some location might feel Excessive, while the Yin pulse at the same location feels Deficient, or vice versa. This situation can be treated by using the Source/Connecting Point (Yuan/Luo) treatment. For example, if the Earth Yang pulse is Excess and the Earth Yin pulse is Deficient, then the diagnosis is Stomach Excess and Spleen Deficiency. To treat this condition, the first pair of needles should be inserted in the Luo Point of the Deficient Meridian (SP 4) in the Tonifying direction, and the second pair of needles should be inserted in the Source Point of the Excess Meridian (ST 42) in the Sedating direction. The needles are removed when the pulses show a return to balance in the Earth Element.

These examples of using the Yin and Yang pulses along with both constitutional and conditional pulse diagnosis illustrate the thinking behind many of the cases to be presented in Chapter 19. The rules for using the Creative and Control Cycles, as well as the Source/Connecting Point relationship, should be reviewed by the reader until they are completely clear, before trying to understand the cases in Chapter 19.

In summary, I should emphasize that the Cun, Guan, and Chi pulses (both Yang and Yin locations) are very important guides to the current state of energetic imbalance, a teaching that is at the core of all texts on traditional acupuncture. Often there will be a similar energetic finding at the constitutional level, but not always. For example, the conditional pulses may indicate Spleen Deficiency as the present imbalance, but the constitution might indicate Liver Excess as the root, even if the examination does not indicate an imbalance at the left Guan position (Liver). In such a case it would usually be more helpful to Tonify the Spleen, rather than to Sedate the Liver. Of course, it is possible to do both, and this is a common practice in KCA, where the presence of Fu Organ disturbances[5] in people who have Liver Excess constitutions are treated with a protocol that Sedates the Liver and Tonifies the Spleen. FEA also chooses the treatment based on both the constitution (CF) and the condition as it is reflected in the pulses at Cun, Guan, and Chi. I am not really presenting anything radically new in this discussion, merely trying to shed some light on the underlying dynamics that are employed in several approaches to traditional acupuncture practices.

---

5   For example, indigestion, dysmenorrhea, or dysuria.

CHAPTER 14

REINTERPRETING MINISTERIAL FIRE

Having presented some novel ideas about Yin/Yang theory, I would like to take this opportunity to discuss my thoughts about a rather thorny issue in Five Element theory: the nature of Ministerial Fire. I have previously published some preliminary ideas on this topic in the *Journal of Traditional Acupuncture*,[1] and I have also alluded to the notion that, in some contexts, one must think of Six Elements rather than Five. What I have to say on this issue is based on a combination of doctrines learned from my teachers (especially Kuon Dowon) and on my own clinical experience.

Since the 1984 journal article may not be easily accessible, I will summarize what I had to say then: If one is thinking in terms of Five Element theory, then the right Chi pulse position reflects the Fire Element, including the Officials of the Triple Heater, Pericardium, Circulation/Sex, and Vital Gate. This is an energetic association or resonance. If, however, one is thinking in morphological terms, then the right Chi pulse position reflects issues of the Lower Heater (Jiao), which are traditionally assigned to the Kidney Official, including abnormalities of Kidney Fire and Kidney Water, such as chills, fatigue, diarrhea, edema, pallor, and low libido (Deficient Kidney Yang), as well as fever, nightsweats, insomnia, and constipation (Deficient Kidney Yin). It seems clear to me that the assignment of the right Chi pulse to the Kidney is part of the Yin/Yang tradition, which in turn is more emphasized in herbal medicine than is the Five Element tradition. Since the Kidney Official is responsible for storing the Original Fire and Original Water, it is easy to see how confusion can

---

1   Eckman, P., "The Third House on the Right, Kidney Fire—A Study." *Journal of Traditional Acupuncture*, 7 (3), 1984, pp.13–15.

arise as to whether the right Chi pulse reflects the Fire Element (Pericardium, Circulation/Sex, Triple Heater, Vital Gate), or the Water Element (Kidney Yang, Kidney Yin, Urinary Bladder, Vital Gate). In fact, the descriptions of the Triple Heater in the classics refer to mists, marinades, and drains, which are all fluid terms.[2] In my mind, there is a sense in which Ministerial Fire shares aspects of both the Fire and the Water Elements. In inorganic nature, Fire rises and Water sinks, while in living organisms, Fire (Imperial, from the Heart/Shaoyin) is made to descend to warm the lower body, while Water (from the Kidney/Shaoyin) is made to ascend to moisten the upper body. How does this inversion happen? I believe it is due to Ministerial Fire (Triple Heater/Shaoyang), which performs this alchemy of interchanging Fire and Water, while partaking of the characteristics of both.

In FEA, as taught by Worsley, the right Chi pulse reflects the Circulation/Sex and Triple Heater Officials, which are clearly part of the Fire Element. I use the term Ministerial Fire to distinguish these Officials from the Small Intestine and Heart, which are classified as Imperial Fire Officials. However, there is a separate usage of the term Ministerial Fire in the classical literature, referring to Fire functions or syndromes of various other Organs, such as the Liver, Gall Bladder, etc. In the present text, this second meaning of Ministerial Fire is not employed, unless specifically indicated. I wish to emphasize this point because the ensuing discussion is specifically concerned with the relationship of Imperial and Ministerial Fire.

In KCA as originally presented by Kuon, the Fire Element is not represented by any of the constitutional types; however, it is treated when employing the Auxiliary Formulae. In fact, what Kuon called the "Psyche" Auxiliary Formula is always directed at one of the Meridians of the Fire Element. Kuon never explained how he derived these Formulae, but he clearly thought very deeply about the nature of the Fire Element, and even published a monograph on the topic called *Pyrologos*,[3] situating Fire as the origin of all life. Even now, much of Kuon's interpretation, as presented in that monograph, is obscure to me, but there is another side of Kuon's work that is much clearer—his clinical recommendations, which are based on more than 50 years of extensive acupuncture practice.

In Kuon's approach, if an Element is Excessive, both its Parent and Child Elements will also tend towards Excess, while its Grandparent and Grandchild Elements will tend towards Deficiency. In order to apply such thinking, one must know which aspect of the Fire Element, Imperial or Ministerial Fire, is implicated. It turns out that, for Kuon, it is always Imperial Fire that

---

2   *Lingshu* 18 uses the terms Wu, Ou, and Du for the Upper, Middle, and Lower Heater, which I have rendered in colloquial English. Character numbers from Mathews, R. H., *Mathews' Chinese-English Dictionary*. Cambridge, MA: Harvard University Press, 1979: 7199, 4819, and 6518.

3   Kuon Dowon, *Pyrologos: A New Theory of Life and the Universe*. Yonsei University Press, 2002.

follows this rule. As for Ministerial Fire, there is no fixed doctrine about its tendencies towards Excess or Deficiency with regard to the situations of the other Elements. There is, however, one interesting finding with regard to how Kuon uses the Ministerial Fire Meridians: The Greater Yin and Lesser Yang constitutions never employ Sedating Ministerial Fire, but may Tonify it, whereas the Greater Yang and Lesser Yin constitutions never employ Tonifying Ministerial Fire, but may Sedate it. One of Kuon's findings that seems to bear on this topic is that caffeine is deleterious to the health of Greater Yang and Lesser Yin types, while it may be beneficial, in moderation, in Greater Yin and Lesser Yang types. Interestingly, caffeine has been found to be a stimulant of both the Sympathetic and the Parasympathetic Nervous Systems, and there has been much speculation about the possible correlation of Ministerial Fire with these two parts of the Autonomic Nervous System. It is easy to envision a relationship of the Central Nervous System with the Heart, Kidney, Small Intestine, and Bladder (Shaoyin and Taiyang), and likewise a relationship of the Autonomic Nervous System and Ministerial Fire (Shaoyang and Jueyin), thus possibly accounting for the use of Ministerial Fire in connection with syndromes of the Liver and Gall Bladder, as previously mentioned.

Let me take this analysis one step further. If there is no fixed relationship of Ministerial Fire to the situations of the other Elements' Officials, it is possible to think of Ministerial Fire as outside the Creative and Control Cycles (Xiang Sheng and Xiang Ke), which as I mentioned employ Imperial Fire whenever the Fire Element is in play, at least in Kuon's methods. Staying with Kuon's model, let's examine the case where the constitution involves an Excess Imperial Fire Organ, i.e. Heart or Small Intestine (this could be Liver Excess or Stomach Excess, for example). In each case, together with its Parent and Child, there are three Excess tending Organs and two Deficient tending Organs. It seems plausible to me that in such a situation, if Ministerial Fire (Pericardium or Triple Heater) were to also tend towards Deficiency, the constitutional configuration would be a more balanced one, with three Excess and three Deficient tendencies. The same reasoning can be applied, with a reversal of polarity, to constitutions involving a Deficient Heart or Small Intestine, such as, for example, Liver or Stomach Deficiency. As it happens, this hypothesis fits Kuon's treatment recommendations, as exemplified in the following cases.

Kuon's Greater Yin Zang constitution is called Hepatonia, or Liver Excess. The Liver belongs to the Wood Element, so its Mother and Daughter, the Kidney and Heart (Water and Imperial Fire), will also tend toward Excess. Its Grandmother and Granddaughter, the Lung and Spleen (Metal and Earth), will tend towards Deficiency. This asymmetric association leaves three Excess Meridians and two Deficient Meridians. Kuon discovered that in Hepatonia patients, the Pericardium Meridian successfully treats "Psyche" conditions, if the Pericardium is Tonified. Thus there are three Excess and three Deficient

Meridians, leading to a balanced Meridian system. Of course, I am leaving out the Fu Meridians, but these have the same tendencies as their Zang coupled Meridians in KCA. In this case we can see that Imperial and Ministerial Fire have opposite tendencies. If we consider Ministerial Fire to be part of the Fire Element, then we cannot say if the Fire Element is Excess or Deficient in individuals of Hepatonia constitution. Perhaps this is adequate reason to consider the possibility that, in this context, Ministerial Fire might represent a "Sixth Element."

Continuing this analysis, Kuon's Lesser Yin Fu constitution is called Vesicotonia, and is characterized by a predominant tendency for the Stomach to become Deficient. Its Parent and Child, the Small Intestine and Large Intestine, will also tend towards Deficiency, while its Grandparent and Grandchild, the Gall Bladder and Bladder, will tend towards Excess. To balance this situation, one might expect that Ministerial Fire, in this case the Triple Heater, would tend towards Excess, and this is exactly the basis of Kuon's Psyche Formula for the Vesicotonia constitution. Once again, we see that Imperial Fire and Ministerial Fire have opposite tendencies. Is this always the case? Let us look at one of the 24 constitutions that Kuon did not discuss.

According to Puramo, the Lesser Yin Fu constitution also includes a variant where the dominant tendency is towards Gall Bladder Excess. The Fundamental Formula he uses to treat this constitution Sedates Small Intestine and Gall Bladder, while Tonifying Stomach. Now we have a problem, as there are already two Excess Organs, and theoretically there are two more Organs that should tend towards Excess, namely Bladder as the Parent, and Triple Heater as the expected expression of Ministerial Fire in Lesser Yin Fu constitutions. Puramo does not discuss this issue, but he does include Sedation of the Triple Heater as the Psyche Formula for this constitution. This is a case where both Imperial and Ministerial Fire seem to share the same polarity, a tendency towards Excess, but as this leads to four Excess Organs and two Deficient ones, I suspect that it contains an error. I therefore believe that Puramo is probably mistaken in this instance, and that Imperial Fire is Deficient, while Water and Ministerial Fire are Excess in Lesser Yin Fu constitutions. I can say that I've treated Gall Bladder Excess individuals with KCA style methods that included Sedating the Triple Heater, and the successful outcome in one such individual will be included in the case history chapter.[4] My most current research suggests to me that the following modification of Kuon's theory is necessary:

1. Each constitutional type consists of three Excess and three Deficient tending Elements (considering Imperial and Ministerial Fire as separate Elements).

---

4   See Case 22 in Chapter 19.

2. Kuon's original types that included treatment of Ministerial Fire for the Psyche Auxiliary Formula (Greater Yin Zang, Greater Yang Zang, Lesser Yin Fu and Lesser Yang Fu) have their Elements correctly described by his theory.

3. Kuon's original types that did not have Auxiliary Formulae for Ministerial Fire, need correction of their Psyche Formulae to address this situation. These new Ministerial Fire Formulae appear to me to be the correct Psyche Formulae for these constitutions, and are as follows: Greater Yin Fu constitutional types have Excess Ministerial Fire (in addition to Excess Imperial Fire). The same is true for Lesser Yang Zang constitutional types. The exact opposite is true for Greater Yang Fu and Lesser Yin Zang constitutional types, which have Deficient tendencies in both Ministerial and Imperial Fire.

4. I believe Kuon expected the Zang and Fu variants of each constitution to share the same tendency in Ministerial Fire, and since this appears to me not to be the case, it is likely to be the reason Kuon didn't propose Ministerial Fire treatments for half his constitutional types.

We are still left with the question of what the Officials of Ministerial Fire actually do. The Triple Heater is said to be the conduit that channels Original Energy (Yuan Qi) from its storehouse in the Kidneys to the Source Points of the 12 Meridians. Thus it brings the Original Fire and Original Water to each of the Officials. If caffeine causes an Excessive release of this Original Energy in individuals who already tend to release too much Yuan Qi, this could easily be understood. Such individuals suffer from relying on Original Energy to perform functions that should be the responsibility of their Normal Energy (Zheng Qi). They might be expected to show symptoms of hyperactivity of the Autonomic Nervous System. Conversely, individuals with sluggish Autonomic Nervous Systems might simply be lacking the spark supplied by Original Energy, which would enable them to produce the necessary amount of Normal Energy. If they consume caffeine, that might release enough Original Energy via the Triple Heater to allow them to reestablish production of Normal Energy in adequate amounts. This interpretation suggests that the Autonomic Nervous System is a precondition for the proper functioning of the major Organs, and that Ministerial Fire has a crucial role in every constitution. I must report that one of Worsley's teachings that I remember quite clearly was that he thought virtually everyone could benefit from proper treatment of the Triple Heater and Circulation/Sex Officials. From the perspective of ensuring that the correct amount of Yuan Qi is being transported to all the Officials, Worsley's suggestion makes sense, as does a possible correlation of Ministerial Fire with a normally functioning Autonomic Nervous System (which evolutionarily preceded the development of a Central Nervous System), and might further explain why Ministerial Fire might not always obey Creative and Control Cycle rules that apply to the other Elements and Meridians.

CHAPTER 15

CHAKRA PULSE DIAGNOSIS

Since I do not believe that I have encountered a useful seven type model of constitutions, I think this would be a good place to introduce one of the less well-known approaches to conditional treatment formulation, as it is based on the Seven Chakras of Ayurvedic medicine (see Figure 15.1). I am greatly indebted to John Cross, a physiotherapist whose training at the British College of Acupuncture was roughly contemporaneous with my own at the College of Traditional Chinese Acupuncture, in England in the 1970s. Cross' doctoral thesis was on the use of the Chakras in acupuncture treatment, and a detailed presentation of his findings was finally published in 2008.[1] I have experimented with his methods and am still in the process of deciding how useful such an approach would be in treating the current condition, and in what circumstances to employ it. Cross' work is very nicely presented, and I encourage others to read his book, to which I can only make passing reference here. Cross associates each of the Seven Chakras with one of the Five Elements, except for two Chakras, each of which he assigns to two Elements.[2] My opinion is slightly different, and is based on the association of the Doshas and the Elements as described in Chapter 3. My belief is that each of the Seven Chakras is associated with one of the Five Elements, and that this Element will appear

1   Cross, J., *Acupuncture and the Chakra Energy System*. Berkeley, CA: North Atlantic Books, 2008.

2   Cross associates the Solar Plexus Chakra with both the Stomach and the Liver. Since both of these Organs manifest imbalance via either a Kapha or a Pitta/Vata Vikruti, treatment of one can help balance the other. He also associates the Sacral Chakra with both the Spleen and the Pericardium. This represents a more irreconcilable difference between our models, and awaits further clarification based on experience, although conjoined treatment of Pericardium and Spleen is quite common in many styles of acupuncture, to say nothing of their use in both Chong Mai and Yin Wei Mai treatments.

in its Dosha correspondence in the Vikruti. The associations I have seen are as follows:

Crown Chakra	Fire (Ministerial)	Vata or Pitta/Kapha
Brow Chakra	Wood	Kapha or Pitta/Vata
Throat Chakra	Metal	Pitta or Vata/Kapha
Heart Chakra	Fire (Imperial)	Vata or Pitta/Kapha
Solar Plexus Chakra	Earth (Stomach)	Kapha or Pitta/Vata
Sacral Chakra	Earth (Spleen)	Kapha or Pitta/Vata
Base Chakra	Water	Vata or Pitta/Kapha

It is possible to visualize a rationale for this arrangement, although my choices are ultimately determined by pulse examination and clinical response to treatment. The Base Chakra is associated with the Water Element, whose essential nature is to flow down to the depths. Likewise, the Crown Chakra is associated with the Fire Element, whose essential nature is to blaze upwards. The blazing up aspect of the Fire Element is particularly associated with Ministerial Fire, which resonates with the climatic linkage of Fire with Shaoyang. In the center of the Chakras is the Heart Chakra, which is also associated with the Fire Element, but in this case with Imperial Fire (Shaoyin), whose place is in the center, the source of life carried by the Spirit, or Shen. The Brow Chakra is associated with the Wood Element, resonating with the knitted brows of an angry or frustrated individual. The Throat Chakra is associated with the Metal Element, which rules the Lungs and the Qi, which are the source of our vocal abilities, expressed via the throat. The Solar Plexus Chakra is associated with the Earth Element, and especially the Stomach, as it is located right over this organ. The more Yin Spleen/Pancreas Chakra is located below it (Yin), as the Sacral Chakra.

This expansion of the Five Elements into Seven Chakras is not as obscure as it might appear. The Chakras are Energy or Qi Centers, and in Oriental medicine there has been a history of associating both the Earth and Fire Elements with the Center in human physiology. The standard association is with the Earth Element, and there are numerous references to the unusual importance of the Stomach, it being more important than the other Fu Organs. Some traditions even switch the correspondences of the Earth Organs, with the Stomach reflected in the deep pulse at the right Guan position, and the Spleen in the superficial pulse at the same location. Thus, a separate Chakra for each of them is not unreasonable. Similarly, the Fire Element is already conveniently double

(Heart/Small Intestine and Pericardium/Triple Heater). We also commonly think of the Heart as the Center, at least in its role as Supreme Controller. Many styles of acupuncture have adopted various strategies to treat the Heart by using either the Spleen or the Pericardium instead, so this double presence of the Earth and Fire Elements seems plausible to me.[3]

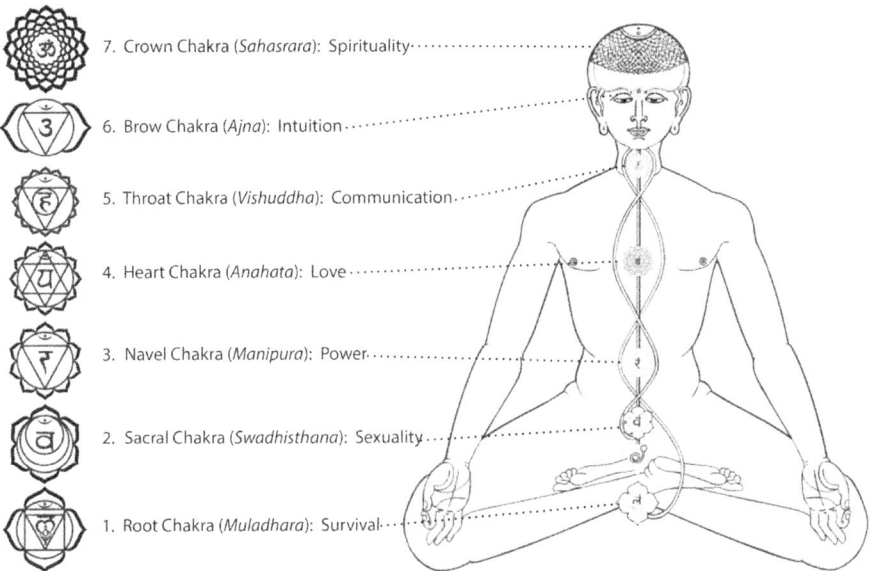

7. Crown Chakra (*Sahasrara*): Spirituality

6. Brow Chakra (*Ajna*): Intuition

5. Throat Chakra (*Vishuddha*): Communication

4. Heart Chakra (*Anahata*): Love

3. Navel Chakra (*Manipura*): Power

2. Sacral Chakra (*Swadhisthana*): Sexuality

1. Root Chakra (*Muladhara*): Survival

Figure 15.1 The seven main Chakras[4]

---

3   In his text, *Acupuncture* (Moulins Les Metz: Maisonneuve, 1982), J. Kespi distinguishes the Center-Source of life (Fire Element) from the Center-Place of life (Earth Element).

4   Image: Neal White and Elisabeth Waller-White. Based on images by © victoria/shutterstock.com and unmeshpatel/shutterstock.com. This chart uses the terms Root Chakra for Base Chakra, and Navel Chakra for Solar Plexus Chakra. The functions associated with each Chakra make sense in terms of the Chinese Elements to which I've correlated them. Survival relates to the "Will to Live," sexuality is consistent with SP 6 being its focal point, power relates to the Stomach's function of providing Qi as the "Sea of Grains and Water," love is certainly associated with the Heart, communication is most directly associated with the voice and related to the Lungs, intuition relates to the Spiritual Soul (Hun) of the Liver, and Spirituality must then be assigned to the only other possibility: Ministerial Fire. I alluded earlier to the idea that Ministerial Fire is the vehicle by which the Zang/Fu get their Yuan Qi via the Triple Heater. In a sense, therefore, Ministerial Fire precedes the activities of the other Organ systems, and consists of functions without a form. The aim of many spiritual practices, typified by meditation, is to detach oneself from identification with one's ego and physical body. Since Ministerial Fire is already without physical form, it is an ideal conduit for the return to an egoless state, and perhaps what is signified by a return to the Dao.

As for how the Chakras are used in treatment, my own belief is that they occupy a system of relative blocks to Five Element treatment, analogous to Aggressive Energy, Husband/Wife, Possession, or Entry/Exit blocks. If a Chakra is in an imbalanced state, it might limit Elemental treatments from having their full effects, because the Qi is stuck in this Chakra, and will not easily allow movement. As Energy centers, the Chakras are likely to have profound effects on an individual's energy level when they are not functioning properly. This idea explains the powerful effects I have seen from Chakra treatments, and at the same time accounts for the close association of the symptomatology with the Organs and endocrine glands at the various anatomical levels in the body, although Chakra treatment is not limited to local Organ pathology. The most common situation where I have found Chakra treatments to be indicated is when the Vikruti is the same on both wrists, but does not correspond to the person's Prakriti. I commonly see this pattern in individuals with chronic fatigue syndrome, an illness that fits the symptomatology to be expected from a blocked Chakra. Cross treats chronic fatigue syndrome via the Solar Plexus, Sacral, and Spleen Chakras,[5] while my own experience is that any of the Chakras may be the site of blockage in chronic fatigue syndrome. I have at least found such blockages in the Crown and Brow Chakras, as well as in the Sacral Chakra using the diagnostic indicators given above.[6]

I should also mention that Cross describes the treatment of 21 Minor Chakras as especially effective for pain relief.[7] Very few sources even mention these Minor Chakras, although they are part of the Ayurvedic description of the human energy system. Again, I have had occasional excellent results upon incorporating these Minor Chakra treatments, but not enough to make them a routine part of my therapeutic strategy. The protocols for treating the Chakras are given by Cross, and the reader should consult his text for specific details. As I have already explained, I use several other treatment strategies that balance the Doshas independently of the Chakras. In summary, the Chakra treatments are for addressing blocks, while the Dosha balancing protocols are analogous to balancing the Elements by various strategies including transfers via the Creative and Control Cycles, which they also employ. Cross gives two Point protocols for treating each Chakra, one using Points on the front of the body and the other using back Points. The ventral Points are mostly selected for Organ dysfunctions and mental/emotional problems, while the back Points are mostly selected to treat musculoskeletal problems, but this rule is not absolute, and both sets of Points can be used in the same treatment, either simultaneously or in succession. These treatment protocols are reminiscent of

---

5   The Spleen Chakra is one of the Minor Chakras.

6   See Case 34 in Chapter 19 for an example of such use in chronic fatigue syndrome.

7   Cross, 2008.

Point combinations and treatment strategies that I learned from the Korean teacher whom I apprenticed with for over ten years, Chae Lew. In these Chakra treatments, the needles are inserted, and left in situ for 10 to 20 minutes. As usual, the patient should be reevaluated after treatment via signs and symptoms (including the pulse), to confirm that there has been an improvement.

PART THREE

PULSE DIAGNOSIS IN THE CLINIC

CHAPTER 16

BEFORE APPLYING THE MODEL

Constitutional considerations are not necessarily the best place to begin treatment. Worsley's synthesis of FEA proposed a number of situations that required other treatments, prior to addressing the CF. These include Aggressive Energy, Demonic Possession, Husband–Wife imbalances, Akabane imbalances, and Entry/Exit Blocks. I believe these same precautions are appropriate in applying the model I have described, although I would not agree that clients with these conditions cannot benefit from constitutionally based treatment; however, their response may be limited, and so clearing these "blocks" is a prudent approach. The protocols in FEA are not the only way to clear these blocks. As an example, I might cite the writings of Jacques Lavier, the teacher from whom Worsley learned about Aggressive Energy (AE). Lavier taught that an alternative to draining AE via the Back Shu Points was to drain it from the Five Shu (Transport) Points, also known as the Five Element Points, on each Meridian. Additionally, the literature of Chinese medicine abounds with other treatment protocols than the Seven Dragons for dealing with Demonic Possession.

Concerning the topic of Demonic Possession, I'd like to propose a reinterpretation of this diagnosis, which relates not only to diagnosis and treatment, but is an attempt to incorporate this subject within the dominant paradigm of TOM, and demystify it at the same time. My starting point for this discussion is Chapter 8 of the *Lingshu*, which describes the coming into being of a new individual at conception. This moment of conception is composed of two factors: the uniting of the Essences (Jing) of the sperm and ovum, and the entry of the Spirit (Shen), which these combined Essences make possible. This dependence of the Spirit on the Essence is a situation that endures throughout the life of the individual. Should anything disturb the individual's Essence later in life, it would be expected to impact the Spirit also, which no longer has its fully functional material substrate. The Essence, in turn, is composed of two parts: the inherited portion (Xian Tian Zhi Jing) and the acquired (from the most refined aspects of food, drink, etc.) portion (Hou Tian Zhi Jing). These two parts of the Essence continually interact and are metabolized slowly over the individual's lifespan. What would happen if either of these components of the Essence became pathologically compromised? As indicated, the Spirit would no longer be fully supported, and some disturbance of the higher faculties might be expected, either in the realm of the emotions, the mental faculties, or the spiritual state itself.

The Inherited Essence is cared for by the Kidney and Water Element, and includes the brain as a part of the Sea of Marrow. If we look at the Points of the Seven External Dragons treatment, we can see that these all relate to the Water Element and the Kidney's functions. DU 20 is a Point of the Sea of Marrow, whose secondary name is "Ghost Gate"; UB 11 is the Meeting Point of Bone (another Kidney function), whose secondary name is "100 Exhaustions," echoing the name of DU 20, and implying a tendency towards Deficiency which needs Tonification; UB 23 is the Associated Point of the Kidney, whose secondary name "Jing Palace" implies its function of storing the inherited Essence; and UB 61 is the "servant"[1] who puts this protocol into action (its secondary name is "Pacify Devils"), reinvigorating the inherited Essence, and thereby allowing the Spirit to settle more fully into its proper role as commander of the individual's life. It has been my experience that people who benefit by use of the External Dragons protocol typically have a Vata Vikruti, even if that is not reflective of their Prakriti (constitution). I have also found that their pulses[2] at all positions tend to be biggest at the deepest level, corresponding to the Kidney according to the *Nanjing*. Such individuals are typically cold, slow in their thinking, and easily tired. This pattern is frequently seen in chronic fatigue syndrome, and in many cases of depression. I have often found this protocol helpful in treating such people. Interestingly, the Master Point, DU 20, is one of the main Points recommended by Maciocia for treating chronic fatigue syndrome.[3] In my experience, these individuals do best if the seven needles are Tonified. My understanding of this is that these Points work through strengthening the Yang Official of the Water Element, the Bladder, and Tonifying the Bladder increases Pitta and Kapha, while decreasing Vata, thus leading to a more balanced state. Theoretically, a patient may need Sedation of these Seven Dragons Points if

---

1   Worsley, J., *Traditional Chinese Acupuncture, vol. 1. Meridians and Points*. Tisbury: Element Books, 1982, translates the traditional name of UB 61 as "Servant's Aide."

2   In the Yang locations of Cun, Guan, and Chi.

3   Maciocia, G., *The Practice of Chinese Medicine*. Edinburgh: Churchill Livingstone, 1994, pp.648–653.

they present with a Vikruti of Pitta/Kapha, but I have not seen anyone whose condition and treatment would validate this hypothesis as yet.

On the other hand, if the acquired Essence is compromised, the same Spirit level disturbances might be expected, but the acquired Essence is under the domain of the Earth Element, which is responsible for post-natal nourishment. Here, the Points of the Seven Internal Dragons come into play. Aside from the Master Point, they are all on the Stomach Meridian, and the Stomach is known as the Sea of Food and Water. Ren 15, whose secondary names include "Spirit Palace" and "Spirit Storehouse," has many Spirit level indications such as hysteria, incoherent speech, and mad walking and singing, and is located at the top of the Middle Heater, where food is transformed. ST 25 (secondary name is Repairing Sources), ST 32 (indicated for ghost talk and possession by devils), and ST 36 (secondary name is Ghost Evil) and ST 41 (indicated for mania, agitation, speech troubles, and convulsions) are all also powerful Points for affecting the digestive process. Again, in my experience, most patients who benefit from the Seven Internal Dragons protocol need these Points Sedated, and present with a Pitta/Vata Vikruti. Many mental, emotional, and spiritual indications are listed as indications for these Points, with the classic description being someone who takes off their clothes and dances on tables. This is clearly an Excess Heat pattern that is reminiscent of a manic episode. Sedating the Stomach will decrease Pitta and Vata, while Tonifying Kapha, to achieve a more balanced state and improve the post-natal Essence. I have also found that these individuals tend to have all their pulses most prominently at the middle (nine bean) level which corresponds to the Spleen according to the *Nanjing*. I have had one client who presented with all pulses strongest at the middle depth, and who had an unusual Kapha Vikruti pulse. Following this line of thought, I Tonified the Internal Dragons Points with good results. I believe these experiences are strongly supportive of my hypothesis about the rationale for the Dragons treatments, but hope to hear from the experiences of other practitioners who try to duplicate my findings.

Using pulse diagnosis makes accessing the Dragons treatments much easier, but in no way contradicts the teachings of J. R. Worsley, who used the evaluation of the Spirit (Shen) in the eyes as his principal diagnostic indicator. I would also like to remind the reader that the history of Chinese medicine is of a continual addition of new paradigms to the old ones, rather than a replacement of the old ones by the newer ones. Thus the approaches I am presenting to the interpretation and treatment of "Possession" should not be taken as evidence that demonic possession by spiritual entities does not exist. I have heard many stories from FEA practitioners that purport to have clients spontaneously talk about feeling released from the Devil, or similar notions after such treatment, despite the absence of any explanation of the Dragons treatment by their practitioner. I am merely adding an explanation at the energetic and physiological level of how these treatments might work. I believe that assertions about the reality of spiritual possession are inherently impossible to either prove or disprove, and I believe that the long history of traditional Chinese medicine favors including the notion of possession in its epistemology.

In my experience, I have also found that there are other situations that may diminish response to, or complicate, constitutional treatment. I believe Kiiko Matsumoto teaches an analogous idea, and discusses a number of conditions that are a priority in treatment formulation. For the present, I would like to mention one condition that stands out in this regard, and has been alluded to in every historical period since the *Neijing*, namely the treatment of the Eight Extraordinary Meridians (EEM), which was presented in Chapter 11. It has been my experience that distortions at the level of the EEM are a possible hindrance to satisfactory responses to constitutional treatment, although they do not seem to present a complete blockage of the response to such treatment. My teacher of Korean Hand Acupuncture, Yoo Tae Woo, used to demonstrate this in class by twisting a Kleenex box and then asking if the students could still follow the natural contours of the original box. I believe what he meant to show was that distortions of the EEM (which regulate the coordinative architecture of the energetic body) had the potential to confuse signaling along the Principal Meridians.

I would also like to say a few words about using the Ayurvedic Vikruti pulse to assist in the choice of Principal Meridian treatments, alluded to earlier. In principle, it is simple: the Vikruti interpretation is exactly the same as was described for the Prakriti. Thus either a Vata or a Pitta/Kapha Vikruti indicates a need to address either the Fire or Water Element, a Pitta or Vata/Kapha Vikruti indicates a need to address the Metal Element, and a Kapha or Vata/Pitta Vikruti indicates a need to address either the Wood or Earth Element. This knowledge can be particularly helpful in diagnosing Entry/Exit blocks, especially those between Meridians of the same Element. The basic principle is that Tonifying an Exit Point Sedates its Meridian, while Tonifying an Entry Point Tonifies its Meridian. For example, let's say a patient has a Metal CF (Lung Excess, for instance), but their Vikruti pulse is Kapha bilaterally. There must be something going on in either Wood or Earth to produce this Kapha pulse. In order to balance the Doshas, we want to Tonify Vata and Pitta, while sedating Kapha. That is an exact description of the state where there is an Entry/Exit block between Gall Bladder and Liver Meridians. Tonifying the Exit Point of the Gall Bladder (GB 41) sedates Kapha, while Tonifying the Entry Point of the Liver (LV 1) Tonifies Vata and Pitta. The occurrence of this Vikruti in a Metal CF is suggestive that this Entry/Exit block might be present, and the Vikruti should markedly improve right away after the indicated treatment. Of course, this particular block is more likely to be the explanation for the pulse described if there happen to be symptoms or signs in the region of the individual's foot. This is just one example. Others will appear in the case histories.

Akabane imbalances are another type of block that can interfere with otherwise helpful treatments. I have found that the Vikruti pulse can also be important in diagnosing and treating these blocks. Take, for instance, a patient whose constitution is Liver Deficiency. If their Vikruti on the left side is Kapha, while their Vikruti on the right side is Pitta/Vata, they can be suspected of having an Akabane imbalance on the Liver Meridian which can be corrected by Tonifying the Luo Point, LV 5, on the left side. This illustrates a way to use pulses to identify suspected Akabane imbalances, but it is not meant to replace standard Akabane testing at the Jing Well Points, since there are other mechanisms that can lead to such Vikruti findings.

Once having cleared any EEM, Entry/Exit, Akabane, Chakra, or other blocks, it is time to initiate constitutional treatment. However, if during the course of treatment the patient stops responding, it is always worth considering if one of these blocks has recurred, and if so, to treat it again. Any trauma, including physical, mental, emotional, or spiritual stress, can create such a block. In my experience, two of the most common etiologies for such blocks are surgery and pharmaceutical treatments. The former are easy to understand, as cutting through the Meridian pathways is apt to interfere with the flow of Qi along them. In most cases, the body learns to reestablish adequate flow in the healing process, but not always. Drugs, on the other hand, are known to have dramatic side effects on the internal organs, and it is not hard to visualize how this can lead to a problem with Qi getting into or out of a Meridian connected to and maintained by such an affected organ.

In the Prologue I raised the question of which side of the body to treat at the selected Point. I believe the Vikruti pulse is also a good guide for making this decision. If the three Doshas will become more even as a result of the chosen Point stimulation on a given side, then it should be beneficial to treat on that side, but one must be clear as to whether the technique is Tonifying or Sedating. As a simple example, in a Metal CF patient who constitutionally has a Large Intestine Deficiency (Jupita), suppose you decide to Tonify a Point on the Large Intestine Meridian. This treatment will be best applied on either side that has a Vata/Kapha Vikruti pulse. It would be better not to treat the Large Intestine on the side that has a Pitta Vikruti pulse. In such a case it would be preferable to Tonify a Point on the Lung Meridian on that side. If only a Vata or a Kapha pulse is felt, treatment of the Large Intestine Meridian on that side may be helpful, but there also may be an Entry/Exit block, as discussed above. Most FEA practitioners have been taught to treat bilaterally except in certain unusual situations such as Akabane imbalances. This bilateral treatment is not necessarily wrong, as it will be effective for improving the Elemental balance, but the advantage of unilateral treatment, where indicated, is that it also improves the Doshic balance at the same time. I have found that in general, when applying transfer strategies, it is most helpful to treat unilaterally on the side that needs Tonification to balance the Doshas, but this must be weighed against other factors. It also appears to be a general rule that treating the opposite side of the body to the location of the most prominent symptoms is preferable. Finally, choosing the side of the body with the greater imbalance between the carotid and radial pulses also seems to be a useful guide. If the findings are in conflict, bilateral treatment is probably safer. In my experience, this approach has been extremely effective. Puramo's treatment style typically involves using two different Four Needle combinations on opposite sides of the body. I have also had good success using this approach, basing the choice of Four Needle Points on the Vikruti and Prakriti findings. Having said that, experience shows that bilateral treatment is quite effective in most cases, and avoids the possibility of inadvertently creating an Akabane imbalance if there has been a mistake in the initial pulse diagnosis.

Having raised the topic of contralateral needling, I'd like to add some information about another Korean style of treatment that also uses contralateral treatment almost exclusively, and will explicate the basis for one of the cases to be presented. I first learned this approach, called "Pyung Chim," from H. B. Kim[4] and later found that it is an adaptation of Sa Am's Four Needle technique for cooling Heat or heating Cold conditions.[5] Some information on this subject can also be found in Byoung Kim's book.[6] This treatment was also taught to me by a Vietnamese teacher many years before either of these Koreans,[7] so I believe it was widespread in traditional acupuncture circles in the past. The basic idea is that most pains and also a number of other conditions that can be clearly assigned to a given Meridian or Organ can be treated by simply Sedating the Fire Point and Tonifying the Water Point of the contralateral involved Meridian. This treatment can be amplified in several ways. The same polarity treatment of the other branch (arm vs. leg) of the same SEL Meridian can be added, if indicated by symptoms. Also the coupled Meridian (Zang/Fu pair) can also be added, if indicated, but the polarity of treatment at the Fire and Water Points must be reversed for the coupled Meridian Points.[8] These needles are all inserted contralateral to the main symptom. It is possible to

4   Kim, H. B., "Korean Acupuncture." Class notes, Los Angeles, 2006.

5   Heat may be assumed if the pulse rate is over 80 beats per minute, while Cold may be assumed if the pulse rate is less than 60 beats per minute. These are general guides, not absolute limits or criteria for these diagnoses.

6   Kim, B., *The Silver Bullet, KOSA*. Buena Park: KOSA of the Americas, 2012.

7   Truong Thin, class on "Vietnamese Acupuncture," Portland, 1996.

8   This method is part of Pyung Chim doctrine, but differs from Byoung Kim's description of Sa Am acupuncture, in which these coupled Meridian Fire and Water Points are treated with the same polarity as the original Meridian, still on the contralateral side. Further study is needed to clarify this disagreement.

add any of these treatment parts on the affected side, but then it must be done with the opposite polarity from the contralateral treatment. I find the simplest treatment is to just treat the involved Meridian initially contralaterally, and only add additional needles if the response is less than anticipated in terms of pulses and other signs and symptoms. These techniques will be illustrated in the case histories, but for now, let me describe a simple example: Suppose someone presents with pain along the Small Intestine Meridian of the left arm. The Pyung Chim treatment would be to Sedate SI 5 and Tonify SI 2 on the right side. If this person also had occasional left side low back pain, I might add UB 60 in Sedation and UB 66 in Tonification on the right side. If instead they had heart disease or angina, I might add HE 8 in Tonification and HE 3 in Sedation on the right side instead. Actually, Sa Am's Four Needle technique, of which this is a truncated version, is much more complex and flexible, and offers many Point combinations to suit different diagnoses. His Heating and Cooling formulae can be found in several references.[9]

At this point, I'd like to say a few words about how I decide the length of time to leave needles in place, and when to decide that any given treatment is finished. There are actually many ways of making these decisions, but ideally they should all be based on a reexamination of the patient, confirming that a change for the better has occurred. These findings may include improvements in the pulses, or any of the signs originally noted to be abnormal, be they color, odor, vocal quality, emotion, bodily posture, tension, etc. Reduced tenderness at Ah Shi, Alarm, or any other places on the body are another form of feedback that the treatment was helpful. This approach uses provocation by the practitioner to bring out the improvement, and needs greater care on the practitioner's part not to cause undue discomfort to the patient. A form of induced feedback that tends to avoid this possibility is applied kinesiology, or muscle testing. I find Omura's bidigital O-ring test to be quite helpful as a form of treatment feedback in this regard (see Figure 16.1).[10]

I usually consider a treatment incomplete if the O-ring test does not show better muscle strength. Finally, the patient's report of a change in their symptoms is not to be ignored. Sometimes a patient feels so much better that there is no question about the treatment being finished successfully. In such a case it is important not to try to "gild the lily" by continuing with more treatment in the quest to balance all the pulses. Such an endeavor may result in a reversion to the initial state, as the ability to change can be overburdened. One's clinical experience should lead one to develop a sense of how much change in the pulses or other signs and symptoms is reasonable to expect in any

9   Lee, J. K. and Bae, S. K., *Korean Acupuncture*. Seoul: Ko Mun Sa, 1974; Yoo Tae Woo, *Koryo Hand Acupuncture*, vol. 1 (ed. P. Eckman). Seoul: Eum Yang Mek Jin, 1988; Kim, H. B., *Minibook of Oriental Medicine*. Anaheim, CA: Qpuncture, 2009; and Kim, 2012.

10   Omura, Y., "O-Ring Test" class, Los Angeles, 1988.

given patient. Jane Grissmer, a FEA practitioner and teacher with many years of experience, has written about the dangers of expecting more change than a person is capable of accomplishing, and thereby losing what was initially a perfect treatment.[11] I am grateful to her for stating this explicitly, as it addresses a temptation to which all practitioners are subject.

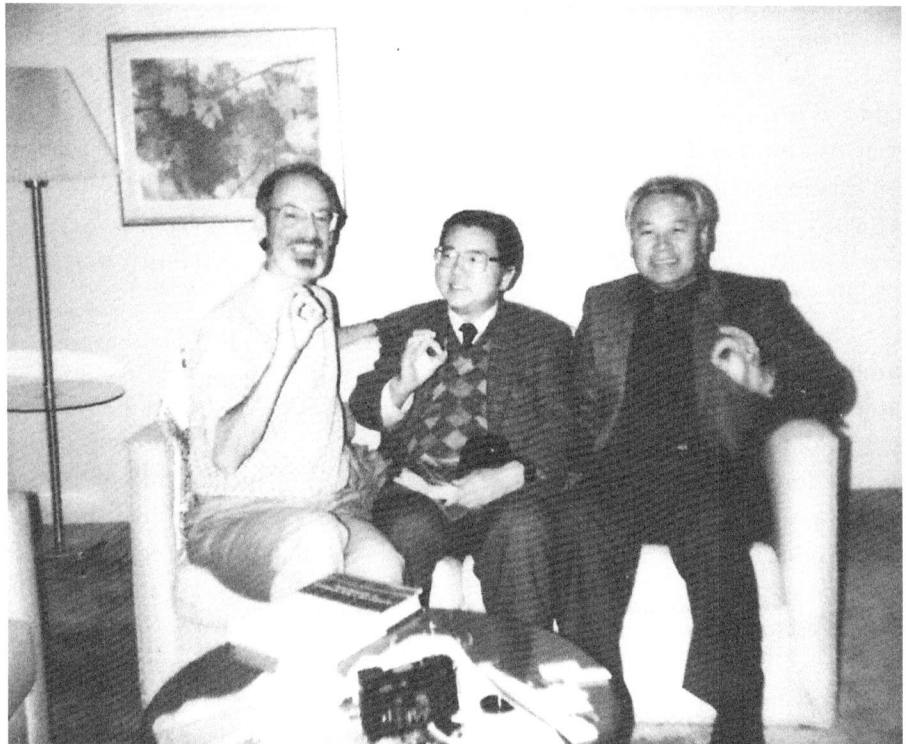

Figure 16.1 Omura's bidigital O-ring Test[12]

---

11   Jane Grissmer, personal communcation regarding her posting on www.taialumni@yahoogroups.com.

12   From left to right: Peter Eckman, Yoshiyaki Omura, and Chae Lew. When I was assisting Yoo Tae Woo at a seminar in New York, he expressed a desire to meet Dr. Omura, so I arranged a get-together. Yoo took this polaroid of the three of us demonstrating Omura's O-ring test, which Yoo adapted for KHA by later manufacturing a strain gauge to quantify finger strength. I find the strain gauge less reliable than the O-ring test, but its one advantage is that it can be used for self-testing.

CHAPTER 17

A FEW MORE WORDS ABOUT TREATMENT

In Chapter 19 I will give some examples of how this constitutional and conditional analysis has been helpful in my own practice. I typically treat patients over an extended period of time, addressing their initial complaints, but always trying to pay attention to their overall state of health and balance. There is insufficient space for me to cover even one patient's complete course of treatment, let alone the variety I'd like to present in order to give a proper feeling for the possibilities inherent in combined constitutional and conditional analyses. Thus the cases, while all describing real individuals that I have treated, have been compressed, and only certain aspects of their treatment are mentioned. Many of these individuals began seeing me well before I had completed the models introduced in this text, so the diagnosis presented in each case reflects my understanding at that time. Working with each of them has been part of the process by which I formulated this constitutional/conditional approach. Not every patient's clinical course has been an unqualified success, but I have learned something from treating every one of my patients, and I'm truly grateful for their trust in my judgment. I began writing up the case histories quite a while before the methods I am now using were in their current state, so the initial set of cases were mainly guided by my work with Ayurvedic Dosha and Korean acupuncture theories. The more recent case histories which follow can be found to include the newer emphasis on Six Level diagnosis, Subdosha considerations, and the introduction of Yin and Yang conditional pulse distinctions.

Do not be discouraged if this methodology seems to give inconsistent results at first. With practice, and the discipline to ask why when treatments are not successful, you are much more likely to make progress. There is one additional word of caution I mentioned before, but I wish to re-emphasize. Should the practitioner incorporate aspects of Ayurvedic medicine into the therapeutic regimen, it should be on the basis of a thorough understanding of both the Vikruti (Superficial, Subdosha, and ideally the tissue or Dhatu level as well) and the Prakriti. I do not know of any Ayurvedic practitioners who treat based on the Prakriti alone.[1]

Although this book is about constitutional/conditional diagnosis, there can be no abstract certainty regarding such a subject. The test of any theory is its utility, which in this matter comes down to treatment and response. Of course by definition, one does not treat the constitution (which is invariant, and cannot change in response to treatment), but one can treat the present condition with respect to the individual's constitution. My suspicion is that many potential readers will have been trained in the Five Element style, in which it is often said that one should not treat symptoms, so I will start the case presentations with examples of how to use the methods taught in this book, while at the same time keeping the focus on the CF. As practitioners of FEA are well aware, merely knowing the CF does not lead automatically to the choice of treatment on any given occasion. I will try to illustrate how knowledge of the Vikruti pulse, reflecting the current energetic state, can help in treatment formulation, especially with regard to emphasis on either the Zang or Fu Meridian/Official in the constitutional Element.

Following the FEA oriented cases, the next set of cases will illustrate how I use Korean Constitutional Acupuncture methods, and attempt to present a rational understanding of how the Auxiliary Formulae can be selected to address specific kinds of illness without discarding either the constitutional perspective nor abandoning the individualization of treatment selection. Since all the Points used in this treatment style are Five Element Points, I will also explain how to "pre-test" a proposed treatment using gold and silver (aluminum) press pellets on KHA hand Points.[2] These Points are easy to locate, and are described in Appendix 1. Some of the more commonly used constitutional formulae, which have been described by either Kuon or his disciples, are to be found in Appendix 2.

---

1   Some authors, however, use the term Prakriti in a similar fashion to the way the word constitution is used in popular speech, KHA, and sometimes in TCM, i.e. to refer to the condition or "acquired constitution." An example of this usage can be found in Svoboda, R., *Prakruti, Your Ayurvedic Constitution*. Wilmot, AR: Lotus Light Publications, 1988. Needless to say, while Svoboda's therapeutic recommendations may be accurate, I believe they are aimed at treating the Vikruti, not the Prakriti. His understanding of the term Prakriti appears to be different than that of the classical texts, and is certainly different than the meaning I'm using in this text.

2   Press pellets can be ordered from the Koryo Institute in Los Angeles among other distributors. The author has no connection with this or any other supplier.

Following the KCA cases, I will show some examples of using the other strategies discussed, including SEL evaluation, Subdosha evaluation, and treatment based on the "Dragons" and the Extraordinary Meridians. Case 29 is one in which I used a Six Level triangular equilibration treatment (from the French Medical Acupuncture tradition),[3] based on the constitution, to deal with an injury that had not responded as well as might be expected to conservative treatment, multiple surgeries, and other acupunctural approaches, and is one in which I later switched treatment to Sa Am's Four Needle technique for taking out Cold. I have included this case to encourage practitioners of other styles of acupuncture to consider whether the methods proposed in this text might be usefully applied in the context of their own traditions. The reader is reminded of Sir Izaak Walton's admonition that "there will still be more new experiments left for the trial of other men that succeed us."

---

3   For a discussion of triangular equilibration, see: Helms, J., *Acupuncture Energetics*. Berkeley, CA: Medical Acupuncture Publishers, 1995, pp.624–628.

CHAPTER 18

THE FOUR NEEDLE TECHNIQUE, FIVE ELEMENTS, AND YIN/ YANG REVISITED

The Four Needle technique, attributed to the Korean ascetic Sa Am, constitutes a high water mark in the history of classical acupuncture theory. Many practitioners are familiar with the most basic of Sa Am's formulae: Tonification and Sedation of individual Meridians. Less well known are his formulae for Dispelling Heat and Cold from individual Meridians, and readers are encouraged to consult the works by Byoung Kim and Yoo Tae Woo for further information on these two applications. Even less discussed are the twentieth and twenty-first-century developments of Four Needle technique thinking originated by Kuon Dowon, and later investigated by Puramo Chong and Lee Dong Woong. I have paid attention to all of these teachers' recommendations, and have tried to organize their thinking into a schema that might help both practitioner and student to better understand the underlying principles. Of course, these are based on the Classics, but there is much room for interpretation in both Five Element and Yin/Yang theory. What I will present in this chapter represents the views of each of the aforementioned teachers, with my own synthesis, based on an analysis of these prior teachings, and my own clinical results.

Sa Am's original formulae for Tonification and Sedation employ the famous law of Mother–Son. According to this law, in order to Tonify a Meridian, one should Tonify its Mother Meridian (by the Five Element Sheng Cycle),[1] and, in order to Sedate a Meridian, one should Sedate its Son Meridian by this same Cycle. This approach is fully compatible with the FEA tradition, as taught by Worsley. The understanding of the Mother–Son law embodied in these examples is based on the notion that the Sheng Cycle of the Elements is unidirectional, always going from Wood to Fire to Earth to Metal to Water to Wood, etc. However, we know that there are other sequences of the Elements that are manifested in nature. The experiences of many practitioners, notably from the Japanese Meridian Therapy school, and the various Korean sources previously cited, demonstrate that Tonifying the Son Meridian also is effective, at times, for Tonifying its Mother Meridian. Likewise, Sedating the Mother Meridian can be effective in Sedating its Son Meridian. What this means is that, depending on circumstances, the Sheng Cycle may be applied in either a forward or a backward direction. Similarly, either the Grandparent Meridian or the Grandchild Meridian can be used in the other half of the Four Needle technique: i.e. to Tonify a Meridian one can Sedate either of these two, and to Sedate a Meridian one can Tonify either of these two. This aspect of Five Element theory can be understood to imply that the Control Cycle (Xiang Ke) can function in either a clockwise (forward) or counterclockwise (backward) direction,[2] or alternatively, one can simply acknowledge the usefulness of both the Control Cycle and the Counteracting Cycle (Xiang Wu)[3] in the second half of the Four Needle technique. All of these alternatives represent possible interpretations of classical passages such as *Nanjing* 50, where the effects of Mother, Son, Grandmother, and Grandson on any given Meridian are discussed.

If one examines all the formulae for variations of the Four Needle technique posited by Sa Am, Kuon, Kim, Chong, and Lee for Tonification and Sedation, they all share the following ideas: For any Meridian, both its Mother and its Son should be treated in the same polarity as the Meridian in question (either by Tonification or Sedation), while that same Meridian's Grandparent and Grandchild should be treated in the opposite polarity. I have mentioned before

---

1   The Mother–Son law is also used in other styles of acupuncture by employing the Horary sequence of the 12 Meridians, in which, for example, the Liver is the Mother of the Lung. It is quite clear that the Four Needle technique is not applicable to this use of the Mother–Son law, as it is an aspect of Five Element theory, and the Horary sequence has no relationship to Five Element theory.

2   It is important to note that the word Xiang in both Cycles does not *mean* cycle. Rather it means mutually affecting, so in a literal way Xiang Sheng means mutually producing and Xiang Ke means mutually controlling, justifying this two way interpretation. The concept of Xiang is very similar to that of Gan Ying (resonance, sometimes referred to as Xiang Ying) that I previously indicated is in my mind one of the foundational concepts in the science of TOM.

3   Mathews, R. H., *Mathews' Chinese-English Dictionary*. Cambridge, MA: Harvard University Press, 1979, no. 7194. Counteracting is the translation used in *The Essentials of Chinese Acupuncture*. Beijing: Foreign Languages Press, 1980, p.19. Other translational choices are Insult Cycle or Violation Cycle.

that Kuon's Formulae are not easy to understand,[4] and in trying to expand his theory to encompass 24 rather than 8 types, I have found this rule to be one of the essential guidelines for discovering the treatment Points for the additional constitutions.

As an example, let us look at the Fundamental formula for Sedating the Liver in an individual of Liver Excess constitution. Kuon's original formula was exactly the same as Sa Am's (Tonify LU 8 and LV 4, and Sedate HE 8 and LV 2). In its more recent incarnation, Kuon changed this Fundamental formula by altering the second half (Tonify LU 8 and LV 4, and Sedate KI 10 and LV 8). This new Fundamental formula was adopted by both Chong and Lee, and has proven useful in my own experience with two provisos: Certain individuals of Liver Excess constitution respond better to Kuon's original formula, while others respond better to his revised formula. Also, these new "Four Needle" formulae are intended to be used only for individuals of each specific constitution, in this case those of Liver Excess constitution (Jupito). For individuals of other constitutional types who happen to have Liver Excess conditions, the internal Elemental makeup of the constitution, presented in Chapter 10, provides a better guide for Point selection to Sedate the Liver. A somewhat more complicated example occurs in the evolution of the Fundamental formula for Tonification in the case of individuals of the Large Intestine Deficiency constitutional type (Jupita). Again, Kuon's original formula was the same as Sa Am's (Tonify ST 36 and LI 11, and Sedate SI 5 and LI 5). At an intermediate step, Kuon changed this to: Tonify UB 66 and LI 2, and Sedate GB 41 and LI 3. One can see that, in this case, Kuon is employing the variant possibilities of both the Sheng and Ke Cycles. In its final incarnation, Kuon changed this Fundamental formula to: Tonify SP 3 and LU 9, and Sedate LV 1 and LU 11. Both Chong and Lee also adopted this new Fundamental formula, but retained Kuon's intermediate teaching as an Immune Strengthening Auxiliary formula for individuals of the Large Intestine Deficiency constitution, most likely following Kuon's usage; however, I have not seen any publication from Kuon describing this new Auxiliary formula. It is easy to see that the final transition in the Points chosen for the Fundamental formula for Large Intestine Deficiency has been the substitution of the corresponding coupled Zang Organ Meridians with their Points of the same Elemental quality, for the Points on the Fu Meridians.

The previous paragraph brings up several issues that may be sources of confusion regarding KCA. In Kuon's use of the Four Needle technique, the order of needling differs for individuals of different constitutional types.

---

4   The problem with Kuon's formulae is not merely one of understanding their structure. Rather, it is a question of how he came to decide which Points to choose for each of the Fundamental and Auxiliary Formulae. He has never commented on this topic, to my knowledge, although the evolution of his Point choices over time is testimony that at least part of his methodology is based on trial and error.

For Greater Yin and Lesser Yin types, the rule is first Tonify and then Sedate, while for those of Greater Yang and Lesser Yang constitutions, the rule is first Sedate and then Tonify. These rules apply to both Fundamental and Auxiliary formulae in all cases. Another confusing issue is the choice of Fundamental formula for individuals of either Zang or Fu constitutions. As was seen above, the Fundamental formula for Liver Excess constitutional types involves treating the Liver Meridian, while the Fundamental formula for Large Intestine Deficiency constitutional types involves treating the Lung Meridian. The rule is that, for Zang constitutions, the Fundamental formula treats the Zang Organ's Meridian, while for Fu constitutions the Fundamental formula treats the Meridian of its coupled Zang Organ of the same Element. From this rule we can see that there is also an aspect of Yin/Yang consideration in KCA, as coupled Organs form a Yin/Yang pair. Also, the Auxiliary formulae for each constitution include treatment of both Zang and Fu Meridians, or in other words both Yin and Yang Meridians. However, in using the Four Needle technique, the Meridians selected for any formula must all be either Zang or Fu; there is no mixing of Points from both Zang and Fu Meridians in any one Four Needle formula. This brings up an interesting question about the Control Cycle: According to Thambirajah and others, the Control Cycle operates from Yang to Yin Meridians and vice versa, while the Four Needle technique clearly uses the Control Cycle from Yang to Yang Meridians and from Yin to Yin Meridians. In FEA, Worsley taught that the Control Cycle only operated from Yin to Yin Meridians, a doctrine that reflected one stage in the teachings Worsley adopted from Jacques Lavier. In my view, there is no correct or incorrect doctrine at stake here, but rather an issue that I first brought up in *Closing the Circle*: When using any aspect of a particular style of traditional acupuncture, it is important to know all aspects of that style. One should not merely pick and choose parts from different traditions and expect that the result will be coherent and effective. As the following case histories will illustrate, each component of the treatments that I will describe can be clearly identified with a particular style of acupuncture, and is supported by the pulse diagnosis and other findings that are germane to that style.

CHAPTER 19

CASE HISTORIES

CASE 1

S. I., a 47-year-old man, came for treatment of chronic sinusitis, which had been a problem ever since he was three years old! In his childhood, the main manifestation had been asthmatic attacks, but these had evolved into recurrent episodes of sore throat, earaches, and fatigue, which continued in spite of occasional Western medical treatment (antibiotics), 20 years of Tai Ji Quan practice, meditation, and the self administration of Chinese herbal remedies, including Yin Qiao San and Bi Yan Wan (he is an alternative healthcare practitioner). He had previously been treated by several Chinese acupuncturists who diagnosed his problem as a combination of Yin Deficiency and Damp Heat resulting from Stomach and Spleen imbalances. Treatments typically brought symptomatic relief of varying degree, but no lasting resolution. The symptoms have usually been bilateral, and feel like blocked Eustachian tubes, with tenderness in both cheeks below the eyes, accompanied by a heavy, clouded, lethargic feeling, but a CAT scan of his sinuses was negative for signs of infection.

Systems review revealed that he was otherwise a healthy individual who had been a vegetarian in the past, but has since been an omnivore for more than 20 years. He tends to have a ravenous appetite, and is benefited by almost any kind of exercise. He was recently divorced, but was already involved in a new relationship.

On initial examination he appeared somewhat anxious, with a blood pressure of 138/82 (elevated); his tongue was red without much coat, but was both stickily moist and cracked at the base. Color, sound, odor, and emotion

(CSOE) led me in the direction of the Wood Element (lack of anger and lack of shouting being the more apparent signs). His body shape (broad flat chest) is typical of the Greater Yang constitution, and his KCA pulse was of the Hespero type. His Prakriti pulse was Kapha. His 12 pulses[1] showed the most normal feeling in the Cun position, wiry and small in the left Guan and wiry and large in the right Guan positions, and weak in both Chi positions.

I chose this as the first case to present because it demonstrates the coherency of the various constitutional diagnostic models I've discussed. In FEA he is a Wood CF. In SCM he is a Greater Yang type, and would probably benefit by a return to a vegetarian/seafood diet (he has reduced his meat intake following my suggestion). In KCA his constitution is Liver Deficiency, for which the basic treatment is the Four Needle technique to Tonify the Liver. This involves simultaneously Tonifying the Kidney (weak Chi pulse) and sedating the Lung (his respiratory system being the locale of his lifelong inflammatory problems with asthma and sinusitis). He has always responded very well to that particular treatment, but of course other treatments have been used to stabilize the Wood Element, with attention to the other Elements as necessary. One interesting aspect of his case is that although his Prakriti is Kapha, his Vikruti pulse is almost always Pitta/Vata, so it is important not to continually Tonify his Liver alone, as that would aggravate both Pitta and Vata. Two ways to remedy this are to also Tonify the Gall Bladder, or to sedate the Stomach, both of which will decrease Pitta and Vata, but this particular presentation can also be indicative of an Entry/Exit block between Stomach and Spleen Meridians. The presence of such a block would explain his exaggerated hunger (Excess building up in the Stomach) and the focus of his prior practitioners on the Stomach and Spleen. I used all of the strategies mentioned, and within a month and a half his blood pressure had returned to normal (119/70), he had only minor symptoms from his sinuses for over a year, and he has begun to look at the psychoemotional issues in his life that have to do with assertiveness, planning, and decision making. He recently volunteered that he has caught up on deferred tasks that he had been putting off for the past two to three years.

CASE 2

N. N., a 32-year-old man, had previously been treated by TCM and FEA practitioners for Meniere's disease, which he had been coping with for 13 years, with only slight improvement. The main symptoms were vertigo (with sweating, nausea, and vomiting when severe), tinnitus, hearing loss, and neck

---

1   This person was treated before I began separately examining Yin and Yang locations for Cun, Guan, and Chi. At the time, the positions I used would be those I now designate as the Yang positions. This was also before I began using the SEL *Maijing* map.

pain, especially on the right side. There was no obvious precipitating etiology, although he had suffered several concussions earlier in life as a result of car accidents. His symptoms began right after high school graduation, when he did a cartwheel in celebration. He works in finance, and is happy with his job. Western medicines including Meclizine and Dyazide were of no help, and although steroids and valium provided some relief, he rarely took them because of their side effects.

Systems review revealed a tendency towards a feeling of fatigue as his only other complaint. He had recently had Lasik eye surgery for myopia, which was successful and uncomplicated. Other than work, the only other stress he experienced was around dating.

On examination his left Guan pulses tend to be the strongest ones,[2] and his Prakriti pulse is Kapha. His left carotid is noticeably bigger than his left radial pulse, whereas they are fairly equal on the right side. On first impression it is tempting to see his constitution as the same as in Case 1, but several findings do not fit, including his "strong" Wood pulses. His body type is between ectomorphic and mesomorphic, but he does not have a particularly broad chest. Finally, his KCA pulse is of the Mercuria type, which would make his constitution Lesser Yin. The only constitutions that fit these findings are Stomach Deficiency and Gall Bladder Excess,[3] but his strong Wood pulses and unremarkable Earth pulses led me to diagnose him as a Wood CF, needing Sedation treatment primarily.[4] He has done well with this approach, and is almost never sweaty, dizzy, or nauseated, but does still have a low level of tinnitus. Finding and dispersing particularly sensitive points on the Gall Bladder Meridian on the head has been helpful, as has a Korean technique called "Pyung Chim" which is a form of Yin/Yang balancing. This consists of Tonifying the Fire Point and sedating the Water Point on his symptomatic side Gall Bladder Meridian, while Sedating the Fire Point and Tonifying the Water Point on his left (contralateral) Gall Bladder Meridian. This is a very useful treatment for one-sided symptoms along a particular Meridian, which is usually employed to treat pain, but is actually helpful for almost any symptom

---

2   This individual was also treated before I began separately examining Yin and Yang position pulses, or the SEL pulses.

3   Gall Bladder Excess is one of the Lesser Yin constitutional types, added by Lee Dong Woong to Kuon's original KCA system.

4   It is interesting to note that the diagnosis of Excess Yang in the Gall Bladder matches his response to Western medications. Diuretics, which deplete fluids, would tend to increase Yang and not help his condition, while both steroids and valium, which act to calm the nervous and immune systems (increasing Yin), were symptomatically effective. Notice also that his symptoms were predominantly right sided, while his carotid/radial diagnosis showed a Yang Excess condition on the left side, exemplifying the rationale for contralateral treatment discussed in the text.

that can be localized to a single Meridian.[5] Although I learned the Pyung Chim technique from one of my Korean teachers,[6] I had previously been taught an almost identical protocol by a Vietnamese teacher,[7] so I suspect that it has its roots in the pre-TCM classical traditions, most likely in the Korean Four Needle technique of Sa Am.[8] During the two years this patient has been in treatment, he has not had a single severe episode of vertigo, in spite of a significant increase in life stress. He was downsized from the job he loved, and is in litigation around that, but has stayed in good spirits and even carried a new relationship through to marriage. After two years in treatment, he moved out of state, and was feeling well.

CASE 3

H. T., a 54-year-old man, initiated treatment because of increasing urinary frequency which his physician had diagnosed as benign prostatic hypertrophy. The symptoms had been gradually increasing over a period of four to five years. In addition, it was often difficult to initiate urination. His PSA test was normal, so his physician had tried prescribing Flomax, an alpha adrenergic blocker, which gave symptomatic relief, but did not eliminate the urinary retention seen on ultrasound. Based on this result, surgery was recommended, but he decided to try alternative means first. He had previously tried acupuncture and herbs with another practitioner for three to four months, without improvement. Over-the-counter Western herbs, including saw palmetto, pygeum, nettle root, and pumpkin seeds, were ineffective, at which point he consulted me. His medical history was entirely benign except for being overweight and having both high cholesterol and high blood pressure for at least four years, although he has had several episodes of fevers of unknown origin over many years that resulted in bouts of fatigue. He is a happily married psychologist with no obvious precipitating cause for his problems.

On examination, his blood pressure was 128/92 (high) and his pulses were particularly strong in the right Guan position, but otherwise fairly even. His body type is between mesomorphic and endomorphic, with a large Middle Heater, and he is typically much colder in the Lower Middle Heater. On the right side

---

5   In retrospect, this approach would make sense for individuals with a somewhat rapid pulse, especially the contralateral component. I did not remark on his pulse rate at the time, and he has since moved out of state. See footnote 8 below for a reference explaining this addendum.

6   H. B. Kim, in 2006.

7   Truong Thin, in 1996.

8   Byoung Kim discusses the history of this approach in *The Silver Bullet, KOSA*. Buena Park: KOSA of the Americas, 2012. Most acupuncturists who are familiar with the Four Needle technique are only aware of its use for Tonification or Sedation, but its originator also described Point prescriptions for treating Hot or Cold conditions, and the Pyung Chim approach is apparently derived from these formulae.

his carotid is clearly bigger than his radial pulse. His KCA pulse is of the Jupita type, although early on I had thought it was of the Jupito type (they are quite similar), and had initially diagnosed him as having a Liver Excess constitution. He did well with Wood sedation treatments, and his urinary symptoms became much less troublesome. Even his blood pressure came down for a while, but eventually it started to increase again, and he developed some minor right sided musculoskeletal complaints. At that point I realized that he could not be of Liver Excess constitution as a result of finding a Jupita KCA pulse, so I changed his constitutional diagnosis to Small Intestine Excess, as I had not yet developed a way to differentiate that constitution from Bladder weakness, and his CSOE presentation seemed more indicative of Fire than Water. Subsequent treatment to Sedate the Small Intestine has resolved these minor complaints, and also brought his blood pressure back down to 120/81 (normal); however, he still had an occasional episode of high fever and fatigue. In the interim, I had incorporated the *Nanjing* depth discrimination to my methodology, and found that his Water pulse was not strongest at the deep level, while his Fire pulse on the left wrist was strongest at its proper superficial level. Therefore I changed his diagnosis again, this time to Bladder Deficiency. Thus he is a Water CF rather than a Wood or Fire CF. Interestingly, Liver Excess, Small Intestine Excess, and Bladder Deficiency are all Greater Yin constitutions, and it has been my experience that treating the correct Sasang (SCM) typology often gives beneficial (though partial) results, even if the exact constitutional type is mistaken. Since changing his diagnosis he has finally begun to lose weight (about 10 pounds), and is now at the lowest he's weighed in 25 years. One other interesting aspect of his treatment is that I have encouraged him to apply heat to the Lower Middle Heater area on a daily basis, as I have found that heating the consistently cold areas of the abdomen has been associated with faster results in many of my patients. Having satisfied myself about the accuracy of his current diagnosis, I restudied his case history to see if I could account for the initial development of his problems. I noticed that both of his parents suffered from heart disease, his mother having had hypertension and his father having died from a heart attack at 77. My supposition is that this patient's problems were a direct result of his genetic constitutional predisposition (Deficient Water and Excess Fire), and that keeping his Fire and Water Elements in balance may ameliorate his familial tendency to develop heart disease.

CASE 4

E. W., a 55-year-old man, initially consulted me because of "stress at work." He had a history of right sided low back pain since childhood, which had been helped in the past by acupuncture and physical therapy, and was told he had two bad discs in his back. For the past few years he had been experiencing erectile dysfunction, helped by Viagra, and had just ended an extramarital affair. The rest of his history was noncontributory.

On examination, his SCM pulse was of the Lesser Yang type. His Prakriti pulse was Pitta/Kapha. The KCA pulse was of the Mercuria type. Putting all these findings together leads to Triple Heater Deficiency as the only possible constitution. Thus he is a Fire CF, but his locus is Ministerial Fire rather than Imperial Fire, as was a preliminary diagnosis in the previous case.

His initial treatment included draining Aggressive Energy from UB 13 and 14, followed by Tonification of PE 7 and TH 4. After that initial treatment, his back pain diminished but, more importantly, he felt calmer, less edgy, and more comfortable with people, a change that has persisted in spite of bouts of pain following trauma and muscle overuse. After a strenuous tennis game, he developed a persistent pain in his left knee, which I chose to treat using one of Richard Tan's balance points, PE 6 on the right side.[9] After a series of such treatments his knee pain resolved. I've included this aspect of his treatment because it illustrates a scenario that often occurs: with Deficiency in a Meridian, the coupled Meridian will sometimes develop an Excess condition. Dr. Tan's treatments involve a deep, strong needling technique, which is Sedating. I have recently resumed Tonifying his Pericardium Meridian because his Vikruti pulse is strongly of the Vata type, and this has alleviated his remaining minor complaints. He has been much happier in his marriage, to which he has recommitted himself. His wife is also a patient of mine, and she recently reported that he is a changed man since treatment ended several years ago, he has felt fine physically, and that their marriage is doing "terrific."

CASE 5

E. F., a 45-year-old man, sought treatment for multiple stress related problems. His main complaint was a feeling of heaviness in his chest, especially on taking a deep breath. He had previously been diagnosed with asthma, but it had been under control until the recent death of his mother. He also experienced bilateral groin pain (with a history of bilateral hernia repair in his teens), periodic constipation (like rabbit pellets), occasional blood in his ejaculate, and poor sleep. He has a brother with cerebral palsy, whose care is divided up among several family members, and the brother also suffers from pancreatitis attacks. His marriage was not doing well because he was too preoccupied by his stress to give it much attention.

On examination, he was extremely anxious, and had the most resistance to abdominal palpation I have ever encountered in any of my patients. He did not

9   Tan, R. and Rush, S., *Twelve and Twelve in Acupuncture*. San Diego, CA: Author, 1991, p.33.

experience pain on palpation, but could not stop the severe involuntary muscle guarding. His Lower Middle Heater was colder than the other Heaters. He had a Vata/Pitta Prakriti pulse of the Jupito type. Thus his diagnosis is either Spleen Deficiency or Liver Excess. Subsequent examination revealed that his proximal SEL Guan pulses were ulnar deviated, thus confirming Spleen Deficiency. His treatment involved counseling and support as a necessary adjunct to the acupuncture. He had a life-long fear of air travel, and was wanting to switch to a less stressful job, but one that would necessitate flying, so that obstacle became a major goal in treatment. With Earth Element Tonification treatments, all of his problems improved, and he was able to travel by plane without much anxiety. Also, the reduced stress greatly improved his relationship with his wife, and he has been essentially asymptomatic for the last two years, in spite of letting the acupuncture sessions lapse. Finally, some mysteriously elevated liver enzymes, that were found on routine testing in the past, have returned to the normal range.

CASE 6

X. N., a 69-year-old man with a complicated medical history, initially sought treatment because of shortness of breath, out of control diabetes, and severe bouts of arthritis, during which he found it hard to get out of chairs or walk any distance. It took some probing to get him to acknowledge that these problems caused him to feel frustrated and short tempered a lot of the time, and he was not enjoying his retired life, in spite of being in good financial, social, and marital status. At the time, he was on Prednisone, Plaquenil, Celebrex, Glucophage, Atrovent, Albuterol, and Claritin on a daily basis. He attributed his breathing difficulties to 30 years of smoking (which he quit seven years before), but had no idea why his joints periodically became swollen and painful, accompanied by laboratory indicators of inflammation (increased ESR). There was no family history of either diabetes or arthritis.

On examination he was significantly overweight, with a body type between mesomorph and endomorph, and he had a prominent umbilical hernia. His blood pressure was 136/70 and his tongue was red, dry, and cracked, but his joints did not appear to be red, hot, or swollen and his lungs were clear. CSOE evaluation suggested an Earth CF (especially fragrant and yellow), and Tonifying his Earth Meridians quickly brought significant relief of all his original complaints. His mood became quite jovial, while his blood pressure dropped to 120/60 in a matter of weeks. He continued treatment for over eight years, and had virtually no trouble with arthritis during that time. His blood sugar returned to the normal range and he rarely had any trouble with his breathing, despite his continued overweight condition and refusal to stop alcohol use. Unfortunately, in his late seventies he suddenly developed bone cancer and was unable to continue acupuncture. I've included his case history because he fits the FEA and 24 constitutions models so perfectly, and showed remarkable improvement in his health and well-being despite the poor shape he was in at first.

Constitutionally, his morphology is typical of Greater Yin types. He has a notably colder Lower Middle Heater, and has felt better from applying heat there, per my suggestion. He has a Jupito pulse and a Vata/Pitta Prakriti. This perfectly describes a Spleen Deficient constitution, which is no doubt the underlying cause of his diabetes, but it is curious that there are no other diabetics in his family. I managed to convince him to eat more sensibly, but was unable to get him to eliminate alcohol completely, although he cut down on his consumption. He and his wife were able to enjoy frequent cruises, where rich food and alcohol are always at hand, and perhaps that was more than acupuncture treatment could compensate.

CASE 7

L. T., a 50-year-old woman, came for treatment because she was "very stressed out." She was working, taking care of a 15-year-old daughter, and going through a house remodeling, which meant living in the garage for several months, all at the same time. She described it as "everything caving in on me, everything drops, and I'm so depressed I want to hide."

Fifteen years ago she had erythema nodosum, diagnosed as an autoimmune problem, and was also diagnosed as being hypothyroid, for which she has been maintained on Synthroid. For the last ten years she has had almost continuous skipping of her heartbeat, but doesn't feel it. Her problems seem to have started when she was pregnant with her daughter and had a fibroid in her uterus at the same time. She almost miscarried at six months after an argument with her husband. Since that time she's felt out of control. She had previously been depressed in her teens, when her parents divorced.

She had successfully used acupuncture in the past for recurrent insomnia, but had not found it effective for back pains. Systems review revealed that she was chronically constipated, usually having bowel movements only every three days. Her father had been abusive, and was described as sad and depressed. He died of emphysema at 77. Her mother was described as narcissistic and attention grabbing. Overall, she felt like she took after her father in most ways.

Diagnostically, she presented quite a challenge. Her voice was laughing in quality, emotion was anger, while color and odor were not clear. Her pulse displayed frequent premature beats, which made interpretation difficult. Her tongue was thin with a red tip, but clearly had an unusual crack in the Lung area. Testing for Aggressive Energy was ambiguous,[10] due to dermatographia, but after leaving those needles in for a while, I began treating her as a Metal CF, because I felt that she was expressing a familial sadness, just like her father. She responded very well to this approach, and I was eventually able to determine the other findings that allowed for a constitutional diagnosis as follows: Vata/Kapha Prakriti and Jupita pulse type. These determine Large Intestine Deficiency as her constitution. She did well in treatment, including the resolution of her irregular pulse and her constipation, and a better sense of well-being, until she found out her husband had been having an affair, at which point all her symptoms returned. He vowed to end the affair, and she tried to salvage the marriage. She was helped by treatments employing both Internal Dragons (IDs) and External Dragons (EDs),[11] and I chose to use a Tonifying technique on all the Points because both the Earth and Water Elements tend towards Deficiency in the Large Intestine Deficiency constitution (Mother and Son Elements). Happily, she was able to save her marriage, but would periodically fall back into depressions after working in the office where her husband had had the affair. Interestingly, she responded best to the ED treatments, as if the office environment was the source of her possession. She is in the process of finding someone else to take over her job there, so as to avoid repeatedly exposing herself to such a toxic situation. When her abdomen presents a Yang Excess pattern (sensitive at ST 25), she responds very well to Tonifying her Lungs (increasing Vata and Kapha), while when her abdomen presents a Yin Excess pattern (sensitive at SP 15), she responds better to Tonifying her Large Intestines (increasing Pitta). This use of the abdominal pattern closely mimics the Vikruti findings on her pulse, which can flip back and forth between Pitta one day, and Vata/Kapha the next. These findings are one reason I believe Ayurvedic pulse diagnosis of both the constitution (Prakriti) and the condition (Vikruti) can lead to more refined acupuncture treatments. She stopped treatment at a time when she was feeling well, and has only recently resumed treatment for a back injury. She reported that she was still feeling fine emotionally, even two years after her last visit, and her irregular pulses have not recurred.

CASE 8

N. M. is a 26-year-old woman who was referred to me by a senior faculty member at the Traditional Acupuncture Institute (FEA style), who had been treating her since about age 12, and needed to find someone in San Francisco to take over her treatment. I'm pleased to include her case, not because the

---

10   See *Footsteps* for a description of this FEA treatment.

11   Internal Dragons and External Dragons are treatments for "Possession" in FEA. See both Chapter 16 and *Footsteps* for a discussion of these protocols.

results were so dramatic, but because it demonstrates the congruity of FEA and the constitutional pulse theory I have described. This young woman had been successfully treated all those years as having a Deficiency in Ministerial Fire. Her complaints were almost always more related to emotional issues than physical ones. I have found her to have Pericardium Deficiency as her constitution (Greater Yin SCM, Jupito KCA, ulnar deviation of the SEL Cun, and Vata Prakriti). I have treated her very intermittently over the last four years, using Ministerial Fire Tonification as the main strategy, but as she is quite high strung, I have found Sedating the Four Gates a helpful adjunct, and she has continued to feel that acupuncture helps her keep her emotional balance.

CASE 9

K. D., a 41-year-old man, was seen for an acute case of low back pain centered in the sacroiliac region on the left side, without radiation. It began after heavy lifting, and he found it hard to walk or stand. The situation had been ongoing for two weeks with minimal improvement from alternating ice and heat, although his impression was that the heat was more helpful, as was the application of pressure in the affected area. He had never had trouble with his low back before, but had occasional problems with a pinched nerve in his upper back. He was otherwise in good health and happy with his life, although he had recently broken off with his girlfriend.

On examination, the pulse findings were as follows: right side carotid bigger than radial, SCM pulse was Greater Yang type, KCA pulse was of the Hespera type, Prakriti pulse was Pitta/Kapha, and the right side radial pulse showed a Dai Mai pattern. These findings are compatible with either Bladder Excess or Small Intestine Deficiency. To distinguish these possibilities, I noted the following: the left Cun pulse was flipped (much deeper than its natural state), while the left Chi pulse was at its correct depth. The symptomatic area was just about at UB 27, the Back Shu Point of the Small Intestine, and there was a distinct nodule there, which responded well to both pressure and heat. Thus I diagnosed this as a case of Small Intestine Deficiency, with compensation by the Dai Mai on the opposite side. After a total of three treatments, including Source Points, Back Shu Points, transfers, and Key Points to release the Dai Mai, the symptoms disappeared completely. He had originally been taking 20 Advil a day for the pain and, along with discontinuing pain medication, he began changing to a vegetarian/seafood diet, which I believe helped his rapid recovery.

CASE 10

X. E., a 78-year-old woman with multiple medical problems, came for treatment of low back and leg pains, which severely limited her ability to walk or go up stairs. MRI revealed that she had advanced arthritis of the spine, and she was also hypertensive and had high cholesterol, diabetes, and chronic obstructive pulmonary disease (COPD). She was on nine different medications at the time, in addition to depending on a portable oxygen tank with nasal catheter. Her main concern was that the pain kept her from doing things, which she found to be quite frustrating, as she had always been very active, being a retired bank manager.

On exam, her pulses showed the radials bigger than the carotids bilaterally, but more dramatically on the left side. Her SEL pulse on the right side was ulnarly displaced in the Chi position, and she had a Lesser Yang Sasang pattern and a Saturno KCA pulse. Her Prakriti pulse was Pitta/Kapha. These findings are compatible with either Kidney Deficiency or Heart Excess, but it was her left Cun pulse that was at an abnormal depth, rather than her left Chi pulse. Thus I treated her as having Heart Excess. Sedating the Heart, opening up the Heart, Kidney, Bladder, and Small Intestine circuit (Shaoyin/Taiyang), and releasing the Chong Mai on the left side have all been helpful. She is able to spend days out shopping again, and her blood pressure and blood sugar are both staying in an acceptable range.

CASE 11

N. T. was a 39-year-old woman when she first came to see me 15 years ago with a chief complaint of anxiety attacks during the preceding six months. She had a history of surgical removal of her left ovary at age 16 due to a teratoma neoplasm. After being married, she was unable to get pregnant for several years, and underwent fertility enhancement treatments with hormones and IVF, which resulted in having twin girls (delivered by C-section) who were then three and a half years old. She described the anxiety attacks as primarily occurring while driving, with feelings of anger over lack of support from her husband, causing her to get dizzy almost to the point of passing out. Other complaints included swelling, pain, and numbness in her hands and feet (worse at night and with any weather change), headaches near the end of her menses, always feeling cold, and watering of her left eye.

The most notable findings on examination were pulses that had a bounding and wiry quality everywhere, except that they were almost imperceptible in the right Chi position. She had a slow pulse (60 per minute) and low blood pressure (90/50). Her left radial was bigger than her left carotid, and her right carotid was bigger than her right radial. Abdominal exam revealed marked tenderness at Ren 5 and some tenderness at ST 25 on the left. My initial impression (based on color, sound, odor, and emotion) was that she had a CF in Ministerial Fire, but I was unsure if it was coming from Excess or Deficiency. By KHA theory, the larger right sided carotid together with the marked tenderness at Ren 5 suggested TH Excess. I decided to test this hypothesis using metallic press pads at the KHA Points. Upon applying an aluminum pad (Sedating polarity) to the right side KHA Point corresponding to TH 10, she immediately reported a decrease in her headache and a decrease in the stiffness of her hands. She never experienced another anxiety attack. Over the years I have treated her mainly by Sedating the TH, and her headaches, swelling, and eye watering all improved or disappeared. When I later incorporated Ayurvedic pulses, SEL pulses, KCA pulses, and SCM pulses in my practice, I found that she was of a Lesser Yin constitution of the Mercuria type, with radial deviation of the Chi position and a Vata Prakriti. These findings are all consistent with, and diagnostic of, TH Excess.

During the years that I have worked with her, her main concerns have been with intimate relationships. She got divorced, and then went through a series of relationships that never quite worked out. She has gradually come to an understanding that being happy in herself is a prerequisite to a good relationship, and is presently in a fulfilling one. Looking back over her case history there are several points of interest. I had mentioned in the text the controversy over the status of the right Chi pulse, and whether it represented the Fire or Water Element. I have treated her TH Meridian as a Fire Meridian, but she clearly has manifestations of Water dysfunctions: swelling of hands and feet and watering of eyes being prominent. Her headaches, however, tend to be along the TH pathway. These findings reinforce my conclusion that Ministerial Fire also has a strong relationship with the Water Element.

CASE 12

I. T., a 36-year-old woman with a 15-year history of bipolar disorder controlled by lithium, came for treatment of left hip pain, which began two years previously after falling on it while rollerblading. She had tried various types of exercise and manipulative therapy without much benefit. She was a retired dentist, married, and had taken up weaving as a second avocation, but her main focus in life was deepening her connection to the Jewish spiritual tradition. Her pulses were remarkable for the Excess quality at the Chi position on the right side. On the right side her carotid was bigger than her radial pulse, she had a Greater Yang SCM pulse and a Hespero KCA pulse, and was convinced that following a vegetarian/seafood diet was most conducive to maintaining her sense of well-being. She also had scars on her back at the L 1 level from herpetic lesions dating back to childhood, and was noticeably tight at the T 4/5 level of her back (L 1/2 corresponds to the Triple Heater and T 4/5 corresponds to the Pericardium). I therefore diagnosed her as having a Pericardium Excess constitution, and treatments to Sedate Pericardium and Triple Heater have helped resolve her hip pain. Her first treatment, however, was an Aggressive Energy tap, which was positive at UB 15 and UB 20. Although she no longer suffers from hip pain, she derives a great deal of comfort on a mental and emotional level from ongoing intermittent treatment based on her constitution.

CASE 13

K. T., a 47-year-old man, was seen initially for an acute flare of pain from a chronic injury to his low back, most likely from a skiing injury seven years before. The acute flare started after lifting, but he was otherwise in very good health except for mildly elevated liver function tests on routine screening, and he was happy with his life. His pulses were unusual in that they were all bounding in quality except for the right Chi position, which was almost imperceptible. His Sasang pulse was of the Lesser Yang type and his KCA pulse was of the Saturna type. His Prakriti was Pitta/Kapha, and his blood pressure was 100/50 (low). FEA style treatment aimed at Tonifying his Triple Heater was successful in alleviating the pain and returning his liver functions to normal.

CASE 14

K. C. is a 66-year-old woman who came for treatment of tinnitus and pressure in her ears for a whole year. This problem started after she was started on a combination of medications for hypertension, high cholesterol, low thyroid function, anxiety, and insomnia. On this polypharmacy regimen, she experienced five episodes of severe nausea and vomiting, and the onset of the ear symptoms, so she stopped most of the drugs, but the ears did not recover. She had a lifelong tendency to sleep poorly, but had otherwise been in good health. On examination, her blood pressure was 130/72 and her pulse rate was 72, with occasional premature beats. Her SCM pulse was Greater Yin type, KCA pulse was Jupita type, Prakriti was Vata, and SEL pulse was radially deviated in the Cun position. These findings are compatible with either Bladder Deficiency or Small Intestine Excess. I wasn't clear about which of these types fit her better, and initially tried Tonifying her Bladder Meridian, because her Water pulses felt the most abnormal in quality. This led to some improvement in her ears, but also resulted in a feeling that her heart was agitated, so I switched to Sedation of her Small Intestine and Heart Meridians. This latter approach got rid of the pressure in her ears right away, and reduced the tinnitus, but did not eliminate it. After several treatments based on a constitutional diagnosis of Small Intestine Excess, she maintained the improvement in her ears, was in a calmer and happier mood, and labwork showed an improvement in her elevated blood lipids.

CASE 15

B. M. is a 59-year-old man I have treated, also about once a month, for the past 17 years. He initially presented with arthritis in multiple joints and psoriasis, but over the years he has come to value the emotional benefits of acupuncture, although at first he was quite skeptical that needles could affect his emotions. He is a Buddhist, and places great importance on the quality of his meditation practice, and he has found that acupuncture has helped him in this regard. It has been many years since he had any serious problems from arthritis, and the psoriasis is also rarely an issue. Interestingly, both his brother and his mother developed arthritis at about the same age as he did. I have treated him mainly as having Heart Deficiency (Lesser Yin SCM, Mercurio KCA, ulnar deviation of SEL Chi, and Vata Prakriti). On his most recent visit he complained of feeling colder than usual (he has a history of hypothyroidism), and his Yin pulses were abnormal in depth at the Heart and Spleen locations. The Heart pulse was biggest at the Earth depth and the Spleen pulse was biggest at the Fire depth. Tonification of HE 7 and SP 2 corrected these abnormalities, and he immediately felt warmer.

Cases 8–15 all have Fire Element CFs, but they are representative of eight different constitutions and involve four different Organs/Officials, displaying varying tendencies towards Excess or Deficiency. In FEA it might be difficult to ascertain these dynamics, even if the Fire CF was correctly identified by color, sound, odor, and emotion. This ability to discriminate constitutions within the same Element is one of the additional benefits of the type of constitutional pulse diagnosis I am proposing.

CASE 16

N. C., a 52-year-old man, presented with persistent right hip pain that originated eight years previously following a fencing injury. Periodic cortisone shots gave marked, but temporary, relief, and he was managing the pain with a combination of ice, stretching, and Vicodin (a narcotic pain medication). He was unable to lie on his right side due to the pain (diagnosed as bursitis), and also experienced back pain and severe respiratory allergies, which occasionally developed into sinus infections.

His past medical history was quite complicated, for someone his age. Following an auto accident 20 years ago, he developed Meniere's syndrome, which was treated surgically by inserting an endolymphatic shunt. For the past 11 years he has had type 2 diabetes, for which he takes multiple medications, with variable success in controlling his blood sugar level. He has also had elevated lipids and coronary artery disease since his thirties, and two years ago had a heart attack with four blocked coronary arteries, treated surgically with stent implants. Finally, he experiences life as very stressful, having divorced six years previously, and is currently studying intensively for the bar exam to become a lawyer. At the time of his first visit, he was on at least ten different prescription medications.

His SCM pulse seemed to be clearly of the Greater Yang type, and he always has a cold Lower Middle Heater. His KCA pulse was of the Hespera type. Initially I thought his Prakriti pulse was Pitta, and treated him as having a Large Intestine Excess, with a Metal CF. This greatly relieved his hip and back pains, and after the first of such treatments he remarked, "It feels good to breathe." However, his blood sugar became more difficult to regulate, which I found puzzling. After rechecking his pulse, I decided that his Prakriti was actually Pitta/Kapha, which would mean that his constitution might be Bladder Excess instead, with a Water CF. Subsequent treatments from that perspective greatly relaxed him and continued to keep his pain at a minimal level, while allowing him to study more effectively, but he was not being very attentive to his diet, and is still experiencing blood sugar swings. I wanted to include his case because it again illustrates the beneficial effects of treating the Sasang typology, even if the exact constitution is still elusive. Both Large Intestine Excess and Bladder Excess are examples of the Greater Yang Sang and, incidentally, since they are both disorders of a Fu Official, are likely to present with right sided symptoms, which this man consistently exhibits. Because his Vikruti pulse is strongly Vata in type, my treatments have been primarily to transfer Qi away from his Kidney, and into his weakest pulse, which has recently been the Spleen. Sedating the Kidney and Tonifying the Spleen should both have the effect of diminishing Vata, and he has done very well with this approach. Tonifying his Spleen also makes sense in trying to address his diabetes. Even though his constitution is Bladder Excess, it would have been a mistake to have focused primarily on transferring Qi out of the Bladder Meridian, as that would have increased Vata even more. Treating both Bladder and Kidney together would be safer, although perhaps not as dynamically effective as focusing on the Kidney alone has been.

His case is one in which I was quite puzzled regarding the CF. From a Five Element perspective, I would say he definitely has a weeping sound in his voice, which probably influenced my original Metal diagnosis, but there is no striking color or odor, and I would say that, although he might display occasional flashes of sadness, they seem appropriate to his situation. He has never shown the slightest indication of inappropriate fearfulness, but perhaps his carelessness with diet might be interpreted as reckless "lack of fear."

I am guessing that there are readers who are saying to themselves, "I have a bunch of clients whose CSOE findings are confusing or difficult to assess, just as in this case," and that is exactly why I am introducing this pulse diagnostic method especially for FEA practitioners. I tried to pick these cases as random examples of the different constitutional types and Elements. However, I do not want to limit the scope of this methodology to FEA practitioners alone. The next series of case histories will gather examples of patients I have primarily treated with Korean Constitutional Acupuncture techniques that I originally learned from Kuon Dowon, but have since expanded as my perspective evolved. Kuon calls his method ECM now, but since I am proposing the existence of 24 constitutions, that terminology would not be the best title for the methods I am about to describe. For that reason, when speaking in general terms regarding such methodology, I will revert to its former acronym, KCA. Again, the reader is encouraged to refer to Appendix 2 for referencing some of the more common treatment formulae, or prescriptions, used in KCA, especially if it becomes difficult to make sense of the case histories that follow.

CASE 17

M. U. is an 85-year-old woman whom I have taken care of for the last 12 years, being the mother of one of my prior patients. Her original complaint was a tremor in her right hand, which had been present for 15 years, following an automobile accident in which she was thrown over the hood of a car, fracturing her pelvis, ribs, and facial bones. It was interesting to note that she had other physical abnormalities which were only revealed by questioning and examination, including moderately severe swelling, numbness, and limitation of movement of both (very cold) feet, heart disease treated by angioplasty but resulting in bouts of tachycardia (treated by beta blocking drugs), and an abnormality in her gamma globulin which was diagnosed as a premyeloma condition. I believe the tremor was her biggest concern because it was the only one of her problems that was visible to the people with whom she normally interacted. Since I began working with her, she has had several accidents in which she has fallen due to poor balance; I suspect this is because she has such poor sensory nerve function in her feet. At this time the balance issue has become her main concern. On exam, she has generalized muscle tightness in addition to the tremor, so that taking her pulses can be challenging.

Nevertheless, she has responded well to treatment based on her constitution, which I have determined to be Gall Bladder Deficiency. Her SEL pulse shows radial deviation in the Chi position, her Prakriti is Pitta/Vata, and she has a Lesser Yang SCM pulse of the Saturna type. I have used various strategies to treat her, in which the Fundamental formula for Gall Bladder Deficiency per Lee Dong Woong has been a mainstay. It is a Four Needle treatment using Sedation at ST 36 and GB 34 and Tonification at SI 5 and GB 38. I treat these Points on her left side because her symptoms are worse on the right side, but also because Fu constitutions are more frequently successfully treated on the left side. Other strategies that I have included in her treatment have been Tonifying the Wind Points on her GB Meridian (GB 20 and 31) and also Tonifying GB 39 which treats the Marrow. The tremor has become less of an issue, and her blood tests indicate that the abnormal gamma globulin level has slowly been diminishing towards normal. I might add that her pulses at the standard positions might be confusing to many, as her Gall Bladder and Liver pulses at the Yang location of the left Guan position are typically Excess in nature. I believe this is an indication that her underlying problem is Gall Bladder Yin Deficiency, showing in the tendency towards tachycardia and muscular tension. Her Wood pulses at the Yin location of the left Guan position more often show this Deficient state.

CASE 18

M. U. is a 51-year-old man who has had Meniere's disease for two years, mainly manifesting as tinnitus, fullness, nausea, and hearing loss in his left ear, accompanied by balance disturbances that vary from wooziness to incapacitating vertigo. These symptoms began at a time of severe stress at work when he experienced an emotional confrontation as being "stabbed in the back." He had only transient relief from Western medications such as Meclizine, and thought they made him feel worse in other ways, but was still taking Valium, Lexapro (an antidepressant), and diuretics. At the time of his first visit he was having a severe vertigo attack at least every other week. His strategy for dealing with stress at work was to "power through it," and his language describing the work situation was full of scatological and other expletives in almost every sentence. He had a past history of hepatitis in childhood following a case of influenza. In describing his childhood, raised by a single mother who was depressed, he called it "bad" and said he suffers from survivor's guilt, and often feels hopeless.

On exam his left carotid was bigger than his left radial pulse, and he had a Vata/Kapha Prakriti and a Jupita KCA pulse type. All his pulses felt either close to normal or more clearly Excess, with a slippery quality. His blood pressure was 110/70 (low). In addition he had a non-tender nodule at LI 4 on the left side. Pulsewise he seemed clearly to fit the Large Intestine Deficiency constitution, and for his first treatment I decided to use a KCA approach. I pre-tested him with gold (Tonifying) and silver (Sedating) press pellets on the KHA Points corresponding to their body acupuncture Points. First I tested the gold pellets at the LI 4 and LU 9 corresponding Points. I used both pulse quality and the strength of Omura's O-ring test (a kinesiology test of muscle strength),[12] and determined that these Points were helpful on the left side, but not on the right. I next tested both the original and revised formulae that Kuon proposed for Jupita types (LI Tonification), and determined that the revised formula was better. Thus his first treatment was as follows: Regular needles were inserted at 45 degrees at UB 66 and LI I2 (Tonifying direction) and GB 41 and LI 3 (Sedating direction) and left in place for 20 minutes. His report the next week was that his energy level had come way up, and that he was back to "feeling like my old self again." His first three treatments followed a similar style, although I added an FEA second part if the pulses did not change enough, but these were all quite simple transfers and the use of Luo Connecting Points. At the end of a month, he had had no further vertigo attacks, and his concern had shifted to the loss of libido he experienced ever since he had been on Lexapro. I rechecked his carotid/radial ratio, which had not changed, and determined that he had a Ren Mai imbalance on his left sided radial pulses. I again used the press pellets and the O-ring test to see if the use of LU 7 (silver) and KI 6 (gold), on the left side, would be helpful, and decided on that as his treatment, using the standard body Points and leaving the needles for ten minutes. He subsequently reported that his sex drive had returned to normal despite continuing the Lexapro, and that his bowel function had also improved, even though he had never mentioned having had a problem with it. He has been in treatment for over six months with only one episode of vertigo, which occurred shortly after I tried dispersing his Liver in an attempt to help with the residual mild tinnitus and the continual state of anger and stress that he exhibited. Returning to LI Tonification quickly stopped the vertigo, and it has not recurred. My thinking is that as long as he stays in a job that is so upsetting and stressful to him, he will be likely to experience some health consequences. We discussed this, and he recognized that it was his choice, and eventually ended up quitting the job and going into business for himself. He has been much happier and less symptomatic ever since.

CASE 19

U. E. is a 38-year-old male investment advisor who suffered from low back pain as a consequence of scoliosis, which he had noticed at least since age 13. He wore a brace until he was 17, and was then diagnosed with spondylolysthesis.

---

12   Omura, Y., "O-Ring Test" class, Los Angeles, 1988; First International Symposium on the Bi-Digital O-Ring Test, Waseda University, Japan, 1993.

The pain was manageable until one year ago when it was aggravated by playing golf. The pain felt localized to his left hip, and at first he couldn't walk more than two blocks, but it had improved with a combination of diet, yoga, and exercise. Radiology revealed that he had a bulging lumbar disc, but no problem with his left hip joint. He had a history of mild hypertension and high cholesterol.

On exam, he had weak pulses in the left Chi and right Cun positions, as well as the right Chi position. The Prakriti was Pitta/Kapha and his KCA type was Saturno. Putting these together pointed to a Kidney Deficiency constitution. I decided to treat him with the in and out type of repetitive needling used in KCA. The Point prescription I chose was based on the disc disease formula: Fundamental (five times), Zang (five times), and Psyche (once).[13] The treatment was given on the right (opposite side), and the only variation was that I substituted Puramo's choice of Psyche Formula Points for Kuon's as follows: Fundamental—SP 3, KI 3 Sedated, LU 8, KI 7 Tonified; Zang—HE 8, SP 2 Sedated, KI 10, SP 9 Tonified; and Psyche—PE 3 Sedated, PE 7 Tonified. The next week he reported that following treatment he had walked for two hours without pain for the first time in two years. I have only treated him a dozen times in the last three years, and similar treatments have been effective at stopping painful flare-ups; however, I have found that Kuon's original Psyche Formula (HE 7 Sedated, HE 3 Tonified) is more reliably helpful for him. Considering that he is a financial investment advisor, he has done remarkably well during the recent extremely stressful economic times.

CASE 20

K. T. is a similar 40-year-old male investment banker who was first seen by me seven years ago for recurrent bouts of low back pain. His problem started at age 17 following a contact sports injury, and he began having attacks of low back pain about every three months, which would last about a week, but had recently worsened and now lasted ten days. Over many years he had had nine MRIs that revealed disc herniations at L 4/5 and L 5/S 1, which he treated with physical therapy and one epidural steroid injection, all of which gave only temporary relief. Attacks of pain were limited to the lumbo-sacral area of his back and did not radiate to his legs, except for one episode after yoga when he developed left sided leg pain along the Bladder Meridian. He also complained of very tight hamstring muscles and sensitivity on the soles of his feet around the insteps. His medical history was otherwise unremarkable except for diminished sexual stamina, but social history revealed that he had switched from journalism to banking, and that his new career was extremely stressful, necessitating waking at 4:00 a.m. in order to keep up with Wall Street.

---

13   See Appendix 2.

On exam his right carotid was larger than his right radial pulse, and straight leg lifting was diminished bilaterally, but worse on the left side. His pulses were weakest in the left Chi position, and he seemed very tense in general, a sign that I interpreted as a likely exaggerated fearfulness. I treated him before I began integrating Ayurveda into my practice, so initially I diagnosed him based on his pulses as having a KCA type of Saturno, with a Kidney Deficiency constitution. I decided to treat him with the in and out type of repetitive needling used in KCA, but decided to apply the Zang Inflammation component on the left side, with the Fundamental and Psyche components on the right side as in the previous case. The points used were: Fundamental—SP 3, KI 3 Sedated, LU 8, KI 7 Tonified; Zang—HE 8, SP 2 Sedated, KI 10, SP 9 Tonified; and Psyche—PE 3 Sedated, PE 7 Tonified. The reason for applying the Zang component on the other side was that I had recently studied with Puramo Chong, a Sasang acupuncture specialist, and this was his style of treatment, and I was curious to test its efficacy. There was no dramatic change after two treatments, so I changed the protocol from Fundamental–Zang–Psyche to Degeneration–Zang–Psyche, taking into account the long period of trauma to his back, as this second protocol is commonly used by both Chong and Kuon for serious degenerative disc disease. The Degeneration formula for Kidney Deficiency constitutional types is HE 8, LU 10 Sedated and KI 10, LU 5 Tonified. After two treatments with this approach he reported that he felt looser, with increased flexibility, and that he was no longer in pain and noticed improved sexual functioning. His wife soon became pregnant, and he has since had two children. He did well (no problems with his back), with essentially the same treatment, on an intermittent basis for four years. At that point he began experimenting with hormonal treatments recommended by a consulting physician who diagnosed him with mononucleosis, and his health subsequently deteriorated, aggravating his initial complaint of uncharacteristic fatigue. I have not seen him recently, but advised him to stop the supplements and to consider a change in his extremely stressful lifestyle (now including two young children in addition to his stressful job), explaining the Water Element's role in compensating for chronic stress. Interestingly, he did not experience any significant recurrence of back pain with the onset of chronic fatigue. It is also interesting to note that the Degeneration formula Tonifies the Lung (Mother of the Kidney), while the Zang Inflammation formula Sedates the Spleen (Controller of the Kidney). Using these components together is an example of the creative use of Five Element theory in KCA. His right sided carotid/radial imbalance is an example of the doctrine of energetic imbalances manifesting in symptoms on the opposite side of the body, but best treated on the side opposite to the symptoms, as well as the doctrine that Zang constitutions generally manifest symptoms predominantly on the left side. Extra Meridian treatment, based on the carotid/radial pulse imbalance, might be helpful in the future.

CASE 21

N. H. is a 49-year-old maintenance worker, who came for treatment because he was developing increasing numbness in his right hand and foot over several months. He was significantly overweight, which he blamed on a voracious appetite his whole life. In the past year he experienced increasing levels of fatigue, even on waking after a normal night's sleep. His blood pressure had been found to be high, so he was on medication that controlled it. He also suffered from erectile dysfunction that worsened if he stopped the blood pressure medication. His pulses showed the following findings: Greater Yang SCM pulse, Hespero KCA pulse, ulnar deviation of the SEL Guan pulse, and Kapha Prakriti pulse. This combination of pulses can only indicate a Spleen Excess constitution. Both his Yang and Yin Chi pulses on the right were notably stronger than any of the others. Both left and right Vikruti pulses showed Vata of the Fire type (two Subdoshas in each).

I decided to treat him with the KCA technique, since he struck me as the sort of person who needed to see rapid improvement if he were to remain in treatment long enough to do him some good. Since his constitution was Greater Yang, I planned to Sedate the TH (Psyche Formula) to calm Vata, and also used the Paralysis Formula for the same reason. From experience, I've found that pairing these two Formulae with the Immune Formula as the component for his constitutional Element is the best choice, and in this case that meant Sedating his Stomach, which would also Sedate Vata. As his symptoms were on the right side, I treated all Points on the left side as follows: SI 5 and ST 41 Sedated and GB 41 and ST 43 Tonified; ST 36 and SI 8 Sedated and UB 66 and SI 2 Tonified; and TH 10 Sedated and TH 2 Tonified. His numbness immediately diminished, and his kinesiology improved. I have used similar treatments on each follow-up visit, with minor variations, and he has steadily improved in all his complaints. The only major changes in treatment have been to move the ST Sedation Formula to the right side after finding a Pitta/Vata Vikruti there, and to discontinue the SI Sedation, as that could be suspect on theoretical grounds in a Greater Yang individual. I encouraged him to adopt a strict vegetarian/seafood diet, and to only eat when he is clearly hungry and stop as soon as he ceases to feel hunger. He feels dramatically better, including better marital relations, but notices an almost immediate return of problems if he eats even a little meat.

More recently, he came for treatment complaining of severe seasonal allergies causing itching of eyes, nose, and throat, sneezing, and a stuffy feeling in his ears. He described his current condition as "miserable." Appendix 2 shows that allergic rhinitis is best treated by KCA Formulae K/F or K/B. In SP Excess constitutions, the Fu Formula Tonifies the KI, while the Antibiotic Formula Tonifies the UB. On examination his left side Vikruti was Pitta/Vata of the Earth type (Samana Vata and Sadhaka Pitta), while his right side Vikruti was Vata of the Water type (Apana Vata). Finding Apana Vata indicated that Tonification of the UB was necessary, while the Pitta/Vata Vikruti indicated that the Immune Formula for Sedating the ST would be more appropriate than the Root Formula (K) which Sedates the Spleen. Since the symptoms showed no laterality difference, I treated him on the right side (appropriate for Zang constitutional types). The Formula was I/B, and the Points were chosen from Puramo's suggestions for Spleen Excess as follows: SI 5 and ST 41 Sedated, GB 41 and ST 43 Tonified, plus SI 5 and UB 60 Sedated, GB 41 and UB 65 Tonified. As soon as this treatment was given, he said the allergy symptoms were 95 percent gone. This case history illustrates how different problems are successfully treated by applying the appropriate Formulae in KCA, but that the Ayurvedic Vikruti can help pick out the most helpful treatment, addressing both constitutional and conditional factors.

CASE 22

F. C. is a 49-year-old CFO of a major Internet company, who has been in my practice for ten years. When first seen, he had a history of back pain for about 30 years, following trauma to his coccyx in elementary school. Over the years he had reinjured his back a number of times, primarily by lifting heavy objects. Imaging studies revealed herniated discs at L 4/5 and L 5/S 1, and he had undergone discectomy and nerve root blocks, which gave only partial relief. He still suffered from back pain, right leg sciatic pain and numbness (Gall Bladder Meridian), and weakness of the right big toe. His work is extremely stressful, but he felt it was the career he really wanted, and accepted that it might be contributing to his back problems. His goal in treatment has been to at least stabilize his back, considering that up until then it had been gradually getting worse over time.

The treatment approach that has proven most helpful is based on an integration of diagnostic findings from FEA, KCA, SEL, and Ayurveda. He is a Wood CF, which was no surprise to me, considering the intense devotion to management behaviors that were clearly causing symptoms along his Wood Meridians. His Prakriti is Kapha, and his Sasang type is Lesser Yin, so he must be of the Gall Bladder Excess constitution. Confirmation was provided by finding a radial deviation of his Chi positions in the proximal SEL pulse locations. This constitution was not one of Kuon's original eight types, so in treating him I decided to use Lee Dong Woong's newer formulae. Although his Prakriti is Kapha, his Vikruti is almost always Pitta/Vata. The combination of Kapha Prakriti and Pitta/Vata Vikruti points to the Wood and Earth Elements. Having a Gall Bladder Excess constitution, such a Vikruti suggests a state of

Liver Excess and Spleen Deficiency in those two Elements. There are several effective combinations of Fundamental and Auxiliary formulae, discovered by Kuon, for treating herniated discs. Among them is the combination of Fundamental, Zang, and Psyche formulae. Using Lee's recommendations, these are the Points to implement such a treatment: Tonify SP 3 and LV 3 and Sedate HE 8 and LV 2 (Fundamental); and Tonify LU 8 and SP 5 and Sedate LV 1 and SP 1 (Zang); Tonify TH 1 and Sedate TH 3 (Psyche). I have treated these Points on his left (contralateral) side, using Kuon's method of rapid in and out shallow needling, repeated four times each. Using this approach once or twice a month has resulted in the desired stabilization. It is possible some other approach might provide more definitive relief, but I suspect that as long as he continues in such a stressful occupation, he will continue to have some degree of pain. Whenever he does take a vacation, his pain level always improves.

CASE 23

S. C. is a 31-year-old woman who was referred to me by a fellow acupuncturist who thought she needed Western medical treatment for parasites (Blastocystis hominis and Endolimax nana), which had resisted prolonged herbal and acupuncture treatment. The parasites were apparently picked up on a trip to India three years previously, and had left her with rashes, food intolerances, abdominal bloating, fatigue, and clouding of her mental acuity. Her previous practitioner had diagnosed a Deficient Stomach as the root of her problems, but my own pulse diagnosis differed. I found a Greater Yang SCM pulse, a Hespera KCA pulse, a radially deviated SEL Guan pulse, and a Pitta Prakriti pulse. These findings point to Large Intestine Excess as her constitution. Since she had been in treatment so long already, I decided to start with pharmaceutical intervention as requested, and prescribed a three-day course of Nitazoxanide but, as this medication was not readily available, I began treating her first with needles. She showed an immediate improvement in her symptoms, which lasted the few weeks until she started the medication. As expected, she felt poorly while on this antibiotic, but fortunately it only needs to be taken for three days, as opposed to many of the more commonly used antibiotics which need longer courses and are as unpleasant and often less effective. On the last day of medication, she had a very strong right side Yang Chi pulse, and a Vata Vikruti on the right with two Subdoshas, indicating a Fire imbalance. Since LI Excess is a Greater Yang constitution, and people of that constitution are prone to Excess of Ministerial Fire, I treated her with Sedation of TH 6. I left the needles (pointed against the Meridian flow) in place for 40 minutes. When that treatment was finished, all the side effects from the medication had resolved. Subsequently her "parasitic" issues had also disappeared.

On her next visit, she had flipped pulses in the Yang Cun and Yang Guan positions on the right: Her Cun was biggest at the Earth (middle) depth and her Guan was biggest at the Metal (superficial) depth. As her constitution is LI Excess, I Sedated LI 11 (Earth Point) and ST 45 (Metal Point), as these are in a Mother–Son relationship. She felt even better after this treatment directed at her constitutional Organ, and her pulses and kinesiology tests also improved. She had already found that a basically vegetarian diet worked best for her, but was eating meat about once a week. I advised her to substitute seafood for the meat component. Since her digestive symptoms and food intolerances were better, she decided to wait about three weeks before repeating testing to see if there were still any parasites. During this interval, she continued to feel quite well, on a more liberal diet. Interestingly, retesting showed that the parasites were still present. Interpreting this scenario presents a challenge. Did the acupuncture help her body accommodate to the presence of the parasites? Should more aggressive antibiotic treatment be pursued? The one possibility that I feel is unlikely is that her positive response was merely placebo induced. My reason for this conclusion is that she had much more acupuncture treatment from her prior practitioner, a colleague in whom she had great faith, without experiencing this degree of improvement. She is pondering the next step at this point.

CASE 24

L. O. is a 53-year-old woman who consulted me for pain in her right foot that had lasted for two years. She had been referred by her podiatrist, who had diagnosed her problem as tarsal tunnel syndrome, but had been unable to resolve it. She had tried osteopathy, Feldenkreis work, and using orthotics, which, if anything, had only made things worse. The pain was in several locations: along the Kidney Meridian between KI 2 and KI 3, on the dorsum of her foot above the MTP joints of her second and third toes, and on the sole of her foot directly below these same joints. Ibuprofen gave no relief, but Lidoderm patches were of temporary help, as was local application of heat. Cold weather seemed to aggravate the pain and was also associated with some swelling in the legs. She noted that her feet had been mildly uncomfortable for "decades," that they didn't feel "adaptable," and that she had previously experienced a similar severe attack of pain in her left foot 12 years ago, which had resolved spontaneously. The present pain was aggravated by standing or walking, and limited both normal activities such as doing errands as well as recreation, although swimming was possible. There was no history of injury to her feet, legs, or back.

She is an extremely amiable and attractive history professor who had an enjoyable life, with the exception of the lack of a satisfying relationship (several failed romances), and lived alone as a consequence. Both of her parents were in good health in their eighties, and she had no other complaints except a recent tendency for her hair to become thinner and fall out more. Her periods were regular, but she consistently experienced night sweats premenstrually, and she often felt uncomfortable in the pelvic area, especially around her menses. On questioning about her emotional life, she stated that she suffered from panic attacks in high school, and that she had used psychotherapy ten years previously to deal with feelings of "being out of control."

Her constitutional pulses showed the following characteristics: Pitta/Vata Prakriti, Lesser Yang SCM type, Saturna KCA type, and radial deviation of the Guan position in the Six Level proximal pulse exam. This combination allows only one possible interpretation: a Stomach Excess constitution. I did not arrive at this diagnosis on my first exam, however, since at that time I had not yet incorporated the proximal Six Level pulse method, and being swayed by the Lesser Yang SCM pulse, the symptoms along the Kidney Meridian, the night sweats, and the history of panic attacks, I thought her constitution was probably Kidney Deficiency.[14] My first treatment consisted of testing for Aggressive Energy (negative),[15] and Sedating the Dragon Points for Internal Devils.[16] She reported less generalized aching in her feet on her subsequent visit. For the next few treatments I Tonified Kidney and Bladder Points, but this eventually seemed to aggravate the pain, although it ameliorated the hair problem. When I finally changed my diagnosis to Stomach Excess, she began to show steady improvement. Simply Sedating ST 45 turned out to be a very helpful treatment, as did transferring Qi from the Stomach to the Kidney using KI 4, UB 67, and LI 11, with Tonification of KI 4. Because of her tendency to develop swelling in cold weather, I have also prescribed Flex CD[17] as a herbal supplement to address that issue. She is now able to walk miles at a time without significant discomfort. Interestingly, she has also developed a romantic relationship that seems to be working out well. On her most recent visit, she was on the fifth day of symptoms of an upper respiratory infection (sore throat, cough, and congestion). To illustrate how I approach treatment of the present condition in the context of the constitution, I will elaborate on this particular session.

---

14 Saturna and Saturno pulses are almost the same, and it is easy to confuse them. I have found the same difficulty with Mercuria and Mercurio pulses.

15 A protocol taught by Worsley for draining Perverse Energy (Xie Qi) involving shallow needling in the Back Shu Points of the Zang Organs.

16 See Chapter 16. The history of panic attacks and subsequent "out of control feelings" suggested that this would be a prudent treatment. Note that almost all the Points are on the Stomach Meridian, and were Sedated.

17 From Evergreen Herbs. I have no financial relationship with this company.

Her Yang pulses showed Deficiency in the left Guan position (Wood) and Excess in the right Guan (Earth), which also showed a "flipped" shape with the widest pulse at the superficial or Metal level. Her right Cun (Metal) was also flipped, with the widest part at the middle or Earth level. Her Yin pulses showed Deficiency in the left Guan (Wood) position. The Vikruti pulses were Pitta/Vata on both sides, but the Subdoshas involved were not the same. On the left they reflected Wood (Udana and Ranjaka), while on the right they reflected Earth (Samana and Sadaka). This pulse presentation could be addressed in at least three ways: First, given the Excess in Earth and Deficiency in Wood, a transfer of Qi per FEA protocol could be used. Second, one could Sedate GB 34 (the Earth Point, which would decrease Pitta/Vata) and Tonify ST 43 (the Wood Point, which would increase Kapha). Finally, one could Sedate ST 45 and LI 11 (the Metal Point of ST and the Earth Point of LI). The first option would balance the Elements and pulse volumes, and the second would balance the Doshas, but I chose the third because, in addition to balancing Elements and Doshas, it uses Points that are also symptomatically indicated. As soon as I put the needles in ST 45 and LI 11, she said the congestion was already noticeably better. I have found that treating the Element within, which is showing in an altered pulse shape, is often the best treatment.

CASE 25

K. S. is a 35-year-old woman who first consulted me for depression. She had developed asthma in childhood, and later discovered accidentally that she had polycystic kidneys (while training to be an ultrasound technician). Her emotional problems apparently began at age 15 when her parents divorced. She described her feelings then as a sense of melancholy and abandonment, which eventuated in a diagnosis of depression. She had been treated with almost every pharmaceutical antidepressant, but had no benefit from any drugs except Adderall (a stimulant), but her doctors refused to keep her on that. She was able to manage the depression until her boyfriend broke up with her shortly before our first session. At that time she said quite plainly, "I want to die."

Before presenting her constitutional pulse picture, I'd like to describe a very unusual finding in her pulses, and how I treated her. All of her Yang pulses (Cun, Guan, and Chi) on both wrists were most prominent (flipped) at the Earth depth; however, all her Yin pulses were at their correct depths. Given her chief complaint, I treated her with the Seven Dragons for Internal Devils,[18] using the variant for depression taught by Worsley. Following that treatment, all her Yang pulses reverted to their normal depths, and on her next visit, she said, "I feel

---

18   Master Point below Ren 15, ST 32, and Master Point below ST 36, ST 41. All needles left in place for 20 minutes.

happy, like my old self again." Over the course of three years she needed this treatment repeated occasionally but survived several unsuccessful relationships without becoming severely depressed, until an impending breakup with a fiancé, shortly before they were to be married. The flipped Yang pulses had reappeared then, and she once again expressed a feeling of wanting to die, and hating herself. The same treatment again corrected the pulse abnormality and improved her mood. During the course of treatment, some of the things she said included, "I don't know how to nurture myself, so I eat when I'm not hungry; I worry about everything; I can't produce; I need support." Practitioners of a FEA background will probably recognize these statements as correlates of the Earth Element, which, however, is not her CF. Her constitutional pulse diagnosis is Saturno, specifically of the Kidney Deficiency type. Her case is a perfect example illustrating the analysis of "Possession" treatments that I presented earlier.[19] Her precipitating trauma was of an emotional nature, and it resulted in an inability to nurture herself on the deepest Spirit level, inhibiting her from properly producing postnatal Jing to nourish her Shen. Even though she has a Water Element CF, the problem that arose from emotional causes affected her postnatal, rather than her prenatal, Essence. The Dragons treatment needed Sedation, because her Earth Element was constitutionally and conditionally in Excess, but this perturbation was correctable with acupuncture. She already shows signs of Kidney problems (elevated creatinine, proteinuria, and elevated blood pressure). I believe these can be reversed if she is treated with consistent Tonification of the Water Element, now that her "Internal Devils" are under control.

CASE 26

W. K. is a 70-year-old woman who has been in treatment with me for a decade. She has had multiple problems including allergies, herpes simplex outbreaks, diverticulitis, bursitis of the hips, low back pain, sciatica, hypertension, hyperlipidemia, coronary artery disease, and arthritis. In general, all of her symptoms have responded well to treatment based on her constitution, which is Gall Bladder Deficiency (Lesser Yang SCM pulse, Saturna KCA pulse, radially deviated SEL Chi pulse, and Pitta/Vata Prakriti). She usually has only slight improvement noticeable at the time of treatment, but then feels considerably better the next day.

During one session, I noted that all of her Yang pulses (Cun, Guan, and Chi) were widest at the deep (Water Element) level, while all her Yin pulses were at their correct depths. On questioning, she related a lifelong history of physical trauma, including whiplash injuries, falls resulting in dislocated joints,

---

19   Chapter 16.

severe sprains, and multiple surgeries, and had just been overstraining herself physically in preparing to move residences. I treated her with the protocol for the External Dragons (DU 20, UB 11, UB 23, and UB 61), all Points being Tonified and then the needles removed without retention. On that visit she had been complaining about her back before treatment started, and as she got up from the table she claimed her back wasn't hurting anymore. All of her Yang pulses had recovered their proper depths. This seems to be a clear case of "External Devils," wherein the repeated physical trauma had disturbed the mechanism whereby her prenatal Essence was able to pattern her Normal (Zheng) Qi, resulting in multiple organ system malfunctions. Since her constitution is Wood Deficiency, it made sense to Tonify the Water (Mother) Element Points on the Bladder Meridian as part of the Dragons protocol. This decision was supported by finding a Vata Vikruti, which would be ameliorated by Tonifying the Bladder. This case, and the previous one, illustrate using the two different Dragons protocols, employing Elements that are not those of the person's CF. When I have found these pulse patterns, such treatments seem especially effective. The patient in this case is a very emotional woman, with extreme levels of stress in her life over an extended period of time. It would have been tempting to treat her with the Internal Dragons protocol, had not this method of pulse diagnosis pointed otherwise.

CASE 27

K. U., a 54-year-old woman, first consulted me 22 years ago for multiple problems which had not resolved despite seeing numerous therapists, including four different acupuncturists. Her main problems at that time were loss of dexterity in her hands (especially her thumbs), burning in her stomach, and constipation. Her digestive issues began soon after her mother suffered a stroke and needed to be placed in a convalescent hospital. My patient was then in her early twenties, and felt at that time as if her digestive tract just "shut down." She subsequently suffered a number of whiplash injuries, and had intermittent back pains and sciatica ever since, including a feeling that her sacrum was swollen. She was also environmentally sensitive, especially to air quality, and couldn't tolerate perfumes or car exhaust.

As a long-term patient, she has received quite a lot of acupuncture treatment from me, so I will just present a few highlights that illustrate treatment approaches that may not have been covered in the previous cases. She is clearly a Metal CF of the Jupita type, which belongs to the Greater Yin category. Her specific constitution is Large Intestine Deficiency, which certainly could explain her issues with loss (grief is the emotion of Metal), constipation, malfunctioning of her thumbs (pathway of the coupled Lung Meridian), and sensitivity to air quality (again, a Lung symptom). An interesting set of diagnostic indicators include her love of hiking in the mountains (clean air), preference for Fall, and especially the time of dusk, which all point to Metal. All of her problems have been greatly alleviated by treatments aimed at Tonifying the Metal Element. Her most resistant symptoms have been the back pain and sciatica, which were not very intense, but which also seemed not to respond strongly to the treatment approach just mentioned. On checking her carotid and radial pulses, I found that she typically had a larger carotid pulse on the right side, while her left sided pulses were fairly equal in size. My KHA teacher used to emphasize that physical distortions, such as are common following whiplash injuries, are best treated as Extraordinary Meridian imbalances, but which Meridians needed treatment? Because her right sided Vikruti pulses showed as Pitta/Vata (Earth Subdoshas in both), I considered using that information as a guide. The Pitta component, equivalent to a Yang Excess marker, could only be treated by the Yang Qiao Mai (see Chapter 8). The Vata component, a Kidney Excess marker, could be treated by either the Du Mai or the Yang Wei Mai. In this case, the Du Mai was not possible, because its Key Points were the same as those for the Yang Qiao Mai, only with opposite polarity, which would have cancelled the effect of that treatment, so the Yang Wei Mai was selected in addition to the Yang Qiao Mai, both on the right side. Her Extra Meridian pulses were confirmatory, with Yang Qiao showing on the Yin locations of Cun, Guan, and Chi, and Yang Wei showing on the Yang locations of Cun, Guan, and Chi. Needles were inserted, and her response was monitored by testing sensitive points on the abdomen, as well as by kinesiology. Both tests showed a positive response, so ion-pumping cords were added and the response stayed positive. I like to use ion-pumping cords with Extraordinary Meridian treatments because they create a very strong polarity, which is necessary for determining which Extraordinary Meridian is being activated when just the two Key Points are treated; however, with this modality of treatment it is essential to monitor the response of the patient after each component of treatment is added.

With this protocol in place, she reported a sense of deep calmness, and at her next visit reported that for the first time her back felt straight, and she had not had any sciatica. All of her other minor symptoms had also improved. This case illustrates my classification of Extraordinary Meridian imbalances as "blocks" that may partially prevent constitutional treatment from having its full beneficial effect. It also challenges the KHA doctrine that each side of the body can only have one of its three "constitutional types" at a time, and therefore can only be treated by one Extraordinary Meridian at a time on that side. Of course, it is possible that only one of the two Extraordinary Meridians I treated was responsible for the improvement, and the other was unnecessary. This is an issue that needs more study, in my opinion.

I would also like to describe her most recent treatment, which illustrates an aspect of my current thinking that includes integrating all the theoretical material presented in the text, to come up with a very simple treatment. She presented with right elbow pain, probably from repetitive stress. Her Vikruti on both sides was Pitta/Vata of the Wood type (Udana and Ranjaka Subdoshas). Her Yang Wood pulses were Excessive and her Yin Wood pulses were Deficient, while her Yang Metal pulses were Deficient and her Yin Metal pulses were slightly Excess. Since her constitution is LI Deficiency, the Vikruti can only reflect Liver Excess, but the left Guan pulses showed it was Liver Yang Excess. The Liver gets its Yang from its Grandfather, the Large Intestine,[20] which was already Deficient. The treatment I used was to Sedate LV 4, the Grandfather Point, which would inhibit any transfer of Yang from LI to LV. After the needles were in place bilaterally for a few minutes, all her pulses were normalized, and the elbow pain had disappeared.

CASE 28

K. N. is a 70-year-old woman who decided to try a short course of acupuncture upon discovering that her blood pressure was dangerously high, as she distrusted Western medications. Indeed, her pressure was 190/90 at the initial visit, she was greatly overweight, and also experienced both Reynaud's syndrome and pain in her left knee and right Achilles tendon. On exam, her right carotid was much bigger than her right radial artery, while on the left side her radial was moderately bigger than the carotid. All her constitutional pulses fit a diagnosis of Liver Excess: Greater Yin SCM, Jupito KCA, ulnar deviation of SEL Cun, and Pitta/Vata Prakriti. She confessed to drinking wine every night, and I explained to her that this was deleterious to her constitutional make-up.

The first treatment was using KHA needles to treat the Yang Qiao and Yang Wei Mai on the right side, as her Vikruti there was Pitta/Vata. I followed that with the Four Needle technique to Sedate the Liver on both sides. This brought immediate relief of her knee pain, and her pressure the next week was 170/92. Her radial and carotid ratios were improved on both sides, so I used a FEA treatment, Tonifying PE 9, UB 13, and UB 38, as her pulses showed the left Guan at the Fire depth on both Yang and Yin pulses, and her right Cun was Deficient with a Pitta Vikruti. By the second week her pressure was 152/80, and she had completely stopped alcohol consumption. I used KCA treatments a few times, employing the Fundamental, Vitality, and Psyche Formulae on the left side, as her left side Vikruti was consistently Vata with Prana and Udana Subdoshas, which is the most typical finding associated with high blood

---

20   See Thambirajah, R., *Energetics in Acupuncture*. Edinburgh: Churchill Livingstone, 2010, for a full explanation of this relationship.

pressure in Ayurveda,[21] and all these components Sedate Vata. At her sixth and final visit, her pressure was 145/80, and all of her initial symptoms had greatly diminished or disappeared. Also, her cholesterol level, which had been elevated, was back in the normal range.

CASE 29

B. C. is a young woman who experienced a severe physical trauma, and whose treatment has involved several methods that I occasionally use in my practice. At age 25, she was working as a stock clerk when a pile of heavy merchandise collapsed and fell on her. She suffered a crush injury that mainly impacted her right shoulder area. Subsequently she developed pain, numbness, and tingling throughout her right arm, and experienced a severely limited range of motion of the right shoulder joint. Over time these complaints worsened instead of diminishing, and she was eventually diagnosed as having reflex sympathetic dystrophy. She underwent nerve blocks and three operations on her shoulder, all without significant benefit. She also was not helped by numerous drugs which had been prescribed. She had previously been healthy, except for having had an ulcer in college. After the injury, she noted that her appetite was less than normal, which was an additional problem, as she was underweight to begin with.

I diagnosed her as an Earth CF, with Stomach Deficiency, which was later confirmed by finding a Lesser Yin SCM pulse, Mercuria KCA pulse, Kapha Prakriti, and a radially deviated Guan SEL pulse. She has responded favorably to FEA treatments aimed at Tonifying her Earth Element, but her symptoms typically returned after a few weeks, probably due to her current job which involves a fair amount of lifting. It is a job that she really loves, working with developmentally disabled children, but it is also both physically and emotionally taxing. I have tried several different alternative treatment strategies including the following: Using Kuon's KCA approach, I used in situ needles on her left side for the Zang, Fundamental, and Psyche Formulae. The Points were LU 8 and LV 4 Tonified, and KI 10 and LV 8 Sedated; SI 5 and ST 41 Tonified, and GB 41 and ST 43 Sedated; and TH 1 Tonified and TH 3 Sedated. I also tried using the French Medical Acupuncture approach of triangular equilibration, starting from the assumption that the Stomach Deficiency was expressing itself as Bladder Excess (Kuon calls this constitution Vesicotonia, implying Bladder Excess as its basic nature). These Points were UB 60, Ren 12, HE 8, KI 25, KI 26, and KI 27, all in situ bilaterally for 20 minutes. These treatments were also effective in consistently reducing her symptoms, but again only temporarily. Presently I have been using Sa Am's Formula for taking out Cold, employing

---

21   Class notes from M. J. Cravatta.

these Points on the left side only: Sedating ST 44, SI 2, UB 66, and PE 3, and Tonifying ST 41, SI 5, UB 60, and PE 8. In this treatment, all the Water Points are Sedated and all the Fire Points are Tonified. This has been the most helpful of all the treatments I have tried and, although her symptoms always recur after a while, I believe that she will never fully recover as long as she keeps overusing the injured area.

CASE 30

M. I. is a 62-year-old man who has been in my practice for over 20 years. His initial complaints were acute and chronic low back pain (from hips to buttocks bilaterally, and beginning at a time of difficult decisions at work), mild hypertension (150/80 for six years), and frequent sore throats and canker sores (worst in spring). At that time in my practice, I had not developed any of the special pulse diagnostic techniques introduced in this book, except for some familiarity with Kuon's KCA. I initially treated him by balancing Akabanes[22] on the Bladder Meridian, followed by a long period during which I used Kuon's Fundamental and Psyche Formulae for Liver Excess (Jupito). The Psyche Auxiliary Formula is recommended for both hypertension and neuralgia. He did well with this approach, almost always showing significantly lower blood pressures after treatments as compared to before treatments. He was also able to continue playing golf, which was his major concern regarding his back pain. I must confess, however, that I was never entirely satisfied with the treatments I was using, as he did eventually need medication to keep his blood pressure well controlled, and over the years he developed a tendency for digestive upsets, lingering coughs following colds, and more recently a marked tremor of his left hand. Using my current panoply of pulse examinations, I changed my mind about his constitution, and decided his type was Lung Deficiency, rather than Liver Excess. This assessment was based on finding a Lesser Yang SCM pulse, a Saturno KCA pulse, an ulnarly deviated SEL Guan pulse, and a Pitta Prakriti pulse. As for his conditional pulses, his Yin right Cun pulse was widest at the Fire depth, and his Yin right Chi pulse was widest at the Earth depth. His Vikruti pulses were Vata (Fire type) on the left and Pitta on the right. These findings are consistent with a combination of Lung and Pericardium Deficiency as his current condition. The treatment selected was Tonification, with needles left in for ten minutes, of LU 9 and PE 7 on the right (contralateral to the tremor). These are Tonification and/or Source Points of their Meridians, but also the Element Points that reflected the altered depth

---

22   The Akabane test is based on heat sensitivity at the Jing/Well Points of each Meridian, and is named after its originator, Kobe Akabane. It is taught in FEA institutions, and is given a historical review in *Footsteps*.

at the Lung and Pericardium pulses, and explained the combination of Vata (Fire) and Pitta (Metal) Vikruti pulses. As soon as the needles were inserted in his right hand, the marked tremor of his left hand virtually disappeared.

This case raises a number of interesting issues for me. The first one has to do with his positive responses to both Liver Excess treatment and Lung Deficiency treatment. Since they represent opposing Elements on the Control Cycle (Wood and Metal) such results are understandable, but the reader might remember that I previously noted that often treatments for different subtypes in the same SCM category are often helpful, even if the exact subtype is mistaken. Here is a case where the SCM categories themselves are different (Lesser Yin and Lesser Yang), yet both treatments are still helpful. This finding, that many different treatment approaches based on different diagnoses can still be helpful, reminded me of a comment made by one of my Korean teachers, Chae Lew, whose treatment style involved many more needles than most of the other practitioners under whom I studied. When I asked him about that, he said, "I learned this from my father, who claimed that the human body loves needles." The implication of such a statement made me think of another problematic issue in acupuncture, the often heard claim that "acupuncture can do no harm, even if it doesn't end up helping."[23] I wish to emphatically put forward the opposite contention, that incorrectly chosen acupuncture treatments can adversely affect the patient's health, an opinion expressed by almost all of my teachers including Kuon and Worsley, but also clearly stated in the classic texts from the *Neijing* onwards. The possibility that numerous treatment strategies can all be helpful does not in any way imply that numerous other treatment strategies can be equally harmful. I believe the answer lies in how well the treatment addresses the actual energetic problems the patient is experiencing. Chae Lew was a Master, in my opinion, of recognizing these energetic imbalances in his patients, and so the multiple needles were all chosen to address a perceived energetic imbalance.

Another reason I'm raising this issue here is that there is a very influential voice in both the Western scientific and Oriental medical circles, claiming that acupuncture is nothing more than a powerful placebo. Unfortunately, this voice belongs to Ted Kaptchuk, a personal friend and one of the most well-known pioneers of acupuncture in the United States.[24] In an article in the *New Yorker* magazine,[25] Kaptchuk, who stopped practicing acupuncture 20 years ago, was quoted as expressing just this conviction, that acupuncture is nothing more than a placebo. In his words, "In the end, it isn't really about the needles. It's about the man." The whole thrust of this book should make it clear that I am diametrically opposed to such a belief, one which relegates Oriental

---

23   Obviously excluding trauma to organs and other vital structures.

24   Kaptchuk, T., *The Web That Has No Weaver*. New York: Congdon and Weed, 1983.

25   Specter, M., "The Power of Nothing." *New Yorker*, December 12, 2011, pp.30–36.

medicine, at least in its use of acupuncture, to a practice that has no valid basis and is "unscientific." Such a view would also support the notion that incorrect treatment can do no harm. This is a very dangerous message in my opinion, and I hope others in the profession will also speak out against it. It surprised me that the *New Yorker* did not publish any rebuttals to Kaptchuk's assertion, but I do not know if they even received any.[26] I wish to make it clear that this is not an ad hominem attack on Kaptchuk, for whom I have very warm feelings and respect, but simply a polemic about the nature of acupuncture, which has crucial implications for both the public and the profession. The case for acupuncture being much more than a placebo could be presented in an entire book itself, but I will simply mention here a recent text by Jean-Marc Kespi,[27] which I think elegantly refutes such a belief, via its large number of case histories. Many of the patients treated by Kespi had no response to multiple treatments based on his initial diagnosis, but when he changed the diagnosis and thus the Points treated (sometimes after two different initial wrong diagnoses), suddenly the patients quickly improved to the point of clinical cure. Even more interesting, to me, was that many of Kespi's patients got dramatically worse after the first one or two treatments, but then progressively got better with each subsequent treatment using the same Points! These patterns of response to treatment are contrary to what a placebo would engender. I will only mention the use of acupuncture to successfully treat babies and animals, again something not explainable by the placebo hypothesis.

CASE 31

S. U. is a 66-year-old man whom I have treated for over a decade for a number of relatively minor complaints, mostly musculoskeletal in nature. Like the previous individual, his constitution is Lung Deficiency, and his most chronic area of discomfort is his left thumb MCP joint, although this problem is rarely an issue anymore. He does have a tendency to develop lingering coughs after catching colds, and recently came to see me because he had been coughing for over a month after his last cold. Upon checking his pulses, I found that on the right side both the Prakriti and the Vikruti showed Pitta patterns, but on his left side the Vikruti was Kapha, with the Earth Subdosha Bodaka. This is consistent with either Spleen Excess or Stomach Deficiency, and an obvious treatment would be to Tonify LU 9, so as to transfer Qi from the Spleen to the Lung. I chose not to do this because I had used the Metal Tonification Points

---

26   In the January 9, 2002 issue of the *New Yorker*, "The Mail" column featured three responses to the article with Kaptchuk's comments, none of which challenged his interpretation of the mechanism of acupuncture's efficacy.

27   Kespi, J., *Acupuncture: From Symbol to Clinical Practice.* Seattle: Eastland Press, 2012.

many times in the past, and this problem presented in spite of that. As a pre-test, I asked him to take a deep breath. Every time he tried, he would start a bout of coughing.

I wanted to choose a treatment that would both affect his Lung directly, and at the same time address the Kapha Vikruti. For those reasons, I chose the Entry Point of the Lung, LU 1, and did a quick in and out Tonification. Then I asked him to take a deep breath again, and there was no coughing at all, regardless of how many times he tried this. Why did I choose the Entry Point instead of the Back Shu Point, which also can Tonify Lung Deficiency? The Back Shu Points are on the Bladder Meridian, and would also Tonify the Bladder, thus increasing Pitta and Kapha. That is exactly the opposite direction suggested by his Vikruti, which was already Pitta on one side and Kapha on the other. Tonifying an Entry Point acts to Sedate the preceding Meridian in the Horary Cycle, in this case the Spleen, and thus reduced the Kapha Dosha. Had he not responded so fully to such a simple treatment, I would have also treated the Exit Point of the Spleen to reinforce the effect, but there was no need to do so in this case. I wanted to include this treatment session as I had mentioned using Ayurvedic information in considering Entry/Exit problems.

CASE 32

I also mentioned Entry/Exit issues between the two Meridians of the same Element. D. M. was a 90-year-old man who presented with trigeminal neuralgia, an extremely painful condition affecting the right side of his face, which had been present for 25 years. He had used Tegretol for the preceding five years for partial symptomatic relief, but disliked taking it because it made him feel unsteady. The illness had started suddenly for no apparent reason, but he had been on multiple medications prior to that time for high blood pressure, high cholesterol, and hypothyroidism, all of which he was still taking. His pulses indicated a Stomach Deficiency constitution, but his Ministerial Fire pulses (right Chi) were the weakest. This is a Lesser Yin constitution, which should have strong Ministerial Fire according to Kuon. His Vikruti pulse on the left was Pitta/Kapha, and on the right it was Vata. Since the painful area included the TH Meridian, it occurred to me that there might be an Entry/Exit problem within Ministerial Fire. The Vikruti on his symptomatic side was Vata, and the extreme pain suggested an Excess in the TH Meridian, along with a Deficiency in the PE Meridian, consistent with his cardiovascular issues, and creating an overall Deficient pulse. Such a situation is consistent with an Entry/Exit block between these two Meridians. I treated him at PE 1 and TH 22, respectively the Entry and Exit Points of their Meridians. Entry Points tend to Tonify, while Exit Points tend to Sedate their Meridians. This treatment led to an immediate disappearance of his pain. He stopped the Tegretol, and with two repetitions of the same treatment he has been without pain for the last two years.

CASE 33

F. I. is a 63-year-old woman whom I had treated over 20 years previously for low back pain. She called for an emergency appointment because she had developed a new problem on the right side, manifesting as pain radiating from the low back to the hip and ankle. The onset of this pain was sudden, and had no apparent cause, and it was severe enough to prevent standing on her right leg or being able to fall asleep. Anti-inflammatory medication gave symptomatic relief, so that when I saw her, she was only in moderate pain. In taking her history, I discovered that she had experienced an episode of shingles in that area of her back five years ago. She worried about a recurrence, so two years later she was injected with a vaccine for preventing shingles. Within a week of getting the vaccination, she developed a second episode of shingles in the same location, which although milder, left her with both numbness and occasional hyperesthesia in the right low back. Her primary doctor told her it was a case of post-herpetic neuralgia, and that there was no treatment indicated for it. Putting all this information together, I suspected that she had a chronic problem with the herpes virus, and that her current pain was probably an exacerbation of the post-herpetic neuralgia. The reason I wanted to include her case here is that it demonstrates the relationship of proximal and distal pulse exams with respect to the SEL and EEM findings.

Her proximal pulses showed an SEL pattern of radial deviation under the index finger ("Cun") on both wrists (Taiyang pattern); however, this radial deviation of the (Yang) Cun pulse in the distal pulse exam was only present on her right wrist. On her left wrist there was a notable Dai Mai pattern instead (very strong Guan pulse on light palpation). In checking her carotid and radial pulses, I found that the carotids were stronger than the radials bilaterally. Abdominal palpation using the KHA test areas revealed no sensitivity, consistent with a diagnosis of Yin Excess syndrome and a Dai Mai imbalance. The pulse suggested that the Dai Mai was in need of treatment on the left side, even though her symptoms were all right sided. I pre-tested her ability to extend her low back (her most painful movement), and found that she was severely restricted. I then needled the Key Points of the Dai Mai on the left side, Sedating GB 41 and Tonifying TH 5, after which I attached an ion-pumping cord to reinforce the polarity of this treatment. Ten minutes later all the pain was gone, she could freely extend her back, and her distal pulses on the left side showed the Taiyang pattern instead of the Dai Mai pattern. This case illustrates my contention that EEM imbalances are reflected in the distal position (Yang location), where they obscure the SEL constitutional pattern, but that this effect is not present in the proximal location for SEL pulse evaluation.

CASE 34

B. I. is a 70-year-old woman who has had chronic fatigue syndrome for the past 28 years. Her symptoms started after a painful relationship breakup, and included exhaustion, myalgia, low grade fevers, and difficulty concentrating. She was initially treated by a practitioner of Medical Acupuncture, who diagnosed her as being Kidney Deficient, and she experienced improvement from his treatments. When I took over her care, I was impressed that she worked full time as a health care provider and legal consultant, in spite of her continuing fatigue and other symptoms. Her pulses confirmed the constitution as Kidney Deficiency (ulnar deviation of the Chi pulse, Lesser Yang SCM, Saturno KCA pulses, and Water Subdoshas frequently appearing in her Vikruti pulses). I'm sure her overworking contributes to the lack of a complete cure, but she loves her work and is highly respected by her professional peers, so she has only managed to slow down a little in response to my suggestions. She responds well to Tonifying Water, and experienced a significant boost in her energy level after starting to take Ling Zhi as a daily supplement on my advice. Kuon has found that Saturno constitutional types are the ones who benefit reliably from this adaptogenic herb.[28] On a recent visit, she showed Pitta/Vata pulses of the Wood type on both wrists. I interpreted that as evidence of a blocked Brow Chakra, and treated her with Cross' protocol: first stimulating DU 4 and SP 6, then needling DU 24.5 and Ren 2.[29] She reported that, after this treatment, she decided to take her dog for a mile and a half walk, something she had not been able to get herself to do for a long time. When seen on follow-up, her energy level had stayed noticeably higher.

CASE 35

I'm including this case in order to give one complete example of not only arriving at the constitutional and conditional diagnoses that this book discusses, but also to demonstrate how the two appendices can be employed to construct treatment protocols based on a creative elaboration of the work of two of my Korean teachers, so that practitioners can discover new and effective acupuncture treatments for the tremendous variety of issues that present

---

28 www.ecmed.org/board/content.asp?bsNo=17&lng=en.

29 Cross' procedures for treating the Chakras involve first stimulating two Points, which he compares to the Key or Opening Points of the EEMs. The next Point is directed at the imbalanced Chakra itself, and the last Point is directed at the Chakra to which it is coupled in Cross' methodology.

themselves to us. Specifically, this case demonstrates how I use KHA metallic pellets to pre-test treatment formulae based on KCA theory. It's an example of how I've been able to rationally select the appropriate Fundamental and Auxiliary Formulae for KCA treatment, even though Kuon did not provide sufficient information to always accurately make this choice. Not only can the treatment Points be chosen rationally, but so can the optimal side of the body on which to stimulate them with the appropriate polarity.

Q.X. is a 65-year-old woman who came for treatment because she had experienced repeated episodes of pneumonia since childhood. Two of these infections had brought her "close to death," the last one only a month prior to her first visit. At the time of her first visit she was already suffering from a respiratory infection that had not yet progressed to pneumonia, a progression that had been her typical scenario in the past. Her constitution was determined to be Kidney Deficiency (ulnar deviation of the SEL pulse, Saturno KCA pulse and Lesser Yang SCM pulse, with a Pitta/Kapha Prakriti). Her Cun, Guan, and Chi pulses showed Deficiency in Yin and Yang at both left Chi positions, but with normal findings at both right Cun positions, and the other positions also felt normal to me. The Vikruti was Vata (Water type) on the left, and Vata (Fire type) on the right. She had a family history of cardiovascular illness on her father's side, but no family history of renal or pulmonary problems. She herself had a mild degree of osteoporosis, which was asymptomatic. The first problem was in determining her constitution. The pulse findings are consistent with either Kidney Deficiency or Heart Excess. She described herself as always fatigued, and closed her eyes without speaking when I wasn't asking any questions during the examination. These clues, together with the osteoporosis, are supportive of Kidney Deficiency rather than Heart Excess. It's also been my experience that Kidney Deficiency is a much more common constitution than Heart Excess, so I made Kidney Deficiency my presumptive constitutional diagnosis.

The next question was what Formulae to consider in order to treat the recurrent pneumonias. Kuon's protocols for such a case (see Appendix 2) would include the Four Needle technique to Tonify the Kidney as the Fundamental Formula, plus a choice between the Zang Inflammation Formula (Spleen Sedation) and the Antibiotic Formula (Small Intestine Sedation) as the Auxiliary component directed at the condition.[30] I decided to modify Kuon's

---

30   In his second publication ("Studies on Constitution-Acupuncture Therapy." *Korean Central Journal of Medicine*, 25 (3), 1973, pp.327–342), Kuon gave examples of successfully treating hepatitis with Fundamental/Zang Formulae (Cases 1 and 2). He also gave an example of successfully treating tuberculosis with Fundamental/Antibiotic Formulae alternated with Fundamental/Fu Formulae (Case 3), because the patient also had digestive disorders. On page 339 he stated, "All diseases which may be implicated in the concept of inflammation…are treated by the Inflammation Formulae…but that in the case of bacterially caused inflammation, the Antibiotic Formulae are applied alternately." Theoretically, pneumonia would be treated using the same formulae as for other Zang infections, as both Liver and Lung are Zang Organs.

recommendations in order to have the treatment respond to her Vikruti findings. Since her Vikruti was Vata on both sides, for the Base (specific form of the Fundamental) Formula I chose instead the Immune Formula (per Puramo), which Tonifies the Bladder rather than the Kidney. Tonifying the Kidney (Kuon's presumptive choice) would have aggravated her Vata Vikruti, whereas Tonifying the Bladder should ameliorate it, by increasing Pitta and Kapha. Certainly, the recurrent infections support the notion that her immune system wasn't functioning well. The Points for the Immune Formula in a Saturno individual are ST 36 and UB 40 Sedated, and LI 1 and UB 67 Tonified. This is simply the Four Needle technique to Tonify the Bladder. Which side should I choose to treat? Kuon recommends treating the right side for Saturno types. I pre-tested this Formula, using metallic pellets, on the KHA corresponding Points[31] (gold pellets on the KHA Points to be Tonified, and silver colored (aluminum) pellets on the KHA Points to be Sedated), first on the left side and then on the right side, checking her pulse to evaluate her response. Pellets on the right hand improved her left Chi pulses, while pellets on her left hand did not. Next I used the same method to pre-test the Auxiliary Formula. I chose the Antibiotic Formula, because it fits the condition being treated, and at the same time it treats the Small Intestine with Sedation, the appropriate response to her Vata (Fire type) Vikruti. The Points are ST 36 and SI 8 Sedated and UB 66 and SI 2 Tonified. This is the Four Needle technique to Sedate the Small Intestine. Pre-testing each side again showed that treating the right side improved her left Chi pulses, but treating her left side didn't. So the actual treatment given was all on the right side,[32] using Kuon's typical needle technique of quickly piercing these Points in succession very shallowly (about 1 mm), and using needle direction to establish Tonification or Sedation. Kuon's protocol for infections is to repeat the Base Formula five times, and the Auxiliary Formula once, which is what I did. The only other modification I used was to repeat the Sedation Points one extra time in the Antibiotic Formula, which Kuon teaches as a way to direct the effect of the treatment to the upper body, where her infection was located.

After treatment, she said she was feeling livelier already, as she left the office. Her "O-ring" kinesiology test had also shown marked improvement. At her first follow-up visit, she said she felt about 80 percent better, and that meant she was feeling the best in at least four years. I repeated exactly the same treatment, and afterwards she said she felt "like her old self," a phrase

---

31   See Appendix 1.

32   I previously alluded to the difference of opinion between Puramo and Kuon concerning which sides to treat with the Fundamental and Auxiliary Formulae. Puramo treats them on opposite sides, while Kuon treats them on the same side. In this case, the pre-testing confirmed Kuon's approach as the more accurate treatment, even though the Subdoshas in the Vikruti showed Fire and Water patterns on opposite sides. At this time I do not think there is a universal rule concerning the appropriate side to treat. Pre-testing is therefore an invaluable practice for researching this question more fully.

that over the years has proven to be a "Golden Key" to having chosen the ideal treatment. It is interesting to note that this treatment, for pneumonia and respiratory infection in general, did not involve any Points on the Lung Meridian, nor any local Points that might impact the Lung. Cases such as this one illustrate the truly radical conceptual difference in Kuon's KCA style of acupuncture. This case demonstrates a model for constructing and pre-testing treatments. The principles involved can be applied to treatment styles other than KCA, so practitioners of virtually any style of traditional acupuncture can benefit from this pre-testing practice, although it still depends on an accurate pulse diagnosis, or other method of feedback to evaluate the protocol being tested.

CASE 36

One of the senior practitioners who reviewed the original draft of this work asked if I might include a more extensive case history that detailed at least the first five treatments, so that the reader might have a clearer idea of how these different pulse findings are applied over time. C.L. is a 49-year-old female psychiatrist, who has been suffering from right sided sciatica for two years. Her symptoms started around the time she began to increase the amount of exercise she was doing, in the hope that more exercise would help her manage her emotional stresses. The pain came on insidiously, and radiated from her low back to her right buttock. Interestingly, Pilates classes seemed to aggravate her pain. An MRI revealed a bulging disc at the L 4/5 level. She tried physical therapy, anti-inflammatory medication, and two epidural injections of steroids with temporary improvement, but the pain always recurred. Sitting or standing for long periods aggravated her pain, while lying down or moving around improved it. The pain radiated between the Gall Bladder and Urinary Bladder Meridians. She had already tried acupuncture and Chinese herbal treatment with two different practitioners without any benefit before coming to see me, on the recommendation of a friend who was a patient of mine.

Her history and systems review revealed that she had been rear-ended in an auto accident five years previously, and had suffered left sided headaches and neck pain radiating towards her shoulder ever since, although these pains were not as severe as the sciatica. Also around five years ago she experienced a series of urinary tract infections for no obvious reason, but was able to stop them by eliminating acidic foods from her diet, including coffee and tomatoes, although she does still get hematuria at times. Her physician diagnosed the cause as interstitial cystitis. She eats a mostly vegetarian plus seafood diet, motivated by her desire to assist her husband in lowering his cholesterol level, but does complain of abdominal bloating, especially after eating dairy products, and is often mildly constipated, having bowel movements only once in three days, but without any resulting discomfort. She did report that in general her pain levels had been greater ever since she decreased the amount of animal protein in her diet. She reported that she was much more prone to feel too cold than too hot. Her only current medication is Lexapro for anxiety, which she has taken for about four years, claiming that it helped her without inducing any side effects except possibly some decrease in libido.

Family medical history revealed that her father died at age 75 from lung cancer, while her mother died at age 88 after a lifelong problem with congenital kidney problems (including stones), arthritis, heart disease, and digestive disorders.

Her social and personal history were non-contributory except for the emotional stress she reported around raising an autistic child. Her marriage and work were seen as very positive aspects of her life. She did report a tendency to be fearful and overly cautious compared to her peers.

Her pulses showed the following findings: Ulnar deviation (SEL) at the Chi position, and Vata Prakriti. The only constitutions compatible with these findings are Heart Deficiency or Kidney Excess, both of which are Lesser Yin SCM types, and her KCA Mercurio pulses confirmed this diagnosis. It felt to me that her Vikruti pulses were Vata of the Fire type bilaterally, but also that the only pulse that was not at its proper depth was her left Yang Chi pulse, indicating a Water Element imbalance. Also, her right Yin Guan pulse (Earth Element) was noticeably Deficient. Her abdominal sensitivity revealed marked tenderness at Ren 5.

Putting all the history and exam findings together, it seemed to me that her constitution was most likely Kidney Excess (mother's congenital kidney disease, excessive fear, and abnormal depth of her Yang Water pulse). I considered using one of the KCA formulae for disc herniation, which would be KZN (see Appendix 2), but decided to start with just the Zang inflammation component, which tonifies the Spleen. The Points are HE 8 and SP 2 Tonified, and KI 10 and SP 9 Sedated. These Points happen to coincidently be Sa Am's Four Needle formula for treating Cold in the Spleen, and her sensitivity to cold together with abdominal bloating suggested that these might be important Points to treat. I inserted these needles on her right side (the normal treatment side per Kuon for Kidney Excess), and left them in place for ten minutes. I also instructed her to increase her meat consumption as per the Kidney Excess diet.

At her second visit, one week later, she reported feeling a lot better. The biggest change had been in her headaches and neck pain, which had essentially disappeared. Her energy level had increased, and her bowel movements had become more regular. The sciatica had improved initially, but was already starting to come back. I decided that this response (seeing that she had been previously unresponsive to acupuncture) confirmed her constitution as Kidney

Excess. In fact, when I checked her pulses, I found that this time her Vikruti was Vata of the Water type bilaterally (Apana Vata). I decided to use a fuller version of the KCA protocol (KZP), and again treated her on the right side with needles in the following Points: SP 3 and KI 3 Tonified, and LU 8 and KI 7 Sedated, plus HE 8 and SP 2 Tonified, and KI 10 and SP 9 Sedated, plus TH 2 Tonified and TH 3 Sedated. Again, the needles were left in for ten minutes. She reported an increased range of motion in her neck right after treatment.

On her third visit (one week later) she reported that many of her friends had told her how much better she was looking and, indeed, her neck had not been bothering her at all, but she had not really improved in regard to the sciatica. She was however very happy with the progress she had made, and said that she felt much better overall. Her pulses this time showed a recurrence of the Vata Fire type Vikruti, and I additionally detected an abnormal depth of her left side Yang Cun (Fire) and Yang Chi (Water), and right side Yang Chi (Fire) pulses. I decided that the treatment of the Triple Heater had not been helpful (new flipped depth there), and started treatment by stimulating the Xi Cleft Point TH 7 on the right with a rapid in and out needling. This immediately improved her back pain. I then used the KCA formula KF for Fu inflammation, hypothesizing that with disturbances in bladder and bowel function, this would be a reasonable approach, especially as it treats the Heart Meridian, which showed a depth abnormality. The Points were: SP 3 and KI 3 Tonified, and LU 8 and KI 7 Sedated, plus SP 3 and HE 7 Tonified, and LU 8 and HE 4 Sedated, again with right sided needle retention for ten minutes. After this treatment she reported that the back pain was completely gone.

On her fourth visit (ten days later) she reported that the back pain was definitely improving. She only noticed it on first getting up in the morning. Her neck and energy lever were staying improved. At this time I decided to switch treatment technique from KCA style to FEA style, although still keeping the diagnosis of Kidney Excess (Water CF). Her Vikruti showed Vata of the Water type on the left and Vata of the Fire type on the right, with abnormal depths on the left Yang Cun and left Yin Chi pulses. I decided to do a simple transfer along the Creative Cycle from Water to Fire using the left side (opposite to the symptomatic side) needling at HE 9 and LV 8. The needle was manipulated for Tonification at HE 9, and then both were removed. Her pulses responded positively, and her kinesiology showed improved muscle strength.

On her most recent visit, she reported feeling even better. The pain on first getting up in the morning was less, but not completely gone; however, in all other ways she felt normal, with good energy, good bowel function, and no restriction in her activities. Once again, her left side Vikruti was Vata of the Water type and her right side Vikruti was Vata of the Fire type, with abnormal depths at the left Yang Chi and right Yin Cun positions. I interpreted this as

Excess of Kidney Yang and Deficiency of Heart Yin. In order to balance the Doshas, the Water and Fire Elements, and Yin and Yang, I used the following treatment: HE 9, LV 8, and KI 4, needled bilaterally, again with rapid Tonification at HE 9 followed by removal of all the needles. The rationale for this treatment is that KI 4 increases KI Yin by pulling it from KI Yang where it showed as Excess, and the rest of the treatment transferred this Excess Yin to the Heart, which showed Yin Deficiency. Again her pulses and kinesiology improved right away, and she has since reported that even the residual morning pain is continuing to diminish.

In addition to wanting to present a more detailed case history, I also chose this case because it clearly demonstrates the benefits of Sedating the Kidney in certain individuals. Although I have found Kidney Excess to be an unusual constitutional type, recognizing it may be crucial to being able to help such individuals with acupuncture. Although I do not know the specifics of this person's previous acupuncture sessions, it would not surprise me if they were based on Tonifying the Kidney, a common approach in treating low back pain and sciatica, but one which would be counter-productive in her case.

CASE 37

I had envisioned these case histories as illustrating at least one example of each of the 24 proposed constitutions. Although I have often Sedated the Lung Meridian for conditional reasons, I have yet to find a clear case of constitutional Lung Excess. In thinking back over the many people I've treated, the only example of the Lung Excess constitution that comes to mind is myself! It is technically difficult to examine one's own pulses, in addition to which there is an increased subjective bias, so I am also relying on other data to support this diagnosis. Every SCM practitioner I have met has unequivocally diagnosed my type as Lesser Yin. Several senior FEA practitioners, based on color, sound, odor, and emotion, have declared me to have a Metal CF, but that is far from unanimous (all the others, Worsley included, have opted for Fire, specifically Small Intestine, with Metal as the "within" Element). The only constitution that fits both Lesser Yin SCM type and Metal Element FEA type is Lung Excess. The basis for my self-diagnosis is in finding a Lesser Yin SCM pulse, a Mercurio KCA pulse, an ulnarly deviated SEL Guan pulse, and a Vata/Kapha Prakriti. Additional support for this diagnosis was provided decades ago, when I was a demonstration case for a pulse diagnosis instrument developed by Hee Soo Back, a Korean researcher who visited the clinic I worked at in Oakland, California.[33] His instrument recorded the vibrations at Cun, Guan,

---

33   Back, H., *How to Read Hee Soo Type Electronic Pulse Wave*. Seoul: Hee Soo Electronic Pulse Institute of Korea, 1978—in Korean and English.

and Chi much like a polygraph recording. Back had extensively studied such recordings, and developed a schema for interpreting the results. In my case, the only abnormality he detected was "stagnation" on the Lung pulse, which would be interpreted as a type of Excess. Over the years I have had a lot of acupuncture treatment, and the best results have been from Sedating the Lung. I also responded positively to Menetrier's oligoelement therapy for Metal imbalances (manganese-copper, although manganese-cobalt for Fire has helped at times as well), and my constitution would be better described as hyposthenic than as dystonic.[34] My interpretation of all this data is that my CF is Metal, and Fire is the Element within. I've noted before that Lee's original SCM theory posited that the different constitutional types were not present in equal proportions in the population. Lee diagnosed himself as having a Greater Yang constitution that was present in only one in a thousand individuals, according to his experience. It is curious that my own synthetic theory of constitutional diagnosis has also come up finding myself as having an extremely "rare" constitutional type. Although our constitutional theories differ, we both found ourselves with Excess Metal as the dominant characteristic of our constitutions. I don't know quite what to make of this coincidence, but I'm happy to be in such good company.

---

34   See Chapter 5.

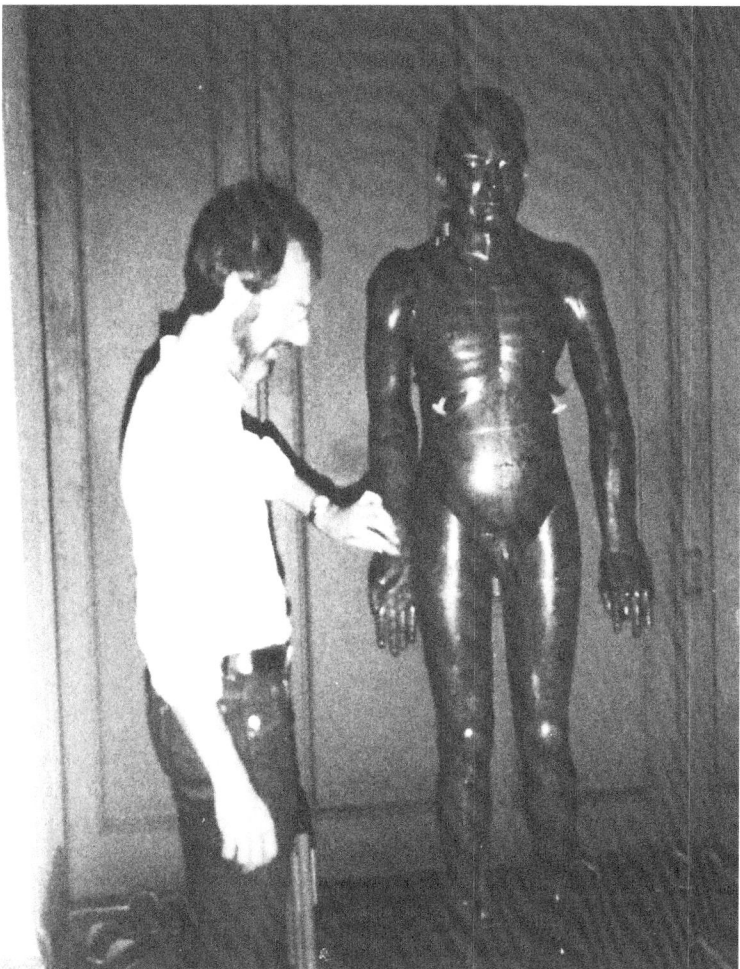

Figure 19.1 Two Metal CFs?[35]

35   I had the rare opportunity to closely examine the bronze acupuncture manikin from China's Song dynasty (960–1279 CE), which was taken to Japan and stored in the basement of their National Museum. A group of American acupuncturists studying in Tokyo in 1982, of which I was a member, were given a private showing of the manikin. I couldn't resist the temptation to indulge my obsession with pulse taking, which apparently existed decades before the idea of writing a book on the subject first crossed my mind.

CHAPTER 20

AN AFTERWORD

I had intended to limit this text to the subject of pulse diagnosis in Oriental medicine, and leave other topics of interest, such as the nature of Oriental scientific thought, for a separate treatise. But I find that there is one topic that begs for a mention, and while it concerns a subject, homeopathy, which is neither an aspect of Oriental medicine, nor based on pulse diagnosis, it has found a way past these limits, in my mind. Most readers are probably not conversant with the work of the contemporary Indian homeopath Rajan Sankaran,[1] but I highly recommend a study of his publications, regardless of whether or not one is trained in homeopathy.[2] In the present treatise I have tried to establish reliable criteria for the various aspects of diagnosis, both constitutional and conditional, as they are encountered in clinic. However, in reality, pulse diagnosis always has a significant subjective component, and there are cases where the methods I have explained may not lead to an unequivocal conclusion. I have found Sankaran's theories to be a help in such cases, so I will very briefly present the most elementary of his ideas, as I apply them, hopefully without distorting what he teaches.

Homeopathic remedies are prepared from materials in nature, and Sankaran has discovered that these natural materials share certain qualities, whether in their natural state or in the form they assume after being used to create the diluted remedies used in homeopathy. It is surprising to me that this idea has not been popularized earlier, for the different materials that the remedies are prepared from represent simply the Three Kingdoms of Mineral, Vegetable, and Animal, which is a familiar system of classification known to every child

---

1   I attended a three-day seminar by Rajan Sankaran on "The Vital Sensation in Homeopathy" in Deerfield Beach, FL, in 2005.

2   Sankaran, R., *The Sensation in Homoeopathy*. Mumbai: Homoeopathic Medical Publishers, 2004, would be my recommendation as a place to start.

who has ever played "Twenty Questions." Sankaran has posited that each of these Kingdoms shares a different "disposition," one might say, which shows up in both the natural source of the remedy and in the individual for whom that remedy is suited. I will present my understanding of these three different "dispositions," but I imagine that the reader might already suspect how I will use this information: Three Kingdoms, following the resonant thinking typical of Oriental medicine, must relate somehow to the Three Doshas that are at the foundation of Ayurvedic medicine. Indeed, it has been my experience that this association is a useful one, and I would offer an hypothesis to homeopaths that they might consider remedies that combine members of two Kingdoms at a time, just as individuals are not restricted to only Vata, Pitta, or Kapha types, but frequently present a mixture of two at a time.

The essential quality or disposition of the Mineral Kingdom relates to structures. Minerals form the building blocks of nature, and individuals who resonate with the disposition of the Mineral Kingdom will experience themselves as primarily lacking something in themselves, or at least are afraid that they may lose something vital in themselves. This latter notion is quite important; such individuals experience their problems as coming from within themselves in the form of a sense of incompleteness.

The essential quality or disposition of the Plant or Vegetable Kingdom relates to a feeling of sensitivity. The feeling is one of being adversely affected by something from outside. We can, of course, see that plants need certain conditions to survive, and every plant has its own optimum environment. This feeling of being affected by something outside of themselves can relate to the weather, the behavior of people they are involved with, the time of day, etc. What's important is that as long as these adverse conditions are absent, such individuals feel quite well.

The essential quality or disposition of the Animal Kingdom is the experience of everything as a struggle of oneself against some adversary. It is not merely some condition that the individual cannot bear, but rather that something from outside themselves is opposing them, and must be defeated. What might be a condition for a "Plant" individual becomes personified as an entity for an "Animal" individual. Typical language that expresses this feeling might be something like, "This toothache is killing me." It is not a feeling of "I have poor teeth" (Mineral) or "my teeth hurt whenever I drink cold beverages" (Plant), but something more personified, and indicative of struggle.

From an Ayurvedic perspective, these Three Kingdoms seem to me to clearly fit the following classification: Mineral = Vata, Plant = Kapha, and Animal = Pitta. There are other ways of relating this to Oriental medicine. The trilogy of Heaven, Earth, and Man can also be seen as Vata, Kapha, and Pitta, with Heaven creating the conditions for existence, Earth providing the sustenance, and Man completing creation. In Ayurveda, Vata is often described as the first of the Doshas, and we can see the two different orders of Heaven/Earth/Man vs. Heaven/Man/Earth in the Doshas. If Plants are of Kapha nature, then they certainly preceded Animals in creation but, as the slowest Dosha, Kapha lags behind Pitta in the pulses. This line of thinking could be extended in much greater detail, but that would indeed carry me away from the purpose of this text. I have merely presented this additional way of looking at the world as a final check on diagnosis, if it is needed. In that regard, I might add the following conclusions: Mineral individuals (Vata) will have either Fire or Water Element constitutions; Plant individuals (Kapha) will have either Wood or Earth Element constitutions; while Animal individuals (Pitta) will have Metal Element constitutions. As for the combined types, Mineral/Plant will be Metal Element; Mineral/Animal will be Wood or Earth Element; and Plant/Animal will be Fire or Water Element.

Sankaran is quite clear that these essential qualities of the Three Kingdoms are only reliably displayed at the deepest level at which an individual experiences life but, at this deep level, all experiences will display this typical quality. At the more superficial levels, individuals may display aspects of all Three Kingdoms, so it is quite easy to get led up the garden path. I have found this type of corroborative analysis to be most useful in understanding my long-term clients, and do not usually apply it in the initial diagnostic session. I would be curious to know if others either corroborate or refute this analysis.

MERIDIAN AND POINT LOCATIONS FOR KHA

In general, the Yin Micromeridians are on the palmar surface and the Yang Micromeridians are on the dorsal surface of the hand. There are two exceptions to this rule for the zone where the Command Points are located on the ring and little fingers of each hand: the Stomach Micromeridian runs on the palmar surface and the Kidney Micromeridian runs on the dorsal surface. The Command Points for these two Micromeridians have their locations in spots analogous to the other Micromeridians on the same surface of the hand. The order of the Points is the same as in body acupuncture. For Yin Meridians, the Wood Point is located just below the fingernail, the Fire Point is located halfway to the DIP joint crease, the Earth/Source Point is located on the DIP joint crease, the Metal Point is located halfway between the DIP and PIP joint creases, and the Water Point is located on the PIP joint crease. The Connecting Point is located halfway between the Earth and Metal Points. For Yang Meridians, the Metal Point is located just below the fingernail, the Water Point is located halfway between the nail and the DIP joint crease, the Source Point is located on the DIP joint crease, the Wood Point is located halfway between the DIP and PIP joint creases, the Fire Point is located halfway between the Wood Point and the PIP joint crease, and the Earth Point is located on the PIP joint crease. The Connecting Point is located halfway between the Wood Point and the DIP joint crease.

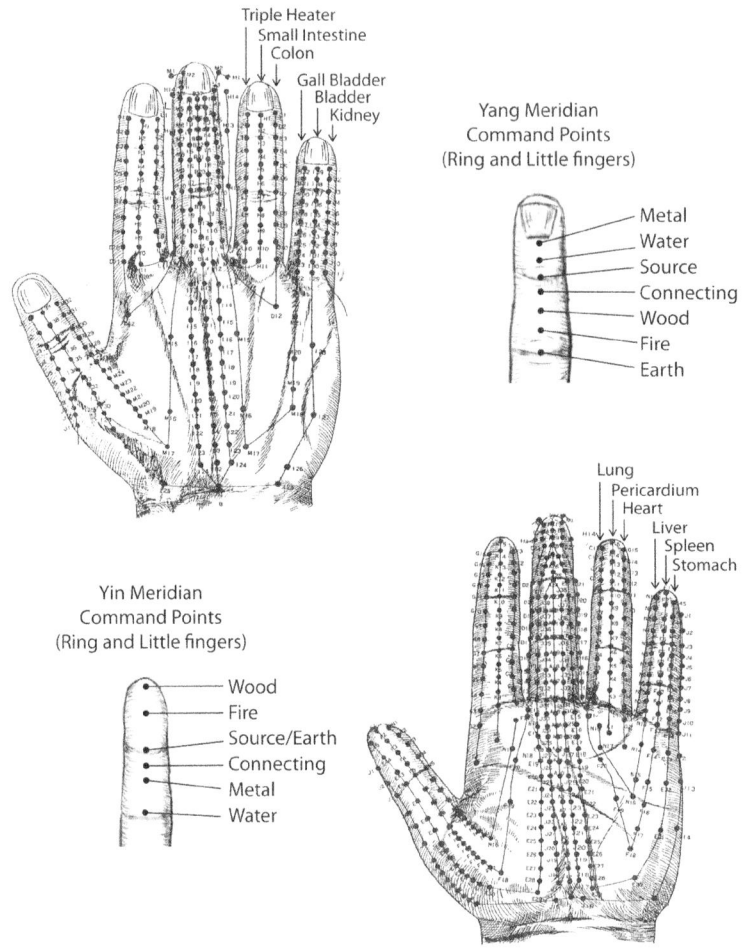

Figure App.1.1 Micromeridian and Point locations in KHA[1]

For pre-testing a treatment, place either a gold (Tonifying) or silver (Sedating) press pellet on the Point on the same side of the body as the proposed treatment. Always use only the ring and little fingers for these Command Point pre-tests. It is quite permissible to use multiple pellets at the same time, either of the same color or of opposite colors. For example, when pre-testing any Four Needle pattern, you will always use both gold and silver pellets on the same hand. The modality chosen for feedback as to whether the proposed treatment is desirable or not depends on the practitioner's choice. One can look for improvements in pulses, abdominal pressure sensitivity, O-ring strength, blood pressure readings, or any other abnormal sign or symptom.

---

1   Image: Neal White and Elisabeth Waller-White. Based on original figures by Yoo Tae Woo.

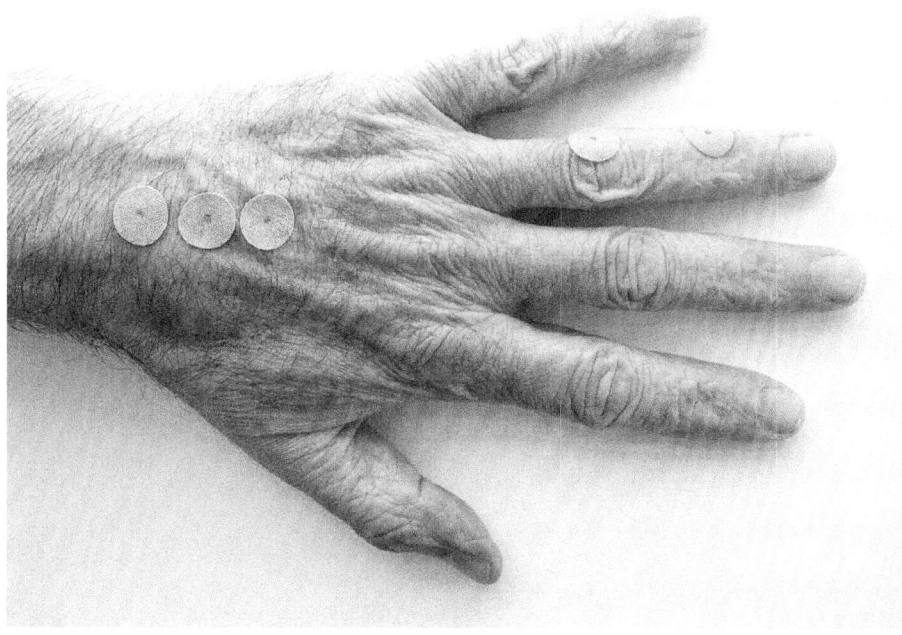

Figure App.1.2 Using Press Pellets in KHA[2]

---

2   Image: Marina Chentsova Eckman. In addition to the pellets on the dorsum of the hand, one can see
     pellets on the ring finger at Points that correspond to LI 4 and LI 11.

TREATMENT FORMULAE FOR KCA

The following list has been compiled from material learned from Puramo Chong. It was communicated to me with the understanding that these were treatment protocols taught in Korean workshops by Bae Cholwan, who at the time was studying under Kuon Dowon, and that Kuon had approved their publication. Many of these treatments are different than the ones I observed at Kuon's clinic in Seoul, and thus differ from the material in Table 8.2, especially with regard to the Formulae for Fu constitutions. Sometimes one of Kuon's Formulae appears to be most accurate and at others one of Chong's appears to work better. A good example can be seen in Case 22, where sciatica due to disc herniation was successfully treated in an individual of a Fu constitution with Chong's Points for the K/Z/N Formulae. In this case I chose Chong's version because it was corroborated by the Ayurvedic Vikruti pulses. This discrepancy in various iterations of the Formulae is a subject that needs clarification, and I think it's a component of KCA that suffers the most from the lack of publication by Kuon himself. The nomenclature for the Root and Auxiliary Formulae uses Chong's terminology as follows:

K = Root, I = Immune, D = Degeneration, P = Paralysis, F = Fu, B = Antibiotic, Z = Zang, V = Vitality, and N = Neuro or Psyche.

The *Root (Fundamental) Formula* K is used to treat fatigue, trauma, sprains, contusions, and pediatric ills.

The *Immune Formula* I is used to treat immunological problems, allergic rhinitis, chronic cough, asthma, skin allergies, diabetes, and neurodermatitis.

The *Degeneration Formula* D is used to treat degenerative and other forms of arthritis, rheumatism, disc disease, sciatica, myalgia, and various unspecified chronic diseases.

The *Paralysis Formula* P is used to treat paralysis, polio, and Bell's palsy.

The *Fu Formula* F is used to treat non-bacterial problems of the Fu Organs, rhinitis, tonsillitis, pleurisy, otitis, conjunctivitis, endometritis, nervous headaches, skin diseases, circulation problems, gynecological problems, ENT problems, epilepsy, insomnia, melancholy, morning sickness, colds, low back pain, shoulder and arm pain, and muscle pain.

The *Antibiotic (Infection) Formula* B is used to treat colds and all other infectious diseases.

The *Zang Formula* Z is used to treat non-bacterial problems of the Zang Organs, tuberculosis, hepatitis, nephritis, cataract, strabismus, hypertension, the sequellae of chronic trauma, disc hernia, osteomyelitis, and joint pain.

The *Vitality Formula* V is used to treat ptosis, hiatus hernia, prolapse, senility, neuralgia, hypotension, enuresis, and nocturia.

The *Neuro (Psyche) Formula* N is used to treat mental ills, autonomic problems, insomnia, headache, neurasthenia, nervous indigestion, and hysteria.

The Points for these Formulae may differ from those listed for Kuon's original Eight Constitutions in Table 8.2. Some of these differences most likely represent an evolution in Kuon's thinking, but it is not clear to me what role, if any, Puramo and his colleagues played in this evolution. The following is a simple presentation of the most recent information about the preceding Formulae, as transmitted to me by Puramo.

For Fu Constitutions (e.g. LI Deficiency), the Root Formula treats its coupled (Yin) Meridian (LU). Staying with Yin Meridians, the Daughter Meridian (KI) forms the Degeneration Formula, the Granddaughter Meridian (LV) forms the Zang Formula, and the Great Granddaughter Meridian (HE) forms the Fu Formula. The Constitutional Meridian (LI) forms the Immune Formula, the Son Meridian (UB) forms the Paralysis Formula, the Grandson Meridian (GB) forms the Vitality Formula, and the Great Grandson Meridian (SI) forms the Antibiotic Formula. The Points selected for each of these Formulae are almost always the ones Kuon listed in Table 8.2 for treating the Meridian concerned, but be careful, as the Formula names have been changed.

For Zang Constitutions (e.g. LV Deficiency), the Root Formula treats its own Meridian (LV), the Mother Meridian (KI) forms the Degeneration Formula, the Granddaughter Meridian (SP) forms the Fu Formula, and the Great Granddaughter (LU) forms the Zang Formula. The Coupled Meridian (GB) forms the Immune Formula, the Father Meridian (UB) forms the Paralysis Formula, the Grandson Meridian (ST) forms the Antibiotic Formula, and the Great Grandson Meridian (LI) forms the Vitality Formula. The same considerations as given above apply regarding the Points in Table 8.2.

The following list designates treatment protocols for various conditions attributed to Bae Cholwan by Puramo:

Allergic rhinitis: K/F or K/B

Anxiety: K/Z or D/V/N

Arthritis or rheumatism: K/F/ N/Z or D/B/N/V

Bronchitis: K/Z

Cholecystitis: K/F/N

Cold Extremities: K/F or K/V

Colds: K/F or K/B

Conjunctivitis: K/B/K/F

Cystitis: K/F/N

Deafness: K/Z/F/P/N

Dermatitis (atopic): K/V/N/F

Diarrhea: K/F/N

Dizziness: K/F or K/Z

Duodenal ulcer: K/F/N

Epilepsy: K/F/K/N

Fatigue: D/B/N

Gastroptosis: K/V

Gout: D/F/N or K/B/N

Headache (tension or migraine): K/F

Hepatitis: K/Z

Hernia: K/V/N

Herniated disc: K/Z/N

Hypertension: K/F/N

Hypotension: K/V/N

Insomnia: K/N or K/Z/K/N

Irritable Bowel Syndrome: K/F/N

Knee pain: K/Z/N

Liver cirrhosis: F/V/B/P/N

Lumbago: K/Z/N

Neuralgia: D/B/N

Prostate hypertrophy: K/V/K/F

Rib pain: K/Z/N

Thyroid disease: K/F/N

Tinnitus: K/Z/F/P/N

Trigeminal neuralgia: K/B or K/B/N

Uterine prolapse: K/V/N

Vaginitis or Ovary/uterine inflammation: K/F

I'm sure most readers will find these prescriptions confusing, since the rules for combining Formulae to match a given clinical presentation are far from complete. My impression is that constitutional energetics are inherently complex and confusing, and the changing nomenclature has made applying this method of treatment even more challenging, but when the treatment is chosen correctly, the results can be remarkable. Also, the reader will note that many conditions are listed with several different Formulae as options for treatment. It is for this very reason that I originally began pre-testing treatments with metallic pellets on the KHA corresponding Points. Any fuller presentation of KCA practice would be both beyond the scope of this text, and test the limits of what I must respect in my relationship to Kuon as my teacher. Let me end by noting that his treatments often involve multiple Formulae from the Auxiliary category, in addition to the Fundamental formula (which is not always used), in each session, and the treatment can be different on the two sides of the body. It is my fervent hope that Kuon will finally publish a text that will make my abridged presentation of KCA obsolete.

REFERENCES

Aihara, H., *Basic Macrobiotics*. New York: Japan Publications, 1985.

Amber, R. and Babey-Brooke, A., *The Pulse in Occident and Orient: Its Philosophy and Practice in India, China, Iran and the West*. New York: Dunshaw Press, 1966.

Athavale, V., *Pulse*. Delhi: Chaukhamba, 2000.

Back, H., *How to Read Hee Soo Type Electronic Pulse Wave*. Seoul: Hee Soo Electronic Pulse Institute of Korea, 1978.

Bertschinger, R., trans., *The Golden Needle and Other Odes of Traditional Acupuncture*. Edinburgh: Churchill Livingstone, 1991.

Chang, J. and Brinkman, M., *Pulsynergy*. Privately published, 1995. Available from Evergreen Herb Company.

Chang, K., "Quakes, Tectonic and Theoretical." *New York Times*, January 15, 2011. Available at www.nytimes.com/2011/01/16/weekinreview/16chang.html, accessed June 18, 2013.

Chen, E., *The Tao Te Ching*. New York: Paragon House, 1989.

CIRET (Centre International de Recherches et Études Transdisciplinaires), "Charter of Transdisciplinarity" 1994. Available at http://ciret-transdisciplinarity.org/chart.php, accessed June 18, 2013.

Cross, J., *Acupuncture and the Chakra Energy System*. Berkeley, CA: North Atlantic Books, 2008.

Eckman, P., "The Third House on the Right, Kidney Fire—A Study." *Journal of Traditional Acupuncture*, 7 (3), 1984, pp.13–15.

Eckman, P., *The Book of Changes in Traditional Oriental Medicine*. Columbia, MD: Traditional Acupuncture Institute, 1988.

Eckman, P., "Korean Acupuncture." *Trad. Ac. Soc. J.* (UK), 7, 1990, pp.1–6.

Eckman, P., "Ayurveda and Korean Hand Acupuncture: A Brief Introduction to Some Similarities between Constitutional Typologies." *Amer. J. Acup.*, 23 (2), 1995, pp.153–158.

Eckman, P., *In the Footsteps of the Yellow Emperor: Tracing the History of Traditional Acupuncture*. San Francisco, CA: Cypress Books, 1996.

Eckman, P., *In the Footsteps of the Yellow Emperor: Tracing the History of Traditional Acupuncture*. Second edition. San Francisco, CA: Long River Press, 2007.

Eckman, P. and Kutchins, S., *Closing the Circle: Lectures on the Unity of Traditional Oriental Medicine*. Fairfax, CA: Shen Foundation, 1983.

The Essentials of Chinese Acupuncture. Beijing: Foreign Languages Press, 1980.

Filliozat, J., *The Classical Doctrine of Indian Medicine*. Delhi: Munshiram Manoharlal, 1964.

Gupta, K., *Science of Sphygmica or Sage Kanad on Pulse*. Delhi: Sri Satguru, 1891.

Hammer, L., *Chinese Pulse Diagnosis: A Contemporary Approach*. Seattle: Eastland Press, 2001.

Helms, J., *Acupuncture Energetics*. Berkeley, CA: Medical Acupuncture Publishers, 1995.

Helms, J., *Getting to Know You*. Berkeley, CA: Medical Acupuncture Publishers, 2007.

Hicks, A., Hicks, J., and Mole, P., *Five Element Constitutional Acupuncture*. Edinburgh: Churchill Livingstone, 2004.

Jarrett, L., *Nourishing Destiny: The Inner Tradition of Chinese Medicine*. Stockbridge: Spirit Path Press, 1999.

Jarrett, L., *The Clinical Practice of Chinese Medicine*. Stockbridge: Spirit Path Press, 2006.

Kaptchuk, T., *The Web That Has No Weaver*. New York: Congdon and Weed, 1983.

Kespi, J., *Acupuncture*. Moulins les Metz: Maisonneuve, 1982 (in French).

Kespi, J., *Acupuncture: From Symbol to Clinical Practice*. Seattle: Eastland Press, 2012.

Kim, B., *The Silver Bullet, KOSA*. Buena Park: KOSA of the Americas, 2012.

Kim, H. B., *Minibook of Oriental Medicine*. Anaheim, CA: Qpuncture, 2009.

Kim, J., *Compass of Health: Using the Art of Sasang Medicine to Maximize Your Health*. Franklin Lakes, NJ: Career Press, 2001.

Kim, S. H., Kim, W. Y., Lee, P. J., Kuon, D. W., and Kim, Y. O., "A Comparison of Nutritional Status Among Eight Constitutional Groups in Relation to Food Preference on the View Point of Constitutional Medicine." *Korean Nutrition Society Journal*, 18, 1985, pp.155–166.

Kuon Dowon, "A Study of Constitution-Acupuncture." *Journal of the International Congress of Acupuncture and Moxibustion*, 10, 1965, pp.149–167.

Kuon Dowon, "Studies on Constitution-Acupuncture Therapy." *Korean Central Journal of Medicine*, 25 (3), 1973, pp.327–342.

Kuon Dowon, *Pyrologos: A New Theory of Life and the Universe*. Dawnting Cancer Research Institute, 1999. Reprinted as IMKS Occasional Paper No. 1, Yonsei University Press, 2002. The original manuscript in Korean was written in 1983.

Kushi, M., *Nine Star Ki*. Becket, MA: One Peaceful World Press, 1991.

Lad, V., *Secrets of the Pulse: The Ancient Art of Ayurvedic Pulse Diagnosis*. Albuquerque, NM: Ayurvedic Press, 1996.

Lad, V., *Textbook of Ayurveda: General Principles of Management and Treatment*, vol. 3. Albuquerque, NM: Ayurvedic Press, 2012.

Lavater, J., *Essays on Physiognomy*. London: G.G.J. and J. Robinson, 1789.

Lavier, J., *Histoire, doctrine et pratique de l'acupuncture chinoise*. Paris: Tchou, 1966.

Lee, D., *Four Constitutional Medicine: Acupuncture, Diet, and Herbs*. Unpublished manuscript, 2013.

Lee, J. K. and Bae, S. K., *Korean Acupuncture*. Seoul: Ko Mun Sa, 1974. Third edition, 1981.

Lee Je-Ma, *Longevity and Life Preservation in Oriental Medicine*. Seoul: Kyung Hee University Press, 1996.

Lee, M. B., *On Constitution-Acupuncture*. Seoul: New Medical, 1973.

Maciocia, G., *The Practice of Chinese Medicine*. Edinburgh: Churchill Livingstone, 1994.

Mann, F., *The Meridians of Acupuncture*. London: Heinemann, 1964.

Mathews, R. H., *Mathews' Chinese-English Dictionary*. Cambridge, MA: Harvard University Press, 1979.

Matsumoto, K. and Birch, S., *Extraordinary Vessels*. Brookline, MA: Paradigm, 1986.

Morin, E., *On Complexity* (ed. A. Montuori). Cresskill, NJ: Hampton Press, 2008.

Morris, W., "Post-paradox: Room for View." *Acupuncture Today*, 13 (8), 2012.

Morris, W. R., "Chinese Pulse Diagnosis: Epistemology, Practice, and Tradition." Dissertation. California Institute of Integral Studies, San Francisco, 2009.

Needham, J., *Science and Civilization in China*, vol. 2. Cambridge: Cambridge University Press, 1956.

Niboyet, J., *Essai sur l'acupuncture Chinoise pratique*. Paris: Editions Dominique Wapler, 1951.

Niboyet, J., *Compléments d'acupuncture*. Paris: Editions Dominique Wapler, 1955.

Nicolescu, B., *Manifesto of Transdisciplinarity*. Albany: State University of New York Press, 2002.

Ninivaggi, F., *An Elementary Textbook of Ayurveda*. Madison, CT: Psychosocial Press, 2001.

O'Connor, J. and Bensky, D., trans. and eds., *Acupuncture: A Comprehensive Text*. Chicago: Eastland Press, 1981.

Requena, Y., *Terrains and Pathology in Acupuncture*. Brookline, MA: Paradigm, 1986.

Requena, Y., *Character and Health*. Brookline, MA: Paradigm, 1989.

Sankaran, R., *The Sensation in Homoeopathy*. Mumbai: Homoeopathic Medical Publishers, 2004.

Scheid, V., *Chinese Medicine in Contemporary China: Plurality and Synthesis*. Durham, NC: Duke University Press, 2002.

Schmidt, H., *Konstitutionelle Akupunktur*. Stuttgart: Hippokrates Verlag, 1988.

Shen, J., *Chinese Medicine*. New York: Educational Solutions, 1980.

Song, I., *An Introduction to Sasang Constitutional Medicine*. Seoul: Jimoondong International, 2005.

Soulié de Morant, G., *L'acuponcture Chinoise*. Paris: Maloine, 1972.

Specter, M., "The Power of Nothing." *New Yorker*, December 12, 2011, pp.30–36.

Svoboda, R., *Prakruti, Your Ayurvedic Constitution*. Wilmot, AR: Lotus Light Publications, 1988.

Tan, R. and Rush, S., *Twelve and Twelve in Acupuncture*. San Diego, CA: Author, 1991.

Thambirajah, R., *Energetics in Acupuncture*. Edinburgh: Churchill Livingstone, 2010.

Upadhyay, G., *The Science of Pulse Examination in Ayurveda*. Delhi: Sri Satguru, 1997.

Upadhyay, S., *Nadi Vijnana (Ancient Pulse Science)*. Delhi: Chaukhamba, 1986.

Van Meter, S., *Jingei Pulse Diagnosis*. Portland, OR: Working Class Acupuncture, 2007.

Walton, I., *The Compleat Angler*. London: J. M. Dent, 1906.

Wang, J. *et al.*, "Cognition Research and Constitutional Classification in Chinese Medicine." *Am. J. Chin. Med.*, 39 (4), 2011, pp.651–660.

Wang Shu-he, *The Pulse Classic: A Translation of the Mai Jing* (Yang Shou-zhong, trans.). Boulder, CO: Blue Poppy Press, 1997.

Wilhelm, R. and Baynes, C., trans., *The I Ching or Book of Changes*. Princeton: Princeton University Press, 1977.

Worsley, J., *Traditional Chinese Acupuncture, vol. 1. Meridians and Points*. Tisbury: Element Books, 1982.

Yoo Tae Woo, *Lecture on Koryo Sooji Chim*. Seoul: Eum Yang Mek Jin, 1983.

Yoo Tae Woo, *Koryo Hand Acupuncture*, vol. 1 (ed. P. Eckman). Seoul: Eum Yang Mek Jin, 1988.

Yoo Tae Woo, *Koryo Hand Therapy*, vol. 1 (second edition). Seoul: Eum Yang Mek Jin, 2001.

FURTHER READING

Birch, S., "Naming the Unnamable: A Historical Study of Radial Pulse Six Position Diagnosis." *Trad. Acup. Soc. J.*, 12, 1992.

Borsarello, J., *Les pouls en médecine Chinoise*. Paris: Masson, 1981.

Borsarello, J., *Pulsologie Chinoise traditionelle*. Paris: Masson, 1992.

Cross, J., *Healing with the Chakra Energy System*. Berkeley, CA: North Atlantic Books, 2006.

Hicks, J., "What is Five Element Acupuncture?" *J. Chin. Med.* (UK), 25, 1987.

Jin, W., *The Practical Jin's Pulse Diagnosis*. Shandong: Shandong Science and Technology Press, 1997.

Kuon Dowon, "Eight-Constitution Medicine: An Overview." IMKS Occasional Paper No. 2, Institute for Modern Korean Studies, Yonsei University Press, 1999, 12, pp.601–623.

Kuon Dowon, "A Theoretical Basis for the Eight Constitution Acupuncture." *Advances in Medicine and Biology*, Nova Science Publishers, 2011, Volume 5, pp.243–246.

Lavier, J., *Les bases traditionelle de l'acupuncture Chinoise*. Paris: Maloine, 1964.

Matsumoto, K. and Euler, D., *Kiiko Matsumoto's Clinical Strategies*, vol. 1. Natick, MA: Kiiko Matsumoto International, 2002.

Paik, M. J., Kuon, D., Cho, J., and Kim, K. R., "Altered Urinary Polyamine Patterns of Cancer Patients under Acupuncture Therapy." *Amino Acids*, 37 (2), 2008, pp.407–413.

Paik, M. J., La, S., Lee, Y. S., Kim, J. Y. *et al.*, "Therapeutic Monitoring on Urinary Nucleoside and Polyamine Levels of Cancer Patients by CE and GC under Acupuncture Treatment." *Proc. of the Convention of the Pharm. Soc. of Korea*, 1, 2003.

Ros, F., *The Lost Secrets of Ayurvedic Acupuncture*. Twin Lakes, WI: Lotus Press, 1994.

Soulié de Morant, G., *Précis de la vrai acuponcture Chinoise*. Paris: Mercure de France, 1934.

Soulié de Morant, G., *Le Diagnostic par les pouls radiaux*. Paris: La Maisnie, 1983.

Soulié de Morant, G., *Chinese Acupuncture*. Brookline, MA: Paradigm, 1994.

Townsend, G. and De Donna, Y., *Pulses and Impulses*. Wellingborough: Thorsons, 1990.

GLOSSARY

AE: This acronym stands for Aggressive Energy, a concept taught by Worsley as part of his style of Five Element Acupuncture. Worsley adopted this concept from one of his teachers, Jacques Lavier. AE is probably Lavier's terminology for Xie Qi, or Exogenous Perverse Energy. AE is considered one of the blocks to using Five Element treatment, and must be treated before using Five Element Energy transfers.

Akabane test: A diagnostic technique for evaluating the balance between the left and right branches of the Principal Meridians. This test was originated by the Japanese acupuncturist Kobe Akabane, and uses the patient's perception of heat, due to a lighted incense stick applied at the Jing Well Points. The Akabane test, and its treatment implications, were incorporated into FEA by Worsley.

Alojaka: This is one of the five Subdoshas of Pitta Dosha in Ayurveda. Its pulse is felt on the proximal edge of the middle finger. It governs the metabolic changes involved in vision, and is commonly the focus of treatment in any visual disorder. Although not an orthodox teaching, the author associates it with the Chinese Element Water.

Apana: This is one of the five Subdoshas of Vata Dosha in Ayurveda. Its pulse is felt on the proximal edge of the index finger. It governs downward movement, especially of urine, feces, and menses. Although not an orthodox teaching, the author associates it with the Chinese Element Water.

Auxiliary Formulae: In Korean Constitutional Acupuncture (KCA), these Formulae include prescriptions for treating Meridians that are not the Root imbalanced Meridian. They include Anti-inflammatory Formulae for both Zang and Fu Organs, Antibiotic Formulae, Vialization Formulae, Paralysis Formulae, and Psyche or Neuro Formulae. Each of these Formulae consists of a Four Needle technique set of Points, except for the Psyche or Neuro Formulae which use only two Points, and each Formula is specific to its Root constitutional type. In the case histories, the author has added examples of newer Auxiliary Formulae, such as Degeneration and Immune System Formulae, which have not been described in any English publications by this system's originator, Dowon Kuon.

Avalambaka: This is one of the five Subdoshas of Kapha Dosha in Ayurveda. Its pulse is felt between the distal edge and the middle of the ring finger. It provides lubrication to the chest and spine. Although not an orthodox teaching, the author associates it with the Chinese Element Wood.

Avyakta: Pure existence in its unmanifested state, a term in Ayurveda. It is analogous to the term Wu Ji in Chinese medical thought.

Bodaka: This is one of the five Subdoshas of Kapha Dosha in Ayurveda. Its pulse is felt between the proximal edge and the middle of the ring finger. It governs the saliva and lubrication of the mouth, and the sense of taste. Although not an orthodox teaching, the author associates it with the Chinese Element Earth.

Brajaka: This is one of the five Subdoshas of Pitta Dosha in Ayurveda. Its pulse is felt as a simultaneous presence of any two spikes on the middle finger. It governs the skin, especially its color and warmth. Although not an orthodox teaching, the author associates it with the Chinese Element Fire.

CF: This acronym stands for Causative Factor of Disease, a term introduced by Worsley as part of his style of Five Element Acupuncture. The CF is that Element whose state of chronic imbalance is ultimately responsible for the inability of the other Elements to regain normal states of functioning, so it may be thought of as the deepest level of Elemental imbalance, and the Element around which treatment should be selected in order to lead to more than symptomatic relief. Various practitioners trained by Worsley have different opinions about whether the CF is inherited or acquired. The author's opinion is that the CF is an inherited aspect of every individual, and therefore is equivalent to the term (inherited) constitution, as used in this text.

Chakra: There are seven main energy centers along the vertical midline of the body in Ayurveda, called Chakras, starting at the tip of the coccyx and ending at the crown of the head. When any of them are not functioning properly, the normal circulation of the vital force is impeded, leading to different manifestations of ill health.

Chi: The pulse position under the ring finger in Chinese radial pulse examination. It has been translated as Cubit in English. When preceded by the word Yang in this text, it refers to the distal placement of the examiner's fingers, with the middle finger at the apex of the styloid process. When preceded by the word Yin in this text, it refers to a slightly more proximal location where the examiner's index and middle fingers are placed on either side of the apex of the styloid process.

Cholecystonia: One of the eight constitutions in KCA. It is characterized by Large Intestine Deficiency as its Root imbalance. I classify it as a Metal constitution, whereas Kuon associates it with the Wood Element (Jupita, or Wood Yin, even though the Gall Bladder and Large Intestine are classified as Yang Organs in Chinese medicine). It belongs to the Greater Yin category in SCM.

Colonotonia: One of the eight constitutions in KCA. It is characterized by Large Intestine Excess as its Root imbalance. It is a Metal Element constitution (Hespera, or Metal Yin according to Kuon, even though the Large Intestine is a Yang Organ in Chinese medicine), and belongs to the Greater Yang category in SCM.

Control Cycle (Xiang Ke): An aspect of Five Element theory, it describes the restraining effect of one Element on another in the order: Wood, Earth, Water, Fire, and Metal. Although restraining is one of its characteristics, it is also invoked as describing the movement of Qi from any Meridian to its Grandchild Meridian. It was cited in the *Neijing* as the order in which Protective Energy (Wei Qi) circulates through the Zang (Yin) Organs each night. There is controversy about whether it refers to relationships of Yin Meridian to Yin Meridian and Yang Meridian to Yang Meridian, or Yin Meridian to Yang Meridian and

Yang Meridian to Yin Meridian. These two different interpretations are exemplified in the Four Needle Technique and Thambirajah's method of transferring Qi respectively. Worsley taught that it only applied to transfers from Yin Meridian to Yin Meridian.

Creative Cycle (Xiang Sheng): An aspect of Five Element theory, it describes the promoting effect of one Element on another in the order: Wood, Fire, Earth, Metal, and Water. This is the exact order of the Elemental nature of the Five Transport Points on the Yin Meridians. For the Yang Meridians, the sequence is Metal, Water, Wood, Fire, and Earth, which is an identical order, but with a different starting point. This cycle is used for Qi transfers from Yang Meridian to Yang Meridian and from Yin Meridian to Yin Meridian in FEA, and is one example of the Law of Mother–Son.

CSOE: This acronym stands for color, sound, odor, and emotion, which are the diagnostic findings that Worsley used for determining the CF in FEA. They are subtle signals of imbalance emanating from the Element of the CF.

Cun: The pulse position under the index finger in Chinese radial pulse examination. It has been translated as Inch in English. When preceded by the word Yang in this text, it refers to the distal placement of the examiner's fingers, with the middle finger at the apex of the styloid process. When preceded by the word Yin in this text, it refers to a slightly more proximal location where the examiner's index and middle fingers are placed on either side of the apex of the styloid process.

Cun, Guan, and Chi: The three pulses felt on the radial artery under the index, middle, and ring fingers respectively. When preceded by the word Yang in this text, it refers to the distal placement of the examiner's fingers, with the middle finger at the apex of the styloid process. When preceded by the word Yin in this text, it refers to a slightly more proximal location where the examiner's index and middle fingers are placed on either side of the apex of the styloid process.

Dhatu: This term refers to the various tissues that make up the physical body in Ayurveda, of which there are seven: Rasa (plasma), Rakta (blood), Mamsa (muscle), Meda (fat and connective tissue), Asthi (bone), Majja (marrow and nerves), and Shukra (reproductive tissues).

Dosha: Literally, a term meaning impurity in Ayurveda. There are three Doshas: Vata (wind), Pitta (bile), and Kapha (phlegm). The same term is also used to refer to normal physiological functions, with Vata producing movement, Pitta producing heat, and Kapha producing fluidity. The balance of these three Doshas determines a person's constitution and also their current state of health. Each Dosha is composed of two of the five Ayurvedic Elements, which are different than the Chinese Five Elements. Each Dosha is in turn subdivided into five Subdoshas, each with its own function.

ECM: This acronym stands for Eight Constitutions Medicine, a Korean style of treatment developed by Dowon Kuon. Its primary treatment modality is acupuncture, and Kuon first introduced this method as Korean Constitutional Acupuncture (KCA). The author usually uses the original acronym, KCA, when referring to this style of treatment.

EDs: This acronym stands for the "Seven External Dragons" that treat the "Seven External Devils," an acupuncture protocol for treating "Possession" in Five Element Acupuncture, as taught by Worsley. The Points are DU 20, UB 11, UB 23, and UB 61. See Chapter 16 for a detailed presentation.

EEM: This acronym stands for the Eight Extraordinary Meridians (Qi Jing Ba Mai), consisting of Du Mai, Ren Mai, Chong Mai, Dai Mai, Yang Wei Mai, Yin Wei Mai, Yang Qiao Mai, and Yin Qiao Mai.

Eight Principal Patterns (Ba Gang Bian Zheng): This is one translation of the method for differentiating syndromes in the modern acupuncture style referred to as TCM. It has also been translated as Eight Diagnostic Categories, and as Eight Principles.

Entry and Exit Points: These are the Points where Qi enters each Meridian from its predecessor, and leaves each Meridian for its successor, in the Horary sequence described in the Law of Midday/Midnight. The Entry Points are the first Point on the Meridian (except for the LI Meridian, where it is LI 4), whereas the Exit Points are not necessarily the last Point on the Meridian. This connection between sequential Meridians is subject to dysfunction, leading to an Entry/Exit block. Treating these blocks is a preliminary consideration in FEA.

FEA: This acronym stands for Five Element Acupuncture, in the narrow sense of a style of acupuncture systematized and taught by J. R. Worsley. FEA does not include all the methods of acupuncture treatment based on Five Element theory, but is specific to the teachings of Worsley.

Four Needle technique: This acupuncture treatment method was first described by the medieval Korean monk Sa Am. He devised treatments that combined using the Creative and Control Cycles of the Five Elements for Tonification and Sedation of Meridians. These methods are used in both FEA and KCA. He also described some less well-known Point combinations for Heating and Cooling the Meridians.

Fu Organs: The "Hollow Organs" in Chinese medicine which are classified as Yang. They are the Large and Small Intestines, Stomach, Urinary Bladder, Gall Bladder, and Triple Heater. Each has a Principal Meridian of the same name. They are also the Organs which are targeted in KCA by the Anti-inflammatory Fu Auxiliary Formula that treats problems of any of these Organs and also most gynecological, ENT (ear, nose, and throat), and skin problems.

Gastrotonia: One of the eight constitutions in KCA. It is characterized by Stomach Excess as its Root imbalance. It is an Earth Element constitution (Saturna or Earth Yin according to Kuon, even though the Stomach is a Yang Organ in Chinese medicine), and belongs to the Lesser Yang category in SCM.

Guan: The pulse position under the examiner's middle finger in Chinese radial pulse diagnosis. It has been translated in English as Bar. When preceded by the word Yang in this text, it refers to the distal placement of the examiner's fingers, with the middle finger at the apex of the styloid process. When preceded by the word Yin in this text, it refers to a slightly more proximal location where the examiner's index and middle fingers are placed on either side of the apex of the styloid process.

Hepatonia: One of the eight constitutions in KCA. It is characterized by Liver Excess as its Root imbalance. It is a Wood Element constitution (Jupito, or Wood Yang according to Kuon, even though the Liver is a Yin Organ in Chinese medicine), and belongs to the Greater Yin category in SCM.

Hespera: One of several synonyms used by Kuon for classifying the Greater Yang Fu constitutional type. It is also called Colonotonia and Metal Yin by Kuon (even though in Chinese medicine the Large Intestine is classified as a Yang Organ). I prefer Large Intestine

Excess as its designation, in order to accommodate 24 constitutional types, and to indicate its constitutional Element.

Hespero: One of several synonyms used by Kuon for classifying the Greater Yang Zang constitutional type. It is also called Pulmotonia and Metal Yang by Kuon (even though in Chinese medicine the Lung is classified as a Yin Organ). I prefer Liver Deficiency as its designation, in order to accommodate 24 constitutional types, and to indicate its constitutional Element.

IDs: This acronym stands for the "Seven Internal Dragons" that treat the "Seven Internal Devils," an acupuncture protocol for treating "Possession" in Five Element Acupuncture, as taught by Worsley. The Points are Ren 15 (using a Master Point below it), ST 25, ST 32, and ST 41. See Chapter 16 for a detailed presentation.

Imperial Fire: This term refers to the two Organs of the Fire Element whose pulses are felt in the left Cun position, namely the Heart and Small Intestine. In KCA this aspect of the Fire Element is the one treated in all cases except for the Psyche or Neuro Auxiliary Formulae, which Kuon selected from both Imperial and Ministerial Fire Meridians.

Jing: This Chinese term is usually translated as Essence. It is one of the Three Treasures in Daoist alchemy: Jing, Qi, and Shen.

Jueyin: One of the Six Great Meridians, which I translate as Fading Yin. It is also one of the stages of Cold induced illnesses described in the *Shanghanlun*.

Jupita: One of several synonyms used by Kuon for classifying the Greater Yin Fu constitutional type. It is also called Cholecystonia and Wood Yin by Kuon (even though in Chinese medicine the Large Intestine and Gall Bladder are classified as Yang Organs). I prefer Large Intestine Deficiency as its designation, in order to accommodate 24 constitutional types, and to indicate its constitutional Element.

Jupito: One of several synonyms used by Kuon for classifying the Greater Yin Zang constitutional type. It is also called Hepatonia and Wood Yang by Kuon (even though in Chinese medicine the Liver is classified as a Yin Organ). I prefer Liver Excess as its designation, in order to accommodate 24 constitutional types, and to indicate its constitutional Element.

Kapha: One of the three Doshas in Ayurveda. It is often translated as phlegm, and is composed of the Ayurvedic Water and Earth Elements. Physiologically, it provides fluidity to the body, while at the same time being the most inert of the three Doshas, and therefore providing the major influence on the body's structure. It has five Subdoshas: Kledaka, Avalambaka, Bodaka, Tarpaka, and Shleshaka, each of which has a specific role to play in the individual's structure and functioning.

KCA: This acronym stands for Korean Constitutional Acupuncture, a treatment style developed by Dowon Kuon, which he now calls Eight Constitutions Medicine. See ECM above.

KHA: This acronym stands for Korean Hand Acupuncture (Koryo Sooji Chim), a style of treatment developed by Yoo Tae Woo. It treats all problems via Points on the hands, as a microsystem. Its diagnostic procedures, however, include examination of the whole body, with a particular emphasis on abdominal palpation to differentiate the three patterns of Yang Excess, Yin Excess, and Kidney Excess. Yoo teaches this methodology to non-professionals as well as licensed professionals, and recommends non-invasive stimulation of the Points with pressure, magnets and contact pellets of different metals. This non-professional usage is referred to as Korean Hand Therapy (KHT).

Kidney Excess syndrome: One of three patterns revealed by abdominal palpation in KHA. It is characterized by tenderness and hardness at the Points Ren 4 and Ren 5, and indicates any one or more of the following conditions: Excess of Kidney, Liver, Small Intestine, Triple Heater, Stomach, and Lung, or Deficiency of Bladder, Gall Bladder, Heart, Pericardium, Spleen, and Large Intestine.

Kledaka: This is one of the five Subdoshas of Kapha Dosha in Ayurveda. Its pulse is felt on the distal edge of the ring finger. It governs the fluids that are involved in the digestive function of the stomach and its mucous membrane. Although not an orthodox teaching, the author associates it with the Chinese Element Metal.

Luo Mai: The Connecting Meridians, which link the coupled Yin and Yang Principal Meridians of the same Element, and are used in FEA to transfer Qi between them. There are additional types of Luo Mai that are not discussed in this text.

Mercuria: One of several synonyms used by Kuon for classifying the Lesser Yin Fu constitutional type. It is also called Vesicotonia and Water Yin by Kuon (even though in Chinese medicine the Bladder and Stomach are classified as Yang Organs). I prefer Stomach Deficiency as its designation, in order to accommodate 24 constitutional types, and to indicate its constitutional Element.

Mercurio: One of several synonyms used by Kuon for classifying the Lesser Yin Zang constitutional type. It is also called Renotonia and Water Yang by Kuon (even though in Chinese medicine the Kidney is classified as a Yin Organ). I prefer Kidney Excess as its designation, in order to accommodate 24 constitutional types, and to indicate its constitutional Element.

Ministerial Fire: The connotation of Ministerial Fire used in this text is in reference to the Organs whose pulses are felt on the right wrist in the Chi position, under the ring finger. These Organs and their Meridians are the Pericardium and Triple Heater. In KCA these Meridians are only used in some of the Psyche or Neuro Auxiliary Formulae. In FEA they are commonly treated in almost everyone at some juncture in the course of long-term care. It is the author's opinion that these Meridians have a close association with the autonomic nervous system. There is another usage of the term Ministerial Fire in Chinese medicine to refer to Fire syndromes of any of the Organs other than the Heart or Small Intestine.

Officials: This term is taken from *Suwen*, Chapter 8, where the 12 Organs of the body are compared to Officials in a government bureaucracy. This analogical point of view is one example of the underlying concept of resonance (Gan Ying) that is at the heart of Chinese medicine. FEA was developed by Worsley around the concept of the Officials, and does not generally refer to Organs in its terminology.

Oligotherapy: A system of therapeutics that is similar to homeopathy in its usage of minute doses of specially prepared substances, the oligoelements. Also called functional diathetic medicine, oligotherapy was developed by Jacques Menetrier based partly on his exposure to the Five Element theory of Chinese medicine. Some details are presented in Chapter 5.

Opening and Coupled Points: These are the Command Points that activate the Eight Extraordinary Meridians (EEM). The Opening and Coupled Points of each are: Du Mai SI 3 and UB 62, Ren Mai LU 7 and KI 6, Chong Mai SP 4 and PE 6, Dai Mai GB 41 and TH 5, Yang Wei Mai TH 5 and GB 41, Yin Wei Mai PE 6 and SP 4, Yang Qiao Mai

UB 62 and SI 3, and Yin Qiao Mai KI 6 and LU 7. Since each set of Points is shared by two Extraordinary Meridians, the author prefers to use Manaka style ion-pumping cords with them in order to specify which Meridian is to be activated.

O-ring test: The bidigital O-ring test (BDORT) is a kinesiological test developed by Yoshiyaki Omura, a physician and acupuncture researcher. The author learned it from him, and finds it useful in assessing the efficacy of acupuncture treatments, along with other criteria such as pulse changes, changes in tender points, changes in CSOE, and changes in the patient's Spirit and symptoms.

Pachaka: This is one of the five Subdoshas of Pitta Dosha in Ayurveda. Its pulse is felt on the distal edge of the middle finger. It governs the digestive fire (Agni) of the stomach and small intestine. Although not an orthodox teaching, the author associates it with the Chinese Element Metal.

Pancreatonia: One of the eight constitutions in KCA. It is characterized by Kidney Deficiency as its Root imbalance. The author classifies it as a Water constitution, whereas Kuon associates it with the Earth Element (Saturno). It belongs to the Lesser Yang category in SCM.

Pitta: One of the three Doshas in Ayurveda. It is often translated as bile, and is composed of the Ayurvedic Water and Fire Elements. Physiologically, it provides heat to the body, while at the same time being responsible for all manifestations of metabolism and change. It has five Subdoshas: Pachaka, Ranjaka, Sadhaka, Alojaka, and Brajaka, each of which has a specific role to play in the individual's structure and functioning.

Possession: In classical Chinese medicine, Possession was considered one of the miscellaneous causes of illness, and there have been many recommendations for its treatment by both herbs and acupuncture during the long history of Chinese medicine. Worsley chose to include this diagnosis in his system of Five Element Acupuncture, as one of the blocks to treatment that needs to be cleared, before proceeding to Elemental treatment. Worsley taught that the diagnosis of Possession was made by observing the Spirit (Shen) in the patient's eyes and, when present, was treated with either or both of the ID and ED protocols. Worsley learned this component of FEA from the Taiwanese teacher Hsiu Yang-Chai. Possession is one of the categories of classical Chinese medicine that was not included in the modern formalization of Traditional Chinese Medicine (TCM) in China in the 1950s. The metaphysical explanation for Possession is not amenable to verification, but the author offers a more physiologically based interpretation of Possession and its treatment in Chapter 16.

Prakriti: The primary use of this word in this text is to refer to an individual's constitution. In Ayurvedic theory, Prakriti is also described as Primordial Nature or Primordial Substance. In Chinese, the term Tai Ji is used in the same way, and they can be thought of as parallel concepts. The Prakriti is best identified by its reflection in the deepest level of the pulse via the balance of the three Doshas, but can also be discerned by a careful evaluation of a person's physical, emotional, mental, and spiritual characteristics.

Prana: This is one of the five Subdoshas of Vata Dosha in Ayurveda. Its pulse is felt on the distal edge of the index finger. It is analogous to the Chinese term Qi, in that it is a generic term for the vital energy, and also a specific term, here as one of the Subdoshas. It governs the breath, especially inhalation. Although not an orthodox teaching, the author associates it with the Chinese Element Metal.

Pulmotonia: One of the eight constitutions in KCA. It is characterized by Liver Deficiency as its Root imbalance. The author classifies it as a Wood constitution, whereas Kuon associates it with the Metal Element (Hespero). It belongs to the Greater Yang category in SCM.

Purusha: This term refers to pure unmanifested consciousness, and is parallel to the term Shen in Chinese medicine. Purusha is often paired with Prakriti in Ayurveda as the Pure Consciousness and the Primordial Nature that create the phenomenal world. The author sees a parallel here to Chinese medical thought concerning each individual's endowment at creation: Their Spirit (Shen) has no manifest qualities, and no one can say where it comes from. Their Constitution, however, is a product of the parental gametes, and provides their unique endowment of qualities that can be classified by any of the systems described in this text, whether in terms of Three Doshas, Four Images, Five Elements, Six Energetic Levels, etc.

Ranjaka: This is one of the five Subdoshas of Pitta Dosha in Ayurveda. Its pulse is felt between the distal edge and the middle of the middle finger. It governs the metabolic functions of the liver, and is also a contributor to red blood cell production. Although not an orthodox teaching, the author associates it with the Chinese Element Wood.

Renotonia: One of the eight constitutions in KCA. It is characterized by Kidney Excess as its Root imbalance. It is a Water Element constitution (Mercurio), and belongs to the Lesser Yin category in SCM.

Root Formula: This term, also called the Fundamental Formula, is the Four Needle Combination in KCA that treats the constitutional imbalance in each individual. All other targets of treatment in KCA are addressed by the Auxiliary Formulae. Originally Kuon developed KCA by only treating with the Root Formula. As his experience accumulated, he added the Auxiliary Formulae to target specific pathomechanisms in each individual case.

Sadhaka: This is one of the five Subdoshas of Pitta Dosha in Ayurveda. Its pulse is felt between the proximal edge and the middle of the middle finger. It governs the activities of the heart and brain. Although not an orthodox teaching, the author associates it with the Chinese Element Earth.

Samana: This is one of the five Subdoshas of Vata Dosha in Ayurveda. Its pulse is felt between the proximal edge and the middle of the index finger. It governs peristalsis and other movements in the digestive tract. Although not an orthodox teaching, the author associates it with the Chinese Element Earth.

Saturna: One of several synonyms used by Kuon for classifying the Lesser Yang Fu constitutional type. It is also called Gastrotonia and Earth Yin by Kuon (even though in Chinese medicine the Stomach is classified as a Yang Organ). I prefer Stomach Excess as its designation, in order to accommodate 24 constitutional types, and to indicate its constitutional Element.

Saturno: One of several synonyms used by Kuon for classifying the Lesser Yang Zang constitutional type. It is also called Pancreatonia and Earth Yang by Kuon (even though in Chinese medicine the Kidney and Spleen/Pancreas are classified as Yin Organs). I prefer Kidney Deficiency as its designation, in order to accommodate 24 constitutional types, and to indicate its constitutional Element.

SCM: This acronym stands for Sasang Constitutional Medicine, originally a Korean herbal system of therapy based on the *Yijing* subdivisions of Yin and Yang into Greater

Yang, Lesser Yang, Greater Yin, and Lesser Yin. Its modern proponents have developed acupunctural methods to treat individuals of these four types.

SEL: This acronym stands for the Six Energetic Levels, which are the names and states of the Six Great Meridians: Taiyang, Shaoyang, Yangming, Taiyin, Shaoyin, and Jueyin. The pulses reflecting these six are described in the *Maijing*. These Six Great Meridians are the basis for one method of constitutional and conditional analysis.

Shao Yang: The Lesser Yang constitution in SCM (strong Spleen, weak Kidney).

Shao Yin: The Lesser Yin constitution in SCM (strong Kidney, weak Spleen).

Shaoyang: The Lesser Yang Great Meridian composed of Gall Bladder and Triple Heater Principal Meridians.

Shaoyin: The Lesser Yin Great Meridian composed of Kidney and Heart Principal Meridians.

Shen: The Chinese term for Spirit, which is Pure Consciousness, without material form or qualities. It is considered the highest contributor in the make-up of each individual in the FEA tradition, where there is a focus on treating Points that impact the Spirit if an imbalance at that level is detected.

Shleshaka: This is one of the five Subdoshas of Kapha Dosha in Ayurveda. Its pulse is felt as a simultaneous presence of any two spikes on the ring finger. It governs the synovial fluids of the joints. Although not an orthodox teaching, the author associates it with the Chinese Element Fire.

Six Great Meridians: These each have two Principal Meridians composed of an arm branch and a leg branch. They are Taiyang, Shaoyang, Yangming, Taiyin, Shaoyin, and Jueyin.

Subdosha: The Subdoshas are an aspect of the present condition (Vikruti), and are components of each Dosha. The Doshas (Vata, Pitta, and Kapha) appear at different strengths in the superficial part of the Ayurvedic pulse, but within the Dosha's pulse there may be a more prominent impulse (spike) at a certain location on the examiner's finger. It is also possible for one of these locations to feel unusually weak or absent, although such a finding is uncommon. Each Dosha is composed of five Subdoshas, which can be evaluated by feeling for impulses (spikes) at four places on each examining finger (index for Vata, middle for Pitta, and ring for Kapha). The author believes that these Subdosha locations are correlated with the Chinese Five Elements in the following manner: the distal edge of each finger reflects the Metal Element; between the distal edge and the middle of the finger reflects the Wood Element; between the middle and the proximal edge of the finger reflects the Earth Element; the proximal edge of the finger reflects the Water Element; and if any two of these locations are simultaneously showing a stronger impulse (spike) on any finger, that reflects the Fire Element. This order of Metal, Wood, Earth, Water, and Fire is reflected in the following list of the Subdoshas. The Vata Subdoshas are: Prana, Udana, Samana, Apana, and Vyana. The Pitta Subdoshas are: Pachaka, Ranjaka, Sadhaka, Alojaka, and Brajaka. The Kapha Subdoshas are: Kledaka, Avalambaka, Bodaka, Tarpaka, and Shleshaka.

Tai Ji: This Chinese term literally means Great Pole. It is the first manifest state (Single Pole) of creation emanating from the unmanifest state of Wu Ji (Without a Pole), and is similar to the concept of the Dao, from which all of creation flows, and to which it will ultimately return. The familiar Yin/Yang symbol of interlocking fish shapes is also called the Tai Ji symbol, because it is the source of all creation, beginning with the division of everything into Yin and Yang, and proceeding from there to ever more complex states of manifestation. Tai Ji is analagous to the Ayurvedic concept of Vyakta.

Tai Yang: The Greater Yang constitution in SCM (strong Lung, weak Liver).

Tai Yin: The Greater Yin constitution in SCM (strong Liver, weak Lung).

Taiyang: The Greater Yang Great Meridian composed of Urinary Bladder and Small Intestine Principal Meridians.

Taiyin: The Greater Yin Great Meridian composed of Spleen and Lung Principal Meridians.

Tarpaka: This is one of the five Subdoshas of Kapha Dosha in Ayurveda. Its pulse is felt on the proximal edge of the ring finger. It governs the cerebrospinal fluids of the nervous system. Although not an orthodox teaching, the author associates it with the Chinese Element Water.

TCM: This acronym stands for Traditional Chinese Medicine, the version of Chinese medicine formalized under government auspices during the 1950s in China. Many components of the enormous variety of traditional medical practices in China were not included in the official doctrines of TCM; however, over time the limits of what may be included in TCM have become more flexible. There is still a strong determination not to include much of the spiritual teachings which were historically a very important part of Chinese medicine, so that it is unlikely that Possession, for example, will ever be an acceptable diagnosis in TCM.

Three Constitutions Theory (Sam Il Che Jil): The primary methodology in KHA for determining the Excess or Deficient states of the Organs, in order to treat their Meridians with Tonification or Sedation techniques. The three constitutions are differentiated primarily by response to abdominal palpation, but also reflect differences in body structure, Meridian and Point sensitivity, location of symptoms, and preferences for different climates and seasons. This theory is remarkably similar to that of the Three Doshas of Ayurveda.

Ti Zhi: The original term for constitutional type in the *Neijing* and *Shanghanlun*. It literally means body type, and therefore could refer to either the inherited or acquired constitution.

Transfers: Many versions of Oriental medicine share an idea that illnesses stem from an imbalance in the organism's functions, such that some functions are hyperactive while others are simultaneously hypoactive, and that the organism is always trying to restore its balance (homeostasis) in this regard. If it is unable to restore balance, there is a corollary notion that something is stuck or blocked. There are many techniques in the various styles of Oriental medicine to help the organism to address this state of affairs. In FEA one of the most important means of redressing this stuck situation is by transferring Qi from Meridians that are in Excess (hyperfunctioning) to those that are Deficient (hypofunctioning). This methodology is not unique to FEA, but has been described eloquently by Radha Thambirajah, who was trained in China during the Cultural Revolution in a military school, not subject to the restrictions of TCM. Similar ideas can be found in Japanese medicine (personal communication from Kiiko Matsumoto). Qi transfers are accomplished in FEA by using the Five Element relationships of the Creative and Control Cycles, as well as via the Connecting (Luo) Meridians.

Udana: This is one of the five Subdoshas of Vata Dosha in Ayurveda. Its pulse is felt between the distal edge and the middle of the index finger. It governs upward movement in the body, and especially that of exhalation. Although not an orthodox teaching, the author associates it with the Chinese Element Wood.

Vata: One of the three Doshas in Ayurveda. It is often translated as Wind, and is composed of the Ayurvedic Aether and Air Elements. Physiologically, it is responsible for all movement within the body. It has five Subdoshas: Prana, Udana, Samana, Apana, and Vyana, each of which has a specific role to play in the individual's structure and functioning.

Vesicotonia: One of the eight constitutions in KCA. It is characterized by Stomach Deficiency as its Root imbalance. The author classifies it as an Earth constitution, whereas Kuon associates it with the Water Element (Mercuria or Water Yin according to Kuon, even though the Bladder and Stomach are Yang Organs in Chinese medicine). It belongs to the Lesser Yin category in SCM.

Vikruti: This term refers to the patient's present condition in Ayurvedic medicine, and is contrasted with the constitution (Prakriti). The Vikruti is diagnosed in the superficial part of the pulse, while the Prakriti is diagnosed in the deepest part of the pulse.

Vyakta: The Ayurvedic term for the state of coming into being of manifest reality. It is analogous to the Chinese concepts of Tai Ji and Dao.

Vyana: This is one of the five Subdoshas of Vata Dosha in Ayurveda. Its pulse is felt as a simultaneous presence of any two spikes on the index finger. It governs the circulatory movement of fluids, especially the blood. Although not an orthodox teaching, the author associates it with the Chinese Element Fire.

Wei Qi: Defensive Energy, which is said to flow outside the Meridians in Chinese medicine. It warms and protects the body.

Wu Ji: Literally, "Without a Pole," Wu Ji is the absolutely unmanifest state of existence. It is the realm of Pure Consciousness that has no material component. It is analogous to Avyakta and Purusha in Ayurvedic medicine.

Yang Excess syndrome: One of three patterns revealed by abdominal palpation in KHA. It is characterized by tenderness and hardness at the Point ST 25, and indicates any one or more of the following conditions: Excess of Bladder, Liver, Heart, Pericardium, Stomach, and Large Intestine, or Deficiency of Kidney, Gall Bladder, Small Intestine, Triple Heater, Spleen, and Lung.

Yangming: The Yangming Great Meridian is composed of Stomach and Large Intestine Principal Meridians.

Yin Excess syndrome: One of three patterns revealed by abdominal palpation in KHA. It is characterized by tenderness at the Point SP 15, and indicates any one or more of the following conditions: Excess of Bladder, Gall Bladder, Heart, Pericardium, Spleen, and Lung, or Deficiency of Kidney, Liver, Small Intestine, Triple Heater, Stomach, and Large Intestine.

Ying Qi: Nourishing Energy, which is said to flow inside the Meridians in Chinese medicine. It sustains and nourishes the body.

Yuan Qi: The Original Energy that provides each Organ with its characteristic nature. The Yuan Qi is said to be distributed to each of the Organs by the functioning of the Triple Heater, which carries Yuan Qi from its storage in the Lower Heater under the control of the Kidneys, to the Source Point (Yuan Xue) on each Principal Meridian. Yuan Qi is the energetic aspect of the inherited constitution, while Jing is the material aspect of the inherited constitution.

Zang Organs: The Solid Organs in Chinese medicine that are classified as Yin. They include the Heart, Pericardium, Liver, Spleen, Lung, and Kidneys. Each has a Principal Meridian of the same name. They are also the Organs that are targeted in KCA by the Anti-inflammatory Zang Auxiliary Formula that treats problems of any of these Organs, and also many cases of fatigue and pain.

Zheng Qi: Normal or Anti-pathogenic Energy, which is contrasted with Perverse Energy (Xie Qi). Zheng Qi maintains normal bodily functions, while Xie Qi disrupts them.

INDEX